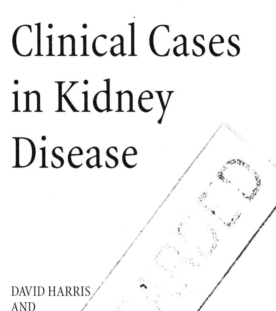

Clinical Cases in Kidney Disease

DAVID HARRIS
AND
COLLEAGUES

D1614485

The **McGraw·Hill** Companies

Sydney New York San Francisco Auckland
Bangkok Bogotá Caracas Hong Kong
Kuala Lumpur Lisbon London Madrid
Mexico City Milan New Delhi San Juan
Seoul Singapore Taipei Toronto

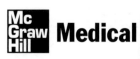 **Medical**

This special edition 2007
Text © 2007 Author
Illustrations and design © 2007 McGraw-Hill Australia Pty Ltd
Additional owners of copyright are acknowledged in on-page credits

National Library of Australia Cataloguing-in-Publication Data

Harris, David C. H. (David Charles Hamlyn).
    Clinical cases in kidney disease.

    1st ed.
    Bibliography.
    Includes index.
    ISBN 9780074717806
    ISBN 9780070158979 (Amgen Edition).

    1. Kidneys - Diseases. 2. Kidneys - Diseases - Case
    studies. I. Title.

    616.6109

Published in Australia by
McGraw-Hill Australia Pty Ltd
Level 2, 82 Waterloo Road, North Ryde NSW 2113
Associate Editor: Hollie Zondanos
Managing Editor: Kathryn Fairfax
Production Editor: Natalie Crouch
Copy Editor: Leanne Poll, Letterati Publishing Services
Proofreader: Tim Learner
Indexer: Russell Brooks
Designer (cover and interior): Jan Schmoeger, Designpoint
Illustrator: Alan Laver, Shelly Communications
Typeset in Minion Pro 10/12 pt by Midland Typesetters, Australia
Printed in China on 80 gsm woodfree by iBook Printing Ltd

Foreword

Caring for patients with kidney disease is a challenge for all clinicians, in part because of the complexities of the relevant basic science, and also because of the difficulties in making a firm diagnosis and applying evidence-based treatment in conditions with such varied manifestations. It is common for medical students and staff at all levels of training to feel some apprehension about tackling these clinical challenges, and clear formats for education in this field are highly valued.

In this context, the current volume will fill a real need. David Harris has drawn together a talented team of expert nephrologists and tasked them with creating self-directed learning exercises based around 32 common problems in nephrology practice. The format is immediately engaging, as the approach is practical and the style interactive. The learner is drawn into thinking about the clinical issues raised by each case scenario, and prompted to respond to multiple-choice questions to which correct answers and accompanying explanations are immediately provided. The key points are then distilled into Clinical Pearls which provide a natural method for breaking up the important learning issues into discrete packages.

A special feature which will widen the range of users to whom the book will appeal is the stepwise development of material in each case at three levels of sophistication, from overall principles at medical student level to current developments of interest to specialist nephrologists. Short listings of key publications enable readers at each level to pursue their interests with reference to selected primary source material.

I congratulate the editor and all contributors for their consistent and disciplined use of this novel format, and warmly recommend the book to all those who wish to deepen their understanding of kidney disease, in the interest of better care for our long-suffering patients.

Michael Field
Professor of Medicine and Consultant Nephrologist
Associate Dean, Northern Clinical School, University of Sydney

Table of contents

About the authors

David Harris, MD, BS, FRACP is Professor of Medicine and Associate Dean of the Western Clinical School of The University of Sydney, at Westmead Hospital. He is a nephrologist, and prior to his appointment as Associate Dean he was Director of Nephrology and Dialysis in Western Sydney.

Mark A. Brown, MB, BS, FRACP, MD
Senior Staff Nephrologist and Professor of Medicine, St George Hospital, University of New South Wales

Fiona Brown, MBBS, FRACP, PhD
Renal Physician, Monash Medical Centre, Clayton, Victoria

Steve Chadban, BMed, PhD, FRACP
Professor, Senior Staff Nephrologist and Director of Kidney Transplantation, Royal Prince Alfred Hospital and The University of Sydney

Shlomo Cohney, PhD, FRACP, MRCP, MBBS
Physician in Internal Medicine, Nephrology and Transplantation, Royal Melbourne Hospital

Nick Cross, MBChB, FRACP
PhD Candidate, Centre for Kidney Research, The Children's Hospital at Westmead

Grahame Elder, MB, BS, PhD, FRACP
Consultant Nephrologist, Department of Renal Medicine, Westmead Hospital; consultant, Bone and Calcium Clinic, St Vincent's Hospital.

Zoltán H. Endre, BSc (Med), MBBS, PhD, FRACP
Professor and Head, Department of Medicine, University of Otago, Christchurch; Adjunct Professor, Centre for Bioengineering, University of Canterbury; Honorary Professor, School of Medicine, The University of Queensland; Consultant Nephrologist, Christchurch Hospital

Randall Faull, MBBS, FRACP, PhD
Senior Consultant in Nephrology, Royal Adelaide Hospital; Dean and Director of the Medical Program, The University of Adelaide

Paolo Ferrari, MBBS, MD, FRACP, FASN
Clinical Professor, The University of Western Australia; Director, Department of Nephrology, Fremantle Hospital; Clinical Director, Medical Division, Fremantle Hospital; Chair, Renal Diseases Health Network, WA Health Network Branch

Carmel M. Hawley, MBBS, M Med Sci, FRACP
Senior Consultant Nephrologist and Director of Haemodialysis, Princess Alexandra Hospital, Brisbane; Associate Professor, School of Population Health, The University of Queensland

Annemarie Hennessy, MBBS, PhD, FRACP, MBA
Professor, Foundation Chair of Medicine, University of Western Sydney; Consultant General and Renal Physician, Campbelltown Hospital, New South Wales

Nicole Isbel, MBBS, FRACP, PhD
Senior Staff Nephrologist, Princess Alexandra Hospital, Brisbane; Senior Lecturer in Medicine, The University of Queensland

David Johnson, MBBS, FRACP, PhD
Professor of Medicine, The University of Queensland; Director of Nephrology, Princess Alexandra Hospital, Brisbane; Chair of Medicine, Princess Alexandra Hospital, Brisbane

Mohammed Omar Kaisar, BMSc, MBBS
Renal Registrar, Royal Adelaide Hospital

John Kanellis, MBBS, PhD, FRACP
Associate Professor, Monash University; Director of Transplantation and Deputy Director Department of Nephrology, Monash Medical Centre, Clayton, Victoria

John Kelly, MB, BS Hons, MD UNSW, FRACP
Associate Professor (Conjoint), St George Clinical School, Department of Medicine, University of New South Wales

Peter G. Kerr, MBBS, PhD, FRACP
Professor/Director of Nephrology, Monash Medical Centre, Clayton, Victoria; Department of Medicine, Monash University

Vincent Weng Seng Lee, MBBS, FRACP
Clinical and Research Fellow, Westmead Hospital

Rob MacGinley, MBBS, BMedSci, MMedSci (Vasc Biol), MMedSci (Epi), FRACP
Senior Clinical Lecturer in Medical Education, Deakin University; Visiting Renal Specialist, Geelong Hospital; Steering Committee Member, CARI Guidelines

George J. Mangos, MBBS, MD, FRACP
Senior Lecturer, St George Clinical School, University of New South Wales; Nephrologist and Obstetric Physician, St George Hospital, New South Wales

Karumathil M. Murali, MD, DNB
Staff Renal Physician, Orange Base Hospital, Orange, New South Wales

Kevan R. Polkinghorne, BHB, MBChB, MClinEpi, FRACP
Consultant Nephrologist, Monash Medical Centre, Clayton, Victoria; Honorary Lecturer, Monash University

Carol A. Pollock, MBBS, PhD, FRACP
Professor of Medicine, The University of Sydney; Senior Consultant Nephrologist, Royal North Shore Hospital, Sydney

Gopala K. Rangan, MBBS, PhD, FRACP
Senior Lecturer (Conjoint) and Staff Nephrologist, Westmead Hospital and Western Clinical School, Sydney West Area Health Service and The University of Sydney

Lena Succar, BSc (Hons)
PhD candidate; Westmead Millennium Institute, Westmead Hospital, The University of Sydney

Kamal Sud, MBBS, MD, DM, DNB, FISN, FRACP
Staff Specialist and Head, Department of Renal Medicine, Nepean Hospital, Penrith, New South Wales

Robert Walker, MB, ChB, MD, FRACP
Professor of Medicine, Head of Department of Medical and Surgical Sciences, Dunedin School of Medicine, University of Otago, Dunedin; Consultant Nephrologist and Head of Department of Nephrology, HealthCare Otago, Dunedin

Angela C. Webster, MBBS, MRCP, MM(Clin Epid), PhD
Senior Lecturer in Epidemiology, School of Public Health, The University of Sydney

Acknowledgments

Authors of this book are nephrologists from Australia and New Zealand, chosen because of their recognised expertise in the subject area of their respective chapters. As editor I would like to thank all the authors for their patience and persistence during the long period required to assemble this book. I am also appreciative of their useful suggestions about other chapters of the book; each chapter was critically appraised by other authors. Thanks are also due to Jeremy Chapman, John Charlesworth, Michael Field, Lukas Kairaitis, David Mudge, Phil O'Connell and Bruce Pussell who kindly assisted in reviewing some of the chapters. Special thanks are due to Peggy Timmins, without whose help this book would not have been possible.

David Harris

Introduction

This book explores important clinical problems in general nephrology, dialysis and transplantation, using a case-based approach. Together the 32 chapters form a comprehensive collection of clinical vignettes in renal medicine. Each chapter covers a separate clinical problem by developing a single case study, posing multiple-choice questions and then providing a detailed explanation for each set of questions. The emphasis is on important and usually common nephrological scenarios. The prime object is to test and impart important contemporary principles of nephrological practice, rather than bald factual knowledge. Clinical Pearls are highlighted throughout each chapter to encapsulate the key issues.

A unique feature of this book is the way in which each case history unfolds. Each case and its associated questions are developed across three levels of increasing complexity. There is a deliberate attempt to push the boundaries of knowledge at each level. In general, Level A questions and explanations are aimed at the level of knowledge expected of a final-year medical student; Level B questions are aimed at that knowledge expected of a basic physician trainee or a general practitioner whose practice includes patients with renal conditions; and Level C questions are aimed at that knowledge expected of an advanced trainee or consultant nephrologist with an interest in the particular subject. Some licence was given to authors in their determination of complexity. Minor differences in levels of complexity reflect the authors' individual expectations. Thus, medical students are advised to confine themselves to Level A questions and explanations, whereas an expert may skip straight to Level C. This advice is intended only as a guide, because an inquisitive student may wish to explore a higher level, and an expert involved in setting exam questions may find each level relevant.

Part A
Fluids and
electrolytes

Case 1
Hyponatraemia

ZOL ENDRE

LEVEL A

Case history

A thin, 74-year-old widow has hypertension. Her weight is 60 kg and blood pressure (BP) is 160/90 mmHg. She began treatment with a diuretic 2 weeks ago. She has been on 40 mg of fluoxetine a day for depression for 6 months following the loss of her husband. Apart from a history of smoking (30 pack years, ceased 20 years previously) she has been well. Friends observed that she has been tired and a little confused for about 1 week, with mildly erratic behaviour including forgetting to feed her cat. She is afebrile, mildly disorientated in time and place, but there are no focal neurological signs. Her current BP is 135/80 mmHg. There is a small postural drop in BP (to 130/75 mmHg). Minimal signs of chronic obstructive pulmonary disease are present (limited chest expansion).

Laboratory data

	Plasma	Reference range
Na^+	111 mmol/L	(136–146)
K^+	3.1 mmol/L	(3.5–5.5)
Cl^-	93 mmol/L	(95–107)
HCO_3^-	22 mmol/L	(22–32)
Urea	7.2 mmol/L	(3.5–7.5)
Creatinine	65 µmol/L	(40–120)
eGFR	57 mL/min/1.73m²	(80–120)
Glucose	6.6 mmol/L	(3.5–7.8)
Urate	0.19 mmol/L	(0.20–0.42)
Osmolality (measured)	248 mosm/kg	(275–297)
Total protein	70 g/L	(63–80)
Albumin	33 g/L	(33–50)
Total globulins	37 g/L	(20–40)
Cholesterol (total)	3.7 mmol/L	(3.9–5.5)
Triglycerides	0.8 mmol/L	(0.6–2.5)

Question 1

Which of the following statements is/are correct?
(a) This lady's total body water (TBW) is approximately 30 L.
(b) The plasma volume is approximately 2.4 L.
(c) Two-thirds of TBW is extracellular.
(d) Sodium is the major effective extracellular fluid (ECF) osmole.

Answer

A, B and D

Explanation

TBW is usually about 60% of body weight, but this is lower in females (~50%) and in the elderly because of reduced muscle mass or increased fat. Infants have less adipose tissue and a higher proportion of body water (70%). TBW is about two-thirds intracellular (ICF). The extracellular fluid (ECF) comprises plasma (about 4% body weight) and interstitial fluid (16% body weight). Effective osmoles are small molecules that are maintained at different concentrations in the ICF or ECF. Sodium (and its accompanying anions) is the principal ECF osmoles; potassium (and its accompanying anions) are the major ICF osmoles which determine the tonicity (effective osmolality) of these compartments. Additional effective osmoles in brain ICF ('brain osmolytes') and renal medullary cells are small organic molecules such as myoinositol, choline-containing compounds (e.g. glycerylphosphorylcholine), phosphocreatine, N-acetyl-aspartate, glutamate and glutamine. The intracellular concentrations of these osmolytes change directly (but slowly) in response to changes in cell volume; this change acts to restore cell volume.

The ECF sodium content will determine the ECF osmotic pressure and therefore the ECF volume. But as Na^+ and water are separately regulated, the concentration of Na^+ in the plasma does not indicate whether the ECF volume is normal, high or low. Within the ECF the concentration of albumin (the colloid oncotic pressure) determines the movement of water from the interstitial to the intravascular space. ICF volume is inversely proportional to the ECF Na^+ concentration since a high ECF Na^+ will shrink cells and a low ECF Na^+ will result in swollen cells. In severe acute hyponatraemia there is therefore a risk of cerebral oedema, uncal herniation and hypoxia from non-cardiogenic pulmonary oedema. This inverse relationship between plasma Na^+ (P_{Na^+}) concentration and ICF volume is not present when other organic solutes in the ECF generate an osmolal gap or when there is an increase in ICF osmoles after seizure or rhabdomyolysis. After a seizure (or with rhabdomyolysis), the movement of water into muscle ICF can cause a rise in P_{Na^+}, obscuring the hyponatraemia which may have caused the seizure.

Clinical pearls

- TBW is reduced in the thin, the elderly and females.
- Effective osmoles are maintained at concentrations that differ in the ICF and ECF.
- Na^+ is the major ECF osmole, K^+ the major ICF osmole.
- ICF volume is inversely proportional to ECF Na^+ concentration.
- An increase in P_{Na^+} immediately after seizure may mask true hyponatraemia.

Question 2

Which of the following statements is/are correct?

(a) The patient's hyponatraemia can be explained by pseudohyponatraemia.

(b) Measured plasma osmolality, $P_{osm\ (measured)}$, is usually low in true hyponatraemia.

(c) The osmolal gap is increased in true hyponatraemia.

(d) $P_{osm\ (measured)}$ is normal after isotonic glycine absorption.

Answer

B and D

Explanation

Pseudohyponatraemia is hyponatraemia with a normal $P_{osm\ (measured)}$; it is a laboratory artefact resulting from the significant total plasma volume occupied by protein or lipid when either is markedly elevated. There is an apparent osmolal gap under these circumstances ($P_{osm\ (measured)} - P_{osm\ (calculated)}$)>15, but P_{Na^+} is normal when measured with ion-sensitive electrodes. $P_{osm\ (measured)}$ is normal since this also reflects only the concentration of ions and small molecules. Additionally, plasma lipid and protein concentrations are normal. Plasma osmolality is reduced in most hyponatraemic patients because it is mainly determined by the plasma sodium concentration and accompanying anions. $P_{osm\ (calculated)}$ is obtained from $2 \times (Na^+ + K^+) + (urea) + (glucose)$, where both ions and molecules are expressed in mmol/L, and equals 244 mosm/L in this example, where there is no significant osmolal gap.

Hyponatraemia with an osmolal gap >15 also occurs in the presence of an additional solute in plasma (such as alcohol, methanol, ethylene glycol or unidentified molecules in ketoacidosis, lactic acidosis and chronic renal failure); and after isotonic glycine absorption during urological or gynaecological procedures (see also Case 2, Acid–base disturbance). In these situations $P_{osm\ (measured)}$ will reflect the contribution of the additional dissolved solutes; in the case of dilution of isotonic plasma with isotonic glycine, measured osmolality will remain normal and there will be an osmolal gap. If isotonic saline could be used as an irrigator for transurethral prostate resection, this would eliminate the frequent occurrence of hyponatraemia accompanying this procedure. However, the electrical conductance of saline has precluded its use until recently. New bipolar resectoscopes under evaluation may allow routine use of isotonic saline for irrigation and eliminate the complication of hyponatraemia. Note that urea is not an *effective* osmole since it readily crosses cell membranes, so that urea usually does not modulate the intracellular volume (ICF).

Clinical pearls

- P_{osm} can be approximated (calculated) by $2 \times (Na^+) + (urea) + (glucose)$.
- The osmolal gap equals $P_{osm\ (measured)} - P_{osm\ (calculated)}$ and is normally <15.
- Hyponatraemia is usually accompanied by a decreased $P_{osm\ (measured)}$ ('no' gap, i.e. <15).
- An osmolal gap of >15 suggests pseudohyponatraemia or the presence of additional plasma solutes.
- In renal failure, effective P_{osm} equals $P_{osm\ (measured)} - (urea)$ since urea is an ineffective osmole.

Question 3

Which of the following statements is/are correct?
(a) The results may be explained by excess antidiuretic hormone (ADH, also known as vasopressin).
(b) ADH is usually increased in chronic hyponatraemia regardless of cause.
(c) She has true hyponatraemia with reduced extracellular fluid volume (ECF).
(d) ECF volume is normal in chronic hyponatraemia.

Answer
A, B and C

Explanation

Hyponatraemia is extremely common and occurs in up to 15% of hospitalised patients. Effective circulating volume depletion and the syndrome of inappropriate ADH secretion (SIADH) are the two commonest causes and both are disorders in which ADH secretion is not suppressed. While some patients with primary polydipsia can (rarely) overcome the excretory capacity of the kidney, this requires ingestion of more than 10 L of fluid daily. Even with psychogenic polydipsia, clinically significant hyponatraemia usually occurs because there is an accompanying impairment of renal water excretion resulting from the failure to suppress ADH. Thus, true hyponatraemia always results from water retention although this may be coupled with a positive or a negative balance for total body sodium. While ADH must usually be present to prevent excretion of excess water, this excretion can also be limited by reduced delivery of filtrate to the distal nephron, such as may occur in reduced osmole excretion with low protein intake (e.g. tea and toast diet in the elderly or anorexia in the young).

ECF volume may be low, normal or increased in chronic hyponatraemia. Since ECF volume is largely determined by the concentration of effective osmoles, ECF volume principally reflects total body sodium. After confirming the presence of true hyponatraemia and assessing the patient's volume status, the next step is to measure the urine sodium and osmolality. Clinical assessment of ECF volume may identify changes in Na^+ balance. Postural hypotension in a patient without oedema and occurring soon after commencing thiazide diuretics suggests ECF volume depletion and strongly suggests that diuretics have contributed to the hyponatraemia. Hypokalaemia associated with hyponatraemia and accompanied by significant urinary K^+ excretion supports the concept that a low ECF volume has stimulated aldosterone release and produced K^+ loss. Nevertheless, the low bicarbonate and urate do not typically support volume contraction and suggest impaired water excretion either as a result of ADH secretion, perhaps induced by volume depletion or nausea, or perhaps because of water retention independent of ADH such as may be associated with reduced renal prostaglandin production after ingestion of NSAIDs. Low creatinine, urea and uric acid have been reported in elderly patients with thiazide-associated hyponatraemia. These features of primary water retention can occur in both SIADH and after thiazide ingestion, especially in the elderly (see also explanation to Question 4).

Clinical identification of subtle degrees of volume depletion or oedema is often difficult. ECF volume may be low, normal or increased in chronic hyponatraemia. While history and clinical examination may be helpful, correct identification of the state of water retention requires quantitative ECF volume determination or tonicity balance. A tonicity balance will explain the aetiology of hyponatraemia. This requires measurement of the water and electrolyte contents of all fluids ingested or lost. Since this may not be possible, laboratory investigations that are helpful (in addition to plasma electrolytes, creatinine and urea) include haematocrit, plasma albumin and urate, plasma and urine osmolality, and urinary sodium, potassium and chloride concentrations. Haematocrit and albumin concentration provide an objective measurement of change in plasma volume in the absence of primary disorders affecting these markers (such as anaemia, cirrhosis, malnutrition and nephrotic syndrome). If patients have a reduced muscle mass (reduced ICF compartment), a smaller positive water balance will cause a greater fall in P_{Na^+}.

Clinical pearls

- Hyponatraemia usually reflects water retention, regardless of volume status.
- ADH is usually increased in chronic hyponatraemia, regardless of cause.
- TBW is 50 to 70% body weight and mostly located in skeletal muscle.
- P_{Na^+} in patients with reduced muscle mass is more susceptible to fluctuation with changes in electrolyte-free water (EFW).

Question 4

Which of the following is/are true regarding the patient's condition?
(a) Urine is maximally dilute in the absence of ADH.
(b) Cardiac failure, nephrotic syndrome and cirrhosis increase ADH secretion.
(c) The patient's water retention can be explained by SIADH.
(d) Hyperglycaemia can cause hyponatraemia with a raised $P_{osm\ (measured)}$.

Answer

All are correct

Explanation

Normally, filtrate emerging from the ascending limb of the loop of Henle is maximally dilute (20 to 80 mosm/kg) and remains dilute as it descends through the medullary collecting duct. When present, ADH binds to basolateral V_2 receptors and initiates cAMP-mediated insertion of type 2 aquaporins (water channels) into the luminal surface of medullary collecting duct cells. This allows water to move out of the filtrate into the hypertonic renal medullary interstitium and to re-enter the ECF (antidiuresis). ADH also stimulates insertion of amiloride-sensitive Na^+ channels (ENaC) into the luminal membrane of cortical collecting duct cells and also promotes urea reabsorption in the inner medullary collecting duct by the urea transporter UT-1, which is important for the generation of the medullary interstitial concentration gradient. Inhibition of ADH secretion or activity allows excretion of EFW (the theoretical fraction of plasma water volume with zero osmolality which would restore dilute plasma osmolality and hence P_{Na^+} to normal). Renal prostaglandins promote water diuresis by inhibiting ADH-mediated water reabsorption in the medullary collecting ducts and are natriuretic by inhibiting sodium reabsorption in the loop of Henle and the cortical collecting tubule.

    True volume depletion will stimulate ADH secretion and produce hyponatraemia if there is accompanying adequate hypotonic water intake (oral or intravenous). Such volume depletion occurs with gastrointestinal or renal fluid loss or surgery, but also after prolonged extreme exertion such as marathon running. Ingestion of non-steroidal anti-inflammatory drugs (NSAIDs) will enhance hyponatraemia in these situations by impairing the prostaglandin-mediated excretion of water (and sodium) described above. Hyponatraemia with 'effective' hypovolaemia occurs even more commonly in cardiac failure, cirrhosis and nephrotic syndrome, although total body Na^+ and ECF including plasma volume may actually be increased (i.e. the increase in EFW is greater than the degree of Na^+ retention). However, ADH secretion is stimulated by reduced carotid sinus baroreceptor sensing of pressure respectively because of reduced cardiac output, peripheral vasodilatation or extravascular redistribution. Thus each of these 'non-euvolaemic' states is associated with increased ADH secretion, which may be regarded as an appropriate physiological response to the non-osmotic stimulus of hypovolaemia, although the usual hyperosmolar stimulus to ADH secretion is absent. Diuretics will increase ADH through volume depletion, but usually only thiazides produce severe hyponatraemia. This may be because loop diuretics prevent the development of the hypertonic medullary interstitium required for ADH to induce water retention and also because they have a shorter duration of action than thiazides.

In contrast, SIADH is a disorder where plasma volume status is normal (no hypovolaemia or oedema) and in which ADH secretion continues inappropriately, since it persists despite the absence of a physiological stimulus and despite a decrease in measured plasma osmolality, which would normally inhibit ADH secretion. The excess ADH prevents the excretion of ingested excess EFW. Partial 'escape' from ADH stimulation occurs secondary to volume expansion. Inhibition of proximal tubular sodium reabsorption, increased glomerular filtration rate (GFR), inhibition of the renin–angiotensin–aldosterone system and increased atrial natriuretic factor all promote a natriuresis which allows sufficient urine output to prevent progressive water retention so that patients are 'euvolaemic'.

SIADH should be suspected when the urine is not maximally dilute in the presence of hyponatraemia and a reduced plasma osmolality. This is usually associated with a urine sodium concentration above 40 mmol/L and the presence of normal acid–base and potassium balance. Patients with intermediate urinary sodium concentrations (20 to 40 mmol/L) will also usually have SIADH and some will have a U_{Na^+} <20 mmol/L if sodium intake is very low. The term SIADH is usually reserved for cases of true hyponatraemia where other pathophysiological settings, such as diuretics, known to stimulate ADH release are absent (see explanation to Question 5). There is some overlap, however. For example, additional treatment or events may induce volume contraction in patients with SIADH. Hyperglycaemia can cause hyponatraemia with a normal or raised P_{osm}: this is clearly excluded in this patient as $P_{glucose}$, P_{osm} and the osmolal gap are not increased.

Clinical pearls

- Effective volume depletion increases ADH secretion regardless of cause.
- Suspect SIADH when U_{osm} is not maximally dilute in the presence of plasma hypo-osmolality.
- SIADH is usually associated with a urine sodium concentration above 40 mmol/L.
- Urine volume may be normal in SIADH (partial escape).

Question 5

Which of the following statements is/are true?

(a) Fluoxetine is a frequent cause of asymptomatic hyponatraemia.
(b) SIADH is caused by ectopic ADH production and central nervous system (CNS) lesions.
(c) ADH action on the kidney is mimicked by lithium.
(d) The correct treatment of hyponatraemia is oral water restriction.

Answer
A, B and D

Explanation

Since ICF volume is inversely proportional to P_{Na^+}, during normal osmoregulation too little water increases P_{Na^+} and tonicity and shrinks hypothalamic osmoreceptor cells. Stimulation of these cells produces two responses: (1) hypothalamic ADH secreting neurons release ADH and (2) stimulation of the hypothalamic thirst centre. Too much water reverses these events. Independent of the prevailing osmolality, drugs may stimulate ADH release or action to cause hyponatraemia. ADH release is stimulated by nicotine, morphine, clofibrate, both tricyclic and selective serotonin re-uptake inhibitor types of antidepressants, carbamazepine, antipsychotics (including chlorpromazine, haloperidol, olanzapine and risperidol), intravenous cyclophosphamide and other antineoplastic drugs (perhaps acting by stimulation of nausea), amiodarone, ciprofloxacin and 'ecstasy' (methylenedioxymethamphetamine, or MDMA). Selective serotonin reuptake inhibitors produce hyponatraemia due to excess ADH in up to 12% of patients with the greatest risk being in elderly females; this usually occurs in the first weeks of treatment and is usually asymptomatic (Fabian et al. 2004). This is therefore unlikely in this patient, who has been on fluoxetine for 6 months.

ADH release is stimulated by 'non-osmotic' factors including pain, nausea, vomiting and anxiety. Pain and nausea probably account for excess ADH associated with major surgery including abdominal and thoracic surgery. Almost all CNS and pulmonary diseases including functional, infective and traumatic conditions have been associated with SIADH through stimulating pituitary ADH release.

ADH effect on the kidney is enhanced by hypoglycaemic agents, methylxanthines including caffeine and aminophylline, analgesics which inhibit prostaglandin synthesis (including aspirin and NSAIDs) and thiazide diuretics.

Exogenous forms of ADH which cause hyponatraemia include administered desmopressin acetate (DDAVP®), vasopressin and oxytocin. Ectopic production of ADH occurs with some tumour cells, especially small-cell carcinoma of the lung but also pancreatic and duodenal carcinoma. The renal actions of ADH are antagonised by lithium and demeclocycline and to some extent by loop diuretics, which inhibit generation of the medullary interstitial hypertonicity.

The appropriate treatment for hyponatraemia depends on whether it is acute or symptomatic and whether the cause can be defined and removed. Since virtually all clinically significant hyponatraemia involves impaired water excretion, oral water restriction is appropriate. Only hyponatraemia present for less than 48 hours can be defined as acute. In this patient the history both of behavioural change and of diuretic ingestion suggest that hyponatraemia has been present chronically. Some experts recommend treatment according to the presence or absence of symptoms rather than the acuity of onset of hyponatraemia. Treatment will be considered further in subsequent sections.

 Clinical pearls

- Physiological stimulation of ADH release is a result of increased osmolality (1% change), or hypovolaemia (aortic baroreceptors responding to a 5 to 10% decrease).
- 'Non-osmotic' stimuli of ADH release are pain, nausea, vomiting, anxiety and hypoglycaemia.
- Non-physiological stimuli which release ADH include pulmonary and CNS pathology and drugs.
- Drugs may cause hyponatraemia by stimulating ADH release or by enhancing ADH renal actions or both.
- ADH actions in the kidney are inhibited by lithium, demeclocycline and loop diuretics.

LEVEL B

Case history continued ...

Additional data are obtained on the patient including the following on her urine:

Na⁺	25 mmol/L
Cl⁻	69 mmol/L
K⁺	45 mmol/L
Osmolality	420 mosm/kg
Volume	1.6 L

Repeat plasma data are unchanged.

Question 6

Which of the following statements are true about this patient?
(a) Plasma ADH is suppressed.
(b) Plasma ADH is increased.
(c) These data can be explained by SIADH.
(d) These data are consistent with thiazide ingestion.

Answer
B, C and D

Explanation

High urine Na^+, K^+ and Cl^- in the setting of hyponatraemia and plasma hypo-osmolality suggests that renal tubular sodium reabsorption (and secondary chloride reabsorption) is inhibited. This occurs in the presence of diuretic therapy and also in SIADH when natriuresis occurs in response to volume expansion secondary to water retention with consequent inhibition of proximal sodium reabsorption, suppression of the renin–angiotensin–aldosterone system, increased GFR and increased atrial natriuretic peptide production. The absence of a maximally dilute urine (let alone a raised urine osmolality as shown here) in the presence of reduced plasma osmolality confirms that ADH is present and acting to facilitate water reabsorption.

By inhibiting sodium reabsorption, diuretics increase Na^+ and Cl^- excretion and secondarily stimulate K^+ excretion so that urine Na^+, K^+ and Cl^- will be >20 mmol/L. Since thiazides do not interfere with ADH action (unlike loop diuretics they do not impair generation of the medullary concentration gradient), thiazides can promote the excretion of urine with a sodium plus potassium concentration higher than that of plasma when ADH is also stimulated by thiazide-induced volume depletion. Thiazides can thus produce hyponatraemia independent of water intake. Older patients with low body weight are at greatest risk of thiazide hyponatraemia, which usually appears acutely. Indeed, if diuretic dose and dietary intake remain constant after initiating therapy, a new steady-state is reached within 2 weeks, after which further sodium and water losses will not occur. At-risk patients (thin, elderly or patients taking NSAIDs) should have plasma electrolytes measured some days after commencing thiazides to detect hyponatraemia. In addition, thiazides can have complex secondary effects on both water and sodium transport. For example, in experimental nephrogenic diabetes insipidus induced by lithium, thiazides have an antidiuretic action secondary to upregulation of aquaporin 2 channels and distal renal Na^+ transporters. Thus reduced water excretion is always present with severe hyponatraemia, since the contraction of ECF volume would otherwise produce circulatory collapse as the presenting symptom. Even with renal Na^+ wasting as the primary cause of hyponatraemia, water ingestion and secondary water retention (due to volume contraction induced stimulation of ADH secretion) must be present for severe hyponatraemia to develop. Consequently, most patients with thiazide-induced chronic hyponatraemia are euvolaemic.

When diuretics are stopped, urine Na^+ and Cl^- will be low (<15 mmol/L) highlighting physiologically appropriate avid tubular sodium reabsorption by the kidney. When hyponatraemia and hypovolaemia have been induced by vomiting, urine Cl^- will be low, but Na^+ may be high (>20 mmol/L) as Na^+ will accompany urinary bicarbonate wasting secondary to the metabolic alkalosis caused by loss of H^+ (and Cl^-) ions. If volume depletion is caused by diarrhoea or laxative abuse, the urine chloride will be high (>20 mmol/L) since bicarbonate is lost in the stools and chloride will replace bicarbonate in the plasma (producing a hyperchloraemic, normal anion gap acidosis).

While the hyponatraemia and volume depletion in this patient may be attributed to thiazides, hyponatraemia to this extent requires a contribution from water retention as outlined. The low uric acid, absence of alkalosis and the raised urinary osmolality confirm water retention and suggest the presence of underlying or associated inappropriate ADH. A patient with SIADH can also have ECF volume contraction from another cause, such as intercurrent diuretic use or diarrhoea (e.g. in HIV-associated SIADH). In this setting urinary Na^+ will tend to be low and when the ECF volume is corrected, urinary Na^+ will increase but hyponatraemia will persist because the underlying stimulus/source of ADH secretion persists preventing a large water diuresis.

Clinical pearls

- Thiazides may cause profound hyponatraemia within 2 weeks of commencing therapy.
- Thin, elderly patients and those on NSAIDs are at greatest risk of thiazide hyponatraemia.
- In the presence of reduced P_{osm}:
  - Na$^+$ deficiency is suggested by low urine electrolytes
  - water excess is suggested by an insufficiently dilute urine.
- Non-renal causes of hyponatraemia generally produce urine low in electrolytes.
- Urine Cl$^-$ indicates the site of GIT loss: high Cl$^-$ = postpyloric loss; low Cl$^-$ = prepyloric loss.
- ECF volume contraction can complicate SIADH.
- Renal Na$^+$ loss hyponatraemia also involves secondary ADH-stimulated water retention.

Question 7

If the same patient was euvolaemic (no postural hypotension) with no history of diuretic ingestion, then likely explanations for her hyponatraemia and clinical findings include which of the following?

(a) Mineralocorticoid deficiency
(b) Addison's disease
(c) SIADH
(d) Remote diuretic use

Answer

C

Explanation

Addison's disease and hypopituitarism (low cortisol) and mineralocorticoid deficiency (low aldosterone) can produce hyponatraemia but are unlikely causes in the absence of hyperkalaemia. In addition, Addisonian patients are usually euvolaemic, while there is usually ECF volume depletion and relatively low urinary K$^+$ (<20 mmol/L) with mineralocorticoid deficiency. In this case the urinary transtubular K gradient (TTKG) can be calculated to assess aldosterone activity and provide indirect evidence regarding primary adrenal insufficiency. Since the urine osmolality is 420 mosm/L, cortical collecting duct (CCD) urinary K$^+$ has been concentrated by ADH-facilitated removal of water to approximately the same extent as the osmolality has increased above plasma (i.e. 420/248 = 1.69). Thus the tubular fluid K$^+$ in the CCD must have equalled the urinary K$^+$/1.69 = 45/1.69 = 26.62 mmol/L. Hence TTKG in the CCD where aldosterone acts must be approximately $26.62/$ plasma $K^+ = 26.62/3.1 = 8.6$, a ratio which suggests significant aldosterone bioactivity is present and this makes primary adrenal insufficiency very unlikely. This could be confirmed with a short synacthen test. Note that the TTKG assumes the presence of ADH and that there is little or no K^+ reabsorption in the medullary collecting duct. This formula is relatively accurate as long as the urine osmolality exceeds that of the plasma (so that the potassium concentration at the end of the cortical collecting tubule can be estimated) and the urine sodium concentration is >25 mmol/L so that sodium delivery is not limiting.

In SIADH there is typically euvolaemia coupled with the high urinary electrolyte excretion and an inappropriately high urine osmolality (lack of adequate dilution) as noted already. It should be noted that with renal failure, there is often an inability to concentrate or dilute the urine resulting in isosthenuria (urine with a plasma-like osmolality). The low GFR in this case is approximately consistent with the patient's age and not a cause for concern. Patients with remote diuretic use may appear euvolaemic but they will have low urine Na^+ and Cl^- consistent with the normal renal response to hyponatraemia, which is to increase Na^+ reabsorption.

Clinical pearls

- Low urine K^+ in the presence of hyponatraemia and ECF volume contraction suggests low aldosterone activity.
- Hyponatraemia due to Addison's disease or mineralocorticoid deficiency can be excluded by a normal TTKG.
- TTKG can be estimated from $U_{K^+}/(U_{osm}/P_{osm})/P_{K^+}$.
- TTKG range: a low value <2 suggests hypokalaemia from a non-renal cause; a high value >7 suggests mineralocorticoid is acting and the renal response is normal.
- Remote diuretic use will result in urine low in Na^+ and Cl^-.
- Chronic kidney disease may impair both dilution and concentrating mechanisms causing isosthenuria.

LEVEL C

Question 8

During treatment of this patient:
(a) diuretics should be ceased
(b) she should initially have oral fluid restricted to 800 to 1000 mL/day

(c) she should receive isotonic saline (0.9% NaCl) infusion

(d) 1 mmol Na^+ per litre TBW (as isotonic saline) will raise P_{Na^+} by 1 mmol/L.

Answer

A, B and D

Explanation

The first question to ask in treatment is: should the patient be treated? Most patients with chronic hyponatraemia are asymptomatic even with a Na^+ <125 mmol/L. Asymptomatic patients are generally thought to be at low risk due to the cerebral adaptation described, which makes brain herniation unlikely. Furthermore, if the condition is due to SIADH with a reset osmostat, then treatment is unlikely to be successful anyway. Symptoms usually become apparent if the Na^+ decreases rapidly or to levels <120 mmol/L. The 4 to 20% mortality data reported for patients with Na^+ less than 110, 115 or 120 mmol/L (not in this order) in various large retrospective studies, reflect data *for treated patients*. The natural history of untreated hyponatraemia has not been studied prospectively. However, even mild hyponatraemia is associated with a higher mortality in a range of disorders such as cardiac failure, cirrhosis and tuberculosis. Symptoms include lassitude, headache, nausea, weakness and then progress to confusion, convulsions, coma and death. Patients with minor symptoms remain at risk of falls and seizures. Furthermore, there is evidence that one of the main risk factors for symptomatic hyponatraemia is preceding asymptomatic untreated hyponatraemia. The consensus is that for chronic hyponatraemia, both symptomatic patients and patients with Na^+ <120 mmol/L should be treated since rapid clinical deterioration may occur.

This patient has chronic hyponatraemia, ECF volume contraction secondary to thiazide diuretics, secondary stimulation of ADH secretion and could have underlying SIADH. ECF volume contraction means that total ECF Na^+ and water are both reduced (Na^+ more than water because water retention has been independently stimulated), but there will be a surplus of water in the ICF. This is an extension of the situation typical of classic euvolaemic SIADH where ECF volume is normal but with a deficit of ECF Na^+. The principles of treatment are similar. In hyponatraemia due to a primary Na^+ deficit, the aim is to replace Na^+ and prevent renal sodium loss (cease diuretics etc.). In hyponatraemia due to water excess (retention), the aim is to restrict water and promote renal water excretion (suppress ADH). In both cases, the rate of Na^+ increase must be carefully controlled to prevent osmotic demyelination syndrome (ODS). In this patient the aim is to lose surplus water (mostly in her ICF) and to retain and replace ECF Na^+. Clearly the thiazide diuretic must be stopped, since this has produced hyponatraemia, hypokalaemia and promoted ADH secretion. However, a loop diuretic and even supplementary ADH may be required during treatment.

Each litre of ECF has lost $140 - 111 = 29$ mmol of Na^+. Her ECF volume is normally 10 L, so she has lost 10 L $\times$ 29 mmol = 290 mmol Na^+. Giving 1 mmol Na^+ per litre of TBW (30 L) will raise plasma Na^+ concentration by 1 mmol/L, but will expand the ECF volume more since water will move out of the ICF into the ECF (the administered Na^+ will stay in the ECF). Thus, the apparent volume of distribution for administered Na^+ will be TBW. The potassium deficit must also be replaced. Note that this will independently raise the plasma Na^+ because Na^+ will exit as K^+ enters cells.

Until treatment is commenced, the osmolality in the ECF and ICF will be the same, and water movement after treatment will again equalise the osmolality in the ECF and ICF compartments. Infusion of a hypertonic solution will shrink the ICF and expand the ECF, while infusion of a solution that is isotonic to the patient will leave the ICF compartment unchanged. Shrinking the ICF too rapidly increases the risk of ODS, while overfilling the ECF runs the risk of producing cardiac failure (especially in patients presenting with an expanded ECF volume). Suppressing ADH secretion will promote a diuresis (of EFW). Such a 'spontaneous' diuresis can accelerate the rise in plasma Na^+ by >2 mmol/L per hour. Such a rapid rise in plasma Na^+ after administration of isotonic saline at an apparently conservative rate of 2 L/day (with KCl 40 mmol/day) has proven fatal from ODS after 6 days following a rise in Na^+ of 12 mmol/L in 18 hours and 41 mmol/L after 41 hours in a patient with profound thiazide-induced hyponatraemia and moderate symptoms (Na^+ = 94 mmol/L: see Lin cited in Sterns 2004). Similarly, a young woman with chronic hyponatraemia due to Addison's syndrome developed ODS after an increase in P_{Na^+} of 9 mmol/L in 4 hours after treatment with isotonic saline, potassium and steroids (Lin et al. 2003). Consequently, it is critical during treatment of chronic hyponatraemia that there is frequent (2- to 3-hourly) monitoring of plasma and urinary electrolytes and of water input and output, so that treatment can be adjusted frequently regardless of the underlying aetiology. Susceptibility to ODS during correction of chronic hyponatraemia is increased in the severely malnourished, patients with cirrhosis and adrenal insufficiency and has been reported with daily increases in P_{Na^+} of 8 to 9 mmol/L. Note that in SIADH isotonic saline will usually worsen the hyponatraemia since it results in some water retention (if the urine osmolality prior to administration is greater than 300 mosm/kg) accompanied by loss of all the administered NaCl in the urine since renal sodium handling is intact.

While adhering to these principles, it must be noted that the ideal strategy for treating chronic hyponatraemia remains controversial. In particular, the use of isotonic, tailored or hypertonic saline (usually 3%) has been advocated. As highlighted above, hypertonic saline is not essential for rapid correction of hyponatraemia even in the presence of symptoms, but is ideal when hyponatraemia is acute or when there is a critical risk of ECF volume overload. Note that 0.9% saline, (NaCl 154 mmol/L, osmolality ~290 mosm/kg) is actually hypertonic relative to the patient's starting P_{osm} of 248 mosm/kg. Therefore, to replace a contracted ECF volume rapidly in a patient in shock without putting the patient at risk of ODS, a solution 'isotonic to the patient not the doctor', to quote Halperin (1988), (i.e. $Na^+ + K^+$ = patient osmolality = 248 mosm/L) should be infused and the rate of increase in Na^+ carefully monitored and controlled. In the event of a large water diuresis, this can be controlled by administering small doses of ADH (e.g. as DDAVP®). Large volumes of this solution will nevertheless put the patient at risk of cardiac failure. Hypertonic saline (3%) has the potential advantage of slowly raising the P_{Na^+} before volume repletion and rapid correction can occur but this similarly requires careful monitoring.

Since there has been chronic hyponatraemia, the daily increase in Na^+ must be limited to 8 mmol/day but should preferably be no higher than 4 mmol/day to reduce the risk of ODS. The rate of rise should be further limited to 0.5 to 1 mmol/L/hour if the patient is not symptomatic or mildly symptomatic. In convulsing patients, increasing the P_{Na^+} by 3 to 6 mmol/L total is recommended. Overexpansion of the ECF compartment can be prevented by concomitant administration of a loop diuretic (frusemide), which may also be useful if the urine remains too concentrated in SIADH (osmolality >500 mosm/kg).

Ideally this patient's ECF volume should be cautiously expanded with 124 mmol/L NaCl solution and this should be followed with a restricted intake of water and carefully controlled promotion of water excretion. Since the urine contains Na^+, urinary Na^+ and K^+ loss will need to be measured and replaced. If isotonic saline is used, use DDAVP® to slow the rate of water excretion if P_{Na^+} rises too quickly. While several formulae exist for interpreting plasma Na^+ concentrations, uncertainty in the estimate of TBW, electrolyte and water intake and excretion and numerous factors leading to unanticipated changes in P_{Na^+} mean that clinicians are better advised to measure P_{Na^+} frequently rather than rely on formulaic predictions. A reasonable alternative strategy in a patient who is relatively asymptomatic (like this one) would be to stop the diuretic and fluoxetine and allow rehydration with eating and drinking to taste while carefully monitoring P_{Na^+} and weight. No further treatment would be required after recovery. If P_{Na^+} continued to fall, oral fluids would be restricted and cautious intravenous fluid therapy and close monitoring instituted as described.

Clinical pearls

- Use TBW as the denominator to predict the increase in ECF Na^+ during administration of intravenous fluids.
- P_{Na^+}, P_{osm} and fluid balance should be measured 2- to 3-hourly during initiation of treatment.

- Aim at a maximal daily increase in P_{Na^+} of 4 mmol/L, except with acute hyponatraemia.
- Limit the hourly increase in P_{Na^+} to 0.5 to 1 mmol/L/hour unless the patient is convulsing.
- Infusion of a solution isotonic (to the patient) will leave the ICF volume unchanged.
- Infusion of a hypertonic solution will shrink the ICF and expand the ECF.
- Replacement of a K^+ deficit will increase P_{Na^+}.
- Urinary electrolyte losses should be replaced with a hypertonic solution to yield net water loss.

Question 9

Which of the following is/are true regarding the patient's condition?
(a) Because diuretics were commenced recently, the hyponatraemia can be regarded as acute.
(b) The risk of ODS is greater in patients with reduced muscle mass.
(c) The P_{Na^+} may be over 120 mmol/L in patients who are fitting.
(d) Brain ammonia levels are associated with hyponatraemia in acute liver failure.
(e) SIADH with a reset osmostat may be present if the urine has a low osmolality.

Answer
B, C, D and E

Explanation

Acute hyponatraemia is limited to decreases occurring in less than 48 hours. There is usually an inverse relationship between P_{Na^+} and ICF volume except when other organic solutes in the ECF generate an osmolal gap or when there is an increase in ICF osmoles, for example after seizure or rhabdomyolysis. In the absence of these events, acute hyponatraemia implies an increase in water in the intracellular compartment. Acute hyponatraemia produces an increase in brain cell volume as the cells swell with water entry. However, within 48 hours brain cells extrude osmolytes, water follows and cell volume returns to normal. If P_{Na^+} is then increased quickly, the cells will not be able to reaccumulate osmolytes rapidly enough to maintain cell volume.

This osmotic shrinkage of oligodendrocytes induces apoptosis and myelin-olysis demonstrable by MRI (or autopsy) and usually affects the central pons (central pontine myelinolysis) but may extend more widely in extreme cases (extrapontine myelinolysis). The typical biphasic clinical course following correction of hyponatraemia in symptomatic patients involves an encephalopathic state that improves with increasing P_{Na^+}. This improvement followed by a deterioration with the development of myelinolysis has been termed ODS. Patients may be asymptomatic but most clinically diagnosed cases present with flaccid then spastic quadriparesis, pseudobulbar palsy and acute changes in mental status, with progression possible to altered levels of consciousness and death. Survival is possible with recovery or varying residual neurologic deficits. Although initial reports were largely confined to chronic alcoholics, the more frequent observation of central pontine myelinolysis in patients after rapid correction of hyponatremia, in patients with cirrhosis who undergo a significant rise in P_{Na^+} after liver transplantation and occasionally in dialysis patients experiencing rapid correction of hyponatraemia in a single dialysis has led to the use of ODS as the generic terminology. The risk of ODS is greater where the ECF volume is smaller (e.g. in thin females with little skeletal muscle where ECF is closer to 50%). The risk is similarly increased where there is potential for a sudden rise in P_{Na^+} when the stimulus to ADH secretion is removed (e.g. following correction of a volume deficit in hypovolaemia) or when there is increased solute delivery to the distal nephron, which allows reabsorption of filtrate and antidiuresis, or simply following the rise in P_{Na^+} itself. While dexamethasone has been reported to prevent demyelination in a rat model of ODS involving correction of hyponatraemia, the occurrence of ODS following correction of adrenal insufficiency and panhypopituitarism, probably through rapid suppression of ADH secretion, suggests a need for caution in using steroids as treatment.

An increase in ICF osmoles will occur after seizure or rhabdomyolysis. This will drive movement of water from the ECF to the ICF, which will increase P_{Na^+} in the ECF. Thus post-ictal P_{Na^+} may be >120 mmol/L even though such high concentrations are not usually the cause of the convulsions. Measurement of brain osmolytes in cirrhotic patients with hyponatraemia has demonstrated that P_{Na^+} concentrations are directly correlated with these osmolytes except for glutamate and glutamine, which correlate with plasma ammonia. Brain ammonia is eliminated by conversion of glutamate to glutamine, so that glutamate accumulation in acute liver failure may be the significant osmole accounting for cerebral oedema. Profoundly low myoinositol in brain cells of cirrhotic patients with modest hyponatraemia may account for the susceptibility of these patients to ODS.

The differential diagnosis of hyponatraemia with a low but not maximally dilute urinary osmolality includes polydipsia in the presence of continuing but low ADH activity (e.g. with psychogenic polydipsia, or intermittent nausea and vomiting), exogenous ADH administration in the presence of continued hypotonic intake or a reset osmostat type of SIADH. A reset osmostat type of SIADH can occur with any cause of SIADH and may account for 25 to 30% of cases overall. This may also occur in hypovolaemic states, psychosis and chronic malnutrition and may also account for the 5 mmol/L lower P_{Na^+} in pregnancy. Hyponatraemia is more commonly milder, P_{Na^+} 125 to 135 mmol/L, stable and asymptomatic. A reset osmostat means that attempting to raise the P_{Na^+} is both unnecessary and likely to be ineffective (due to increased thirst preventing effective fluid restriction). It can be confirmed clinically by observing the response to a water load (10 to 15 mL/kg orally or intravenously). Normal subjects and those with a reset osmostat will excrete more than 80% within 4 hours. Excretion will be impaired in subjects with SIADH. After exogenous ADH administration, subjects with a reset osmostat will increase urine osmolality.

 Clinical pearls

- P_{Na^+} is inversely proportional to ICF volume.
- Acute hyponatraemia is restricted to 48 hours.
- The risk of ODS is greater in elderly patients with a reduced muscle mass.
- P_{Na^+} may be >120 mmol/L in patients after seizure or rhabdomyolysis.
- Cirrhotic patients are at increased risk of ODS.
- Hypertonic solutions should not be used unless the patient is symptomatic.
- SIADH with a reset osmostat is common and usually requires no treatment.

Question 10

Which of the following statements is/are true?
(a) Acute hyponatraemia may occur from self-induced water intoxication.
(b) Neurological symptoms are uncommon in acute hyponatraemia.
(c) Cerebral oedema in acute hyponatraemia leads to death by herniation.
(d) P_{Na^+} in symptomatic patients with acute hyponatraemia should be corrected urgently.
(e) Acute symptomatic hyponatraemia should be corrected by 3 to 6 mmol/L at 1 to 2 mmol/L/hour.

Answer
A, C, D and E

Explanation

Acute hyponatraemia is most frequent in marathon runners who drink excessively during a race, individuals abusing MDMA (ecstasy), hospitalised patients receiving intravenous fluids and institutionalised psychotic patients with self-induced water intoxication. In a sample of 488 runners completing the Boston marathon, 13% had P_{Na^+} <130 mmol/L and 3 (0.6%) had <120 mmol/L and were symptomatic. Since muscle glycogen and triglyceride are oxidised to water and CO_2 during strenuous prolonged endurance activities (sometimes portrayed as releasing 'bound' water), it is important that runners lose weight and do not overhydrate during exercise in order to maintain a normal P_{Na^+}. The consensus recommendations for treating symptomatic runners with hyponatraemia is to use 100 mL 3% saline over 10 minutes to acutely raise the P_{Na^+} and decrease cerebral oedema. This is expected to raise P_{Na^+} by 2 to 3 mmol/L. For persistent or worsening symptomatic hyponatraemia after the patient is hospitalised, a further bolus followed by infusion of hypertonic saline is recommended.

MDMA abuse is particularly risky since this drug stimulates both ADH release and intense thirst, and is frequently consumed during dance parties, an activity which promotes vigorous perspiration and also large volume water ingestion among participants. This is often encouraged by dance organisers 'to avoid dehydration'. As with runners, the intense activity itself can stimulate ADH release. Gastrointestinal motility can decrease with MDMA; an ileus containing a large static volume of EFW which can be absorbed at the end of the physical activity will contribute further to the acute hyponatraemia. In addition women, especially younger menstruating ones, are reported to be at thirty times greater risk of death or permanent neurological damage from non-cardiogenic pulmonary oedema, hypoxia and cerebral oedema associated with acute hyponatraemia. These differences may be hormonal, vascular (increased sensitivity to the vasoconstrictor effects of ADH) or related to reduced muscle mass particularly in young women after surgery and inappropriate hypotonic fluid therapy. Neurological symptoms are relatively common in acute hyponatraemia when the P_{Na^+} falls below 125 mmol/L. Encephalopathic patients usually present with headache, nausea, vomiting, abdominal pain, confusion and seizures. Death from acute hyponatraemia is usually by cerebral oedema and herniation and most reported cases have involved young women and children.

Aggressive therapy with hypertonic saline is indicated in patients with acute severe symptomatic hyponatraemia. Symptomatic patients usually respond to an increase in P_{Na^+} of 4 to 6 mmol/L. There is no evidence that achieving this at a rate of 1 to 2 mmol/L/hour with hypertonic saline is harmful. The complications of hypertonic saline have been identified exclusively in patients with chronic hyponatraemia, where the daily rate of correction has increased 10 mmol/L/day. A large daily increase in acute hyponatraemia is not usually necessary after the acute emergency has been addressed. Urgent therapy with hypertonic saline is usually indicated. This should be supplemented with frusemide when non-cardiogenic pulmonary oedema is present. In less severely symptomatic patients, the administration of a loop diuretic alone may achieve a satisfactory rate of correction of hyponatraemia. It is important to stress that chronic hyponatraemia should not be corrected aggressively and the rate of increase in P_{Na^+} must be monitored frequently and minimised to avoid ODS.

 Clinical pearls

- Avoid overhydrating athletes during strenuous endurance activities.
- Death from acute hyponatraemia is usually by cerebral oedema and herniation; hypoxia from non-cardiogenic pulmonary oedema adds significantly to mortality.
- Acute symptomatic hyponatraemia should be treated acutely.
- Hypertonic saline is indicated with acute symptomatic hyponatraemia.
- Acute symptomatic hyponatraemia should be corrected by 3 to 6 mmol/L at 1 to 2 mmol/L/hr.
- Asymptomatic chronic hyponatraemia may not require treatment.
- Death from chronic hyponatraemia may follow overcorrection and ODS.

Bibliography

Level A

1. Fabian, T.J., Amico, J.A., Kroboth, P.D., Mulsant, B.H., Corey, S.E., Begley, A.E., Bensasi, S.G., Weber, E., Dew, M.A., Reynolds, C.F. & Pollock, B.G. (2004) Paroxetine-induced hyponatremia in older adults: a 12-week prospective study. Arch Intern Med. 164(3), 327–32.
2. Lin, S.H., Hsu, Y.J., Chiu, J.S., Chu, S.J., Davids, M.R. & Halperin, M.L. (2003) Osmotic demyelination syndrome: a potentially avoidable disaster. Q J Med. 96(12), 935–47.
3. Omari, A., Kormas, N. & Field, M. (2002) Delayed onset of central pontine myelinolysis despite appropriate correction of hyponatraemia. Intern Med J. 32(5–6), 273–4.

Level C

4. Halperin, M.L. & Goldstein, M.B. (1988) *Fluid, Electrolyte, and Acid-Base Physiology. A Problem-Based Approach*, 2nd edn. Philadelphia: W.B. Saunders Company.
5. Halperin, M.L., Kamel K.S. & Sterns, R. (2005) Hyponatremia in marathon runners. N Engl J Med. 353(4), 427–8.

6. Sterns, R.H. (2004) Fluid, electrolyte and acid–base disturbances. NephSAP. 3(4), 192–231.
7. Sterns, R.H. & Palmer, B. (2006) Fluid, electrolyte, and acid-base disturbances. NephSAP. 5(1), 10–54.
8. Rose, B.D. (2006) Diuretic-induced hyponatraemia. UpToDate, www.utdol.com, last revised on 10 May 2007.
9. Rose, B.D. (2006) Treatment of hyponatraemia. UpToDate, www.utdol.com, last revised on 9 April 2007.
10. Kalantar-Zadeh, K., Nguyen, M.K., Chang, R. & Kurtz, I. (2006) Fatal hyponatraemia in a young woman after ecstasy ingestion. Nature Clinical Practice. 2(5), 283–8.

Case 2
Acid–base disturbance

DAVID HARRIS

LEVEL A

Case history

A 28-year-old woman is brought into the emergency department by her friends who have noticed that for the past few days she has been confused, generally weak and nauseated. She looks unwell. Her supine blood pressure is 90/60 mmHg. Her pulse is regular and rapid at >100 beats/min and she is afebrile. She has moderate weakness affecting her upper and lower limbs and her trunk. There are no focal neurological signs and examination of her abdomen, chest and precordium is normal. The following arterial blood gas and serum electrolyte results are obtained.

Laboratory data

	Result	Reference range
K$^+$	1.9 mmol/L	(3.2–5.5)
Na$^+$	132 mmol/L	(136–146)
Total CO$_2$	8 mmol/L	(24–31)
Cl$^-$	113 mmol/L	(94–107)
pH	7.10	(7.35–7.45)
PaO$_2$	95 mmHg	(95–100)
PaCO$_2$	35 mmHg	(35–45)

Question 1

Her arterial blood gas results can be explained by which of the following?
(a) Respiratory acidosis
(b) Severe metabolic acidosis with mild respiratory alkalosis
(c) Metabolic acidosis with adequate respiratory compensation
(d) Combined metabolic and respiratory acidosis

Answer
D

Explanation

The patient is acidotic (pH 7.10). Partial pressure of both CO_2 ($PaCO_2$) and serum bicarbonate (total CO_2) are less than normal, indicating a metabolic acidosis (answer A incorrect). With a pure respiratory acidosis, $PaCO_2$ would be elevated, as would serum bicarbonate in anything but an acute respiratory acidosis (answer A incorrect). The respiratory compensation for a metabolic acidosis is hyperventilation causing reduction in blood $PaCO_2$. $PaCO_2$ should fall by 1 to 1.5 times the drop in serum bicarbonate which, with adequate respiratory compensation in this case, would mean that $PaCO_2$ should fall from the normal value of 40 by 1 to 1.5 times (normal bicarbonate –8), or to between 16 and 24 mmHg. Another rule of thumb is that $PaCO_2$ should fall to 100 times (pH – 7.0) or in this case to 10 mmHg. Thus, her $PaCO_2$ has not fallen sufficiently, and so her respiratory compensation is inadequate (answer C incorrect). If she had combined metabolic acidosis and respiratory alkalosis, her CO_2 should have been lower than predicted by the rules of thumb for metabolic acidosis with adequate respiratory compensation (answer B incorrect). The alveolar–arterial (A–a) gradient (FiO_2 – PaO_2 – $PaCO_2 \times 1.2$, which equals 13 in this case) is normal, indicating that her alveolar gas exchange is normal and there is no pulmonary disease. The hypoventilation in this case is probably due to muscle weakness caused by hypokalaemia. Therefore, if this patient did not have any metabolic acidosis, her respiratory acidosis would have been more obvious, and her CO_2 would have been higher than normal due to hypoventilation (despite a near normal PaO_2, which suggests her alveolar gas exchange is normal) (answer D correct).

Clinical pearls

- In metabolic acidosis pH, $PaCO_2$ and HCO_3^- (total CO_2) should all fall.
- The normal respiratory compensation for metabolic acidosis is hyperventilation, causing a fall in $PaCO_2$.
- $PaCO_2$ should fall by 1 to 1.5 times the fall in serum bicarbonate.
- $PaCO_2$ should approximate 100 times (pH – 7.0).
- A–a gradient will be normal (less than 15) with hypoventilation and normal lungs.
- A–a gradient = FiO_2 – PaO_2 – $PaCO_2 \times 1.2$.

Question 2

The plasma anion gap in this case is consistent with:

(a) addition of new anions to the body

(b) pre-pyloric gastrointestinal fluid loss

(c) impaired urinary acidification

(d) inhibition of carbonic anhydrase.

Answer

C and D

Explanation

The plasma anion gap is arbitrarily defined as the difference in plasma concentration between the positive ions sodium and potassium and the negative ions chloride and bicarbonate; most of the normal anion gap is comprised of the negative charge on albumin (and so changes in albumin concentration will alter the gap). The normal anion gap is less than 15. The anion gap in this case is 13. (Note that some definitions of anion gap do not include potassium, in which case the normal value would be lower.)

The most common causes of normal anion gap metabolic acidosis are loss of bicarbonate from the gut (post-pyloric fluids which are alkaline, not pre-pyloric which are acidic, so answer B is incorrect) and proximal (one example of many is answer D) or distal (answer C correct) renal tubular acidosis.

Accumulation of new unmeasured anions in the plasma, giving rise to a raised anion gap (e.g. with renal failure) occurs with addition of new acid from exogenous sources (e.g. toxic alcohols, salicylate) or endogenously (e.g. lactic acid, ketoacid) or failure of renal excretion of the anions of new acids (e.g. with renal failure) (answer A incorrect). This is shown in Figure 2.1.

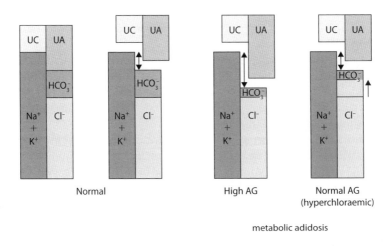

UC = unmeasured cations   ↕ = anion gap (AG)   ↑ = increased Cl concentration
UA = unmeasured anions

Figure 2.1 The anion gap in patients with normal acid–base balance, and those with metabolic acidosis

Clinical pearls

- Plasma anion gap = $Na^+ + K^+ - Cl^- - HCO_3^-$, and is normally <15.
- Normal anion gap metabolic acidosis commonly arises due to gastrointestinal bicarbonate loss or renal tubular acidosis.
- Hypokalaemia with metabolic alkalosis can occur in many conditions, but when hypokalaemia coexists with metabolic acidosis, the cause is usually either diarrhoea or renal tubular acidosis.
- Raised anion gap (>15) metabolic acidosis occurs due to addition of new acid (with a non-chloride anion) or renal failure.

Question 3

The body's defences against this acidosis include:
- **(a)** buffering by intracellular proteins
- **(b)** respiratory hypoventilation
- **(c)** increased renal titratable acid production
- **(d)** increased renal ammonium excretion.

Answer
A and D

Explanation

Intracellular and extracellular buffering occurs immediately. Extracellular buffering is effected predominantly by HCO_3^-/CO_2. While intracellular buffering likewise involves HCO_3^-/CO_2, it also involves proteins and phosphates (answer A correct).

As discussed previously, the respiratory compensation is that of hyperventilation, not hypoventilation, to blow off acid in the form of CO_2 (answer B incorrect).

The kidneys do not produce titratable acids (answer C incorrect); rather, they filter certain ions (mainly phosphates) which titrate H^+ in the tubular lumen, to excrete a total of about 30 mmol per day.

Normal ammonia production and ammonium excretion by the kidney is about 40 mmol per day, and in the case of acidosis this can increase to 200 mmol per day or more (answer D correct). Ammonia is produced from glutamine enzymatically, mainly in the proximal tubular cell; because of the need to make more enzyme, there is a delay of several days before maximum ammoniagenesis can occur.

Clinical pearl

- Body defence against metabolic acidosis includes buffering, hyperventilation and increased renal ammonia production.

Question 4

At this stage, treatment for this patient should include:
(a) artificial ventilation
(b) potassium replacement
(c) dialysis
(d) bicarbonate administration
(e) rehydration with normal saline.

Answer

B and E

Explanation

The patient's potassium needs to be corrected to restore muscle power and normal ventilation (answer B correct). The patient is relatively hypotensive; for adequate intracellular buffering, normal tissue perfusion is required to remove CO_2 from the periphery to the lungs for exhalation. In the case of poor tissue perfusion, CO_2 accumulates within the cells, and so buffering instead involves proteins ('bad' buffering) thereby possibly altering their structure and function. Restoration of tissue perfusion with normal saline permits optimal intracellular buffering (answer E correct).

Acidosis per se, of this severity, is not life-threatening and so there is no need for immediate correction with bicarbonate; moreover, bicarbonate administration may worsen hypokalaemia by driving potassium into cells (answer D incorrect). Bicarbonate therapy could be used after potassium replacement, especially when acidosis is severe. Artificial ventilation is not required at this stage because the patient is not in frank respiratory failure (answer A incorrect). Dialysis would correct the electrolyte abnormalities quickly, but so too would the simpler measures of potassium replacement (to improve ventilation) and volume restoration (to improve tissue buffering by delivering CO_2 to the lungs). Moreover, the normal plasma anion gap indicates that there are no new potentially toxic unmeasured anions (of, for example, a toxic alcohol) to be removed by dialysis (answer C incorrect).

 Clinical pearl

- Emergencies in metabolic acidosis relate to associated derangement of potassium, toxic alcohols and severity of acidosis.

LEVEL B

Case history (continued)

Additional results are obtained on the patient. These include the following.

Plasma creatinine	110 µmol/L	(60–125)
Plasma urea	15 mmol/L	(2.5–6.5)
Plasma osmolality	295 mosm/kg	(275–295)
Plasma glucose	6 mmol/L	(3.6–7.7)
Urinary pH	6.0	

Question 5

Based on these additional results, which of the following is/are likely to explain the pathophysiology of the acidosis?
(a) Ingestion of toxic alcohol
(b) Diabetic ketoacidosis
(c) Rapid metabolism of a toxic alcohol with rapid excretion of its metabolites
(d) Rapid metabolism of a toxic alcohol without excretion of its metabolites
(e) Treatment with ethanol to inhibit metabolism of toxic alcohol

Answer

C

Explanation

Toxic alcohols such as methanol and ethylene glycol are osmotically active and raise the serum osmolar gap. The osmolar gap is the difference between measured and calculated osmolality. The main osmotically active substances in normal serum are electrolytes, urea and glucose. Calculated osmolality is thus the sum of $Na^+ + K^+$ multiplied by two (to account for the accompanying negative ions) plus glucose plus urea. Osmolar gap is normally <15 mosm/kg. The osmolar gap in this case is 6 mosm/kg and so there is nothing to suggest additional osmotically active agents (such as toxic alcohols) in the plasma (answer A incorrect). Toxic alcohols are not acidic but are metabolised by alcohol and aldehyde dehydrogenase to form acidic metabolites that cause the acidosis and can be toxic. If the toxic alcohol were rapidly metabolised, then the osmolar gap might be normal but the anion gap should be raised due to the accumulation of metabolites (new anions); the anion gap is normal in this case (answer D incorrect). However, if the metabolites are rapidly excreted then both the osmolar and the anion gaps could be normal as in this case (answer C correct). Diabetic ketoacidosis is most usually associated with a raised anion gap, though occasionally the plasma anion gap in diabetic ketoacidosis can be normal (answer B unlikely). During the recovery phase of diabetic ketoacidosis, patients can develop a normal anion gap metabolic acidosis by an intriguing mechanism. In the early phase of ketoacidosis, some of the hydrogen of ketoacid is buffered by intracellular buffers and some of the ketoanions are lost in urine. Treatment with saline and insulin converts available ketoanions back to bicarbonate. Some of the newly generated bicarbonate is used to replenish the intracellular buffer so that plasma bicarbonate does not return to normal. Since ketoanions have already been lost in urine, a normal anion gap acidosis results. Treatment with ethanol prevents the metabolism of the alcohol to acidic metabolites and so the osmolar gap should be raised but the anion gap should be normal (answer E incorrect).

Clinical pearls

- Plasma osmolar gap is the difference between measured and calculated osmolality. Calculated osmolality is $2(Na^+ + K^+)$ + glucose + urea (all in mmol/L).
- The normal plasma osmolar gap is <15, as is the normal anion gap and A–a gradient. (The magic gap number is 15!)
- Raised osmolar gap suggests toxic alcohols as the cause of metabolic acidosis.

Question 6

In this case the urinary pH is 6.0. This can be explained by:
(a) bicarbonate wastage
(b) impaired secretion of hydrogen ions into the distal tubular lumen
(c) impaired sodium reabsorption in the distal nephron
(d) impaired potassium secretion in the distal nephron
(e) impaired ammoniagenesis
(f) superimposed metabolic alkalosis.

Answer
B and C

Explanation

The urinary pH is inappropriately high in this case. In proximal renal tubular acidosis due to failure to reabsorb HCO_3^- appropriately in the proximal tubule (see Fig. 2.2), urinary pH varies depending on the amount of HCO_3^- reaching the distal tubule. If its concentration in plasma and therefore glomerular filtrate is low, then despite the defect sufficient HCO_3^- may be reabsorbed in the proximal tubule to prevent the less important unimpaired distal tubular HCO_3^- reabsorption (normally

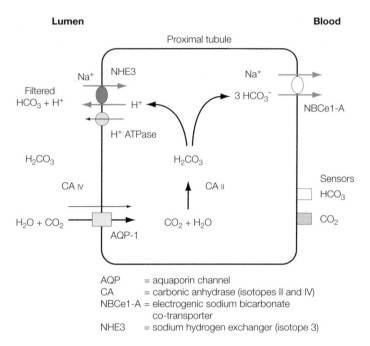

Figure 2.2 Disturbances in H^+ secretion and/or HCO_3^- reclamation by the proximal tubule cell lead to proximal renal tubular acidosis

15% of total HCO_3^- reabsorption) being overwhelmed, thus resulting in no urinary bicarbonate wastage and a low urinary pH. However, if sufficient HCO_3^- leaves the proximal tubule (if the filtered HCO_3^- is high) then urinary HCO_3^- wastage will occur, to buffer H^+ secreted into the distal tubule lumen and raise urinary pH. In this case, plasma HCO_3^- is low and so there should be no HCO_3^- wastage, even in the case of proximal renal tubular acidosis (answer A incorrect).

Impaired Na^+ reabsorption by the principal cells of the distal tubule causes type 4 (distal) renal tubular acidosis because the resultant increased Na^+ concentration in the distal tubule lumen raises luminal positive charge, thus impairing secretion of positively charged ions (H^+ and K^+) into the distal tubular lumen (answer C correct), as seen in Figure 2.3 (a). The impaired secretion of K^+ is thus a consequence of impaired Na^+ reabsorption (answer D incorrect) and results in hyperkalaemia which is typical of type 4 (but not type 1) renal tubular acidosis. Type 1 (distal) renal tubular acidosis occurs due to a defect in the H^+ secretion by intercalated cells (answer B correct), as shown in Figure 2.3 (b). The low luminal H^+ concentration in distal renal tubular acidosis reduces formation of ammonium (NH_4^+) from ammonia (NH_3) and therefore NH_4^+ excretion. In normal kidneys during the acute phase of acidosis, urinary pH would be expected to be 5. However, during chronic acidosis there is time for increased ammoniagenesis and (after buffering of NH_3 by

H⁺ to form NH_4^+) increased luminal NH_4^+ and reduced H⁺ concentration, and so urinary pH may rise. Therefore, impaired ammoniagenesis is unlikely to increase urinary pH (answer E incorrect). In summary, urinary pH is somewhat difficult to interpret and depends not only on H⁺ secretion but also the amount of buffer (bicarbonate, ammonia) reaching the distal tubule.

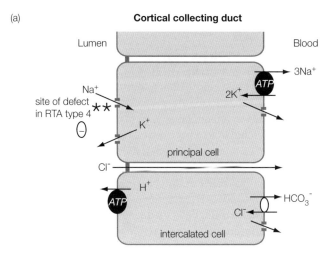

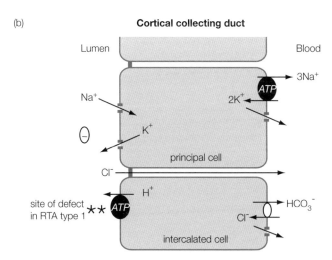

Figure 2.3 (a) Type 4 (distal) renal tubular acidosis occurs due to a defect in Na⁺ reabsorption by principal cells. **(b)** Type 1 (distal) renal tubular acidosis occurs due to a defect in H⁺ secretion by intercalated cells

Mixed acid–base disturbances can be difficult to appreciate. One hint that there might be a superimposed metabolic alkalosis is when the level of serum bicarbonate is not as low as might be expected for the accumulated new anions (whose concentration is equivalent to *calculated minus normal anion gap*). Here, anion gap is normal and so there is no accumulation of new anions (answer F incorrect).

Clinical pearls

- Urinary pH 5 excludes distal renal tubular acidosis; higher urinary pHs are not diagnostically useful.
- Urinary tract infections with urea splitting organisms can produce a high urine pH and should be excluded prior to attributing the high urine pH to renal tubular acidosis.
- Distal renal tubular acidosis can arise due to a primary defect in H^+ secretion or to increased permeability of luminal cell membrane allowing back-diffusion of H^+, or can be secondary to reduced distal tubular Na^+ reabsorption causing a high luminal positive charge which opposes H^+ secretion.
- Impaired distal sodium delivery due to volume depletion leads to distal acidification defect; therefore urine pH >5 should not be considered suggestive of renal tubular acidosis when urinary sodium is <25 mmol/L.

LEVEL C

Case history continued ...

The patient has a normal anion gap and normal osmolar gap metabolic acidosis. The diagnosis is still uncertain. Additional urinary results are received:

Na^+	40 mmol/L
K^+	35 mmol/L
Cl^-	5 mmol/L
Creatinine	5000 µmol/L
Urea	80 mmol/L
Osmolality	510 mosm/kg
Glucose	0 mmol/L

Question 7

True statements about urinary ammonium excretion include which of the following?

(a) It can be measured directly.

(b) It can be easily calculated from the urinary anion gap.

(c) It can be best calculated from the urinary osmolar gap.

(d) If reduced, it is diagnostic of distal renal tubular acidosis.

Answer

A and C

Explanation

Urinary ammonia can be measured directly, but may be falsely elevated in the presence of urea-splitting micro-organisms (answer A correct).

Under some circumstances, urinary ammonium can be calculated from the urinary anion gap. The concept of using urinary anion gap to estimate urinary ammonium excretion assumes that most of the ammonium is excreted as ammonium chloride. The sum of the main urinary cations (Na^+, K^+, NH_4^+) should equal the sum of the main anions (Cl^-, HCO_3^-, sulphate, phosphate) in the absence of new 'unmeasured' anions. Except under conditions of HCO_3^- wastage, urinary HCO_3^- should be very low. Normal sulphate and phosphate excretion totals about 80 mEq/per day. Thus, in the absence of unmeasured anion, $NH_4^+ = Cl^- + 80 - Na^+ - K^+$ (assuming one litre of urine output per day). However, in the presence of unmeasured anions this equation will underestimate the concentration of ammonium (answer B incorrect). A negative urinary anion gap suggests intact ammonia excretion, whereas a positive urinary anion gap may either be because of deficient urinary ammonium excretion or because ammonium is being excreted bound to an anion other than chloride. Therefore, the urinary osmolar gap gives a more reliable estimation (answer C correct).

The equation for calculated urinary osmolality is the same as that for plasma, with the addition of ammonium; that is, calculated $U_{osm} = 2(Na^+ + K^+ + NH_4^+) +$ glucose + urea. Rearranging this equation $NH_4^+ = 0.5 \times$ (calculated U_{osm} – glucose – urea – $2[Na^+ + K^+]$). In the absence of uncharged osmotically active species in the urine, calculated urinary osmolality should approximate measured urinary osmolality. (An unmeasured anion would not alter the difference between measured and calculated urinary osmolality, because anions are accounted for in the equation by doubling the concentration of cations.) Using the calculated urinary osmolality equation, urinary NH_4^+ in this case is 140 mmol/L, suggesting that adequate urinary ammoniagenesis and ammonium excretion (which requires titration of NH_3 by secreted H^+) has occurred and excluding distal renal tubular acidosis. Low ammonium excretion may occur not only due to reduced H^+ secretion (as with distal renal tubular acidosis) but also due to reduced ammoniagenesis, for example with renal failure, and is therefore not diagnostic of the former (answer D incorrect).

Clinical pearls

- When negative, urine anion gap is a good indicator of urinary ammonium excretion but when positive, it can indicate either reduced ammonium excretion or an unmeasured anion in urine.
- Urinary ammonium excretion can be calculated using the equation for calculating urinary osmolality.
- Normal urinary ammonium excretion requires intact proximal ammoniagenesis and distal H^+ secretion.

Question 8

True statements about unmeasured urinary anion include which of the following? In this patient, unmeasured urinary anion is:

(a) low due to poor renal excretion
(b) filtered but almost entirely reabsorbed
(c) filtered and secreted
(d) most likely lactate or ketoacid.

Answer

C

Explanation

Calculating ammonium from the urinary anion gap equation suggests a urinary NH_4^+ concentration of 10 mmol/L, but from the calculated osmolality equation it is 140 mmol/L. Either by solving these two equations simultaneously or by simply looking at the difference, there must be 130 mmol/L (140 – 10) of unmeasured anions in the urine. The plasma anion gap is normal and so there are no unmeasured anions retained in the plasma as they are rapidly cleared by the kidney (answer A incorrect). Renal handling of the anion is best determined by its fractional excretion; or its clearance compared to that of creatinine. Clearance is defined as UV/P, where U and P are the concentrations of the species in urine and plasma respectively and V is the urine volume. Thus, fractional excretion of an anion = (urinary anion/plasma anion) $\times$ (plasma creatinine/urine creatinine) $\times$ 100. In this case, if one assumes plasma unmeasured anion is 1 mmol/L, then fractional excretion of the anion is 286%. If the fractional excretion is 100% then the substance is filtered only with no net flux across the tubule, if it is less than 100% there is impaired filtration or significant reabsorption or if it is greater than 100% it is filtered and secreted. Thus, in this case the anion is filtered and secreted (answer B incorrect, answer C correct). L-lactate is largely reabsorbed and fractional excretion is usually less than 5%; fractional excretion of ketoacids and D-lactate is usually 20 to 80% (answer D incorrect). Hippuric acid, which is a product of the metabolism of toluene, is filtered and secreted and is most likely the unmeasured anion in this case. In other words, the patient is a glue sniffer.

Clinical pearls

- Fractional excretion of unmeasured anions is useful in determining their net handling by the kidney.
- Fractional excretion of 100% suggests filtration without reabsorption or secretion; of less than 100% suggests reduced filtration (e.g. large size or protein bound) or significant reabsorption; of greater than 100% suggests filtration and secretion.

Question 9

Which of the following can occur with metabolic acidosis of glue sniffing?
(a) Raised plasma anion gap
(b) Raised plasma osmolar gap
(c) Distal renal tubular acidosis
(d) Proximal renal tubular acidosis
(e) Endogenous acid production

Answer
A, C and E

Explanation

Toluene is metabolised in the liver to benzyl alcohol by the cytochrome P450 system, benzyl alcohol by alcohol dehydrogenase to benzidine, and benzidine is oxidised to benzoic acid and conjugated with glycine to form hippuric acid. This occurs rapidly within the liver and so plasma alcohol levels should not be elevated and osmolar gap should be normal (answer B incorrect). The negatively charged hippurate is excreted rapidly and drags with it Na^+ and K^+, leading to volume depletion and hypokalaemia. This can cause renal impairment (prerenal azotaemia) which can cause a raised anion gap metabolic acidosis (as has been reported in 10 to 20% of cases) (answer A correct). Distal renal tubular acidosis probably only occurs in the minority of patients (answer C correct). The acidosis is mainly due to the metabolism of toluene and the production of benzoic and in particular hippuric acid (answer E correct).

Other hallmarks of toluene exposure include neuropsychiatric abnormalities, gastrointestinal symptoms, muscle weakness and rhabdomyolysis (due to hypokalaemia), hypophosphataemia and central hypothyroidism.

Bibliography

Level A

1. Field, M.J., Pollock, C.A. & Harris, D.C.H. (eds). (2001) Acid-base balance and regulation of pH. *The Renal System.* Sydney: Church-Livingstone.

Level C

2. Carlisle. E.J.P., Donnelly, S.M., Vasuvattakul, S., Kamel, K.S., Tobe, S. & Halperin, M.L. (1991) Glue sniffing and distal renal tubular acidosis: sticking to the facts. J Am Soc Nephrol 1, pp. 1019–27.

Case 3
Hypokalaemia and metabolic alkalosis

DAVID JOHNSON

LEVEL A

Case history

A 26-year-old female describes a 3-month history of fatigue and leg cramps. Over the last few years, she has had to wake up to go to the toilet approximately twice a night. She describes no other symptoms, denies using any medications or complementary therapies and has no significant past medical history. On examination, she appears well with a seated blood pressure (BP) of 105/60 mmHg, a regular pulse rate of 90 beats/min, a respiratory rate of 16 breaths per minute, a temperature of 36.7°C and a weight of 46 kg. Her jugular venous pressure wave is just visible at the base of her neck when reclined at a 45-degree angle. Pitting ankle and sacral oedema are not observed. Cardiorespiratory, abdominal and neurologic examinations are all normal. The following arterial blood gases and serum electrolyte results are obtained.

Laboratory data

	Result	Reference range
K^+	2.4 mmol/L	(3.2–5.5)
Na^+	133 mmol/L	(136–146)
HCO_3^-	34 mmol/L	(24–31)
Cl^-	91 mmol/L	(94–107)
Mg^{++}	0.50 mmol/L	(0.70–1.00)
Urea	4.5 mmol/L	(3.0–8.0)
Creatinine	40 µmol/L	(70–120)
Osmolality	275 mosm/kg	(275–295)
pH	7.50	(7.35–7.45)
PaO_2	96 mmHg	(100)
$PaCO_2$	46 mmHg	(35–45)

Question 1

Her arterial blood gas results can be explained by which of the following?
(a) Respiratory alkalosis
(b) Metabolic alkalosis with no respiratory compensation
(c) Metabolic alkalosis with at least partial respiratory compensation
(d) Combined metabolic alkalosis and respiratory acidosis

Answer

C

Explanation

The patient is alkalotic (pH 7.50). The partial pressure of CO_2 ($PaCO_2$) and serum bicarbonate concentration are both elevated, indicating that the patient has a metabolic alkalosis. If the patient had a respiratory alkalosis, $PaCO_2$ would be reduced, as would serum bicarbonate if the respiratory alkalosis was of greater than several days' duration (answer A incorrect). The respiratory compensation for a metabolic alkalosis is hypoventilation resulting in an elevation in blood $PaCO_2$. $PaCO_2$ should rise by roughly 0.7 mmHg for every 1 mmol/L increase in plasma bicarbonate. In this case, an elevation in plasma bicarbonate of 9 mmol/L from a normal value of 25 mmol/L to 34 mmol/L would be expected to result in a compensatory increase in $PaCO_2$ from a normal value of 40 mmHg to approximately 46 mmHg (answer B incorrect, answer C correct). Another rule of thumb is that the $PaCO_2$ value should roughly equal the bicarbonate concentration + 15 (e.g. if the plasma bicarbonate is 34 mmol/L, the $PaCO_2$ should be approximately 49 mmHg). This calculation applies principally to bicarbonate concentrations between 10 and 40 mmol/L. Alternatively, the $PaCO_2$ should roughly equal the last two digits of the pH (e.g. for a pH of 7.50, the $PaCO_2$ should be 50). The alveolar–arterial (A–a) gradient ([FiO_2 – PaO_2 – $PaCO_2$] × 1.25, = 10 in this case) is normal (upper limit of normal is approximated by age divided by 4 + 4), suggesting that there is no significant intrapulmonary shunting. Severe hypokalaemia can lead to respiratory muscle weakness and respiratory acidosis, but would be rarely seen at serum potassium levels above 2.0 mmol/L (answer D incorrect).

 Clinical pearls

- In metabolic alkalosis, pH, $PaCO_2$ and HCO_3^- should all increase.
- The normal respiratory compensation for metabolic alkalosis is hypoventilation, leading to a rise in $PaCO_2$.
- $PaCO_2$ should rise by roughly 0.7 mmHg for every 1 mmol/L increase in plasma bicarbonate.

- $PaCO_2$ should roughly equal the bicarbonate concentration + 15 (for serum bicarbonate concentrations between 10 and 40 mmol/L).
- $PaCO_2$ should roughly approximate $100 \times (pH - 7)$.

Question 2

The body's defences against metabolic alkalosis include:
(a) intracellular buffering
(b) hypoventilation
(c) reduced proximal tubular reabsorption of HCO_3^-
(d) increased excretion of bicarbonate by α-intercalated cells
(e) inhibition of H^+ excretion in the cortical collecting duct.

Answer
A, B and C

Explanation

Under conditions of metabolic alkalosis, some intracellular buffering occurs primarily via shifting of H^+ out of cells, although the majority (⅔) of excess base remains in the extracellular fluid compartment (Answer A correct).

As stated in the answer to Question 1, the respiratory compensation for a metabolic alkalosis is hypoventilation resulting in an elevation in blood $PaCO_2$ and a return of blood pH back towards normal (answer B correct). The Henderson-Hasselbalch equation ($pH = 6.10 + \log[HCO_3/(0.03 \times PaCO_2)]$) demonstrates that blood pH is determined by the ratio of HCO_3^- concentration and $PaCO_2$, not by the value of either alone. Thus, in the setting of a metabolic alkalosis where plasma bicarbonate rises, the body compensates by decreasing ventilation rate, which in turn leads to a rise in $PaCO_2$ and a restoration of pH towards normal.

Every day, approximately 65 mmol of bicarbonate per kg body weight (4500 mmol/d) is filtered at the glomerulus (cf. the extracellular bicarbonate space in the body is 350 mmol). Approximately 85% is reabsorbed in the proximal tubule, 10% in the thick ascending limb of Henle's loop and 5% in the cortical collecting duct (titrated against proton secretion). In the proximal tubule, Na^+ transport is linked to acid excretion and HCO_3^- reclamation. For every Na^+ reabsorbed, 1 H^+ is excreted and 1 HCO_3^- is reclaimed (see Fig. 3.1). The reabsorption of bicarbonate is saturable, such that when the plasma HCO_3^- concentration rises above 25 to 26 mmol/L, the transport maximum of the proximal tubule is reached and bicarbonaturia occurs (Answer C correct). Although this represents a theoretical defence against metabolic alkalosis, most cases of metabolic alkalosis are accompanied by volume depletion. This slows the flow of primary urine through the proximal tubule and therefore allows for more avid reabsorption of Na^+ and HCO_3^-, thereby limiting the effectiveness of this defence mechanism.

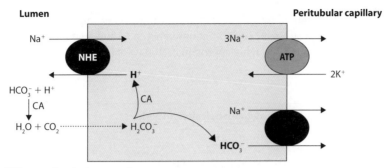

NHE = sodium hydrogen exchanger
CA = carbolic anhydrase

Figure 3.1 Acid–base handling in the proximal tubule

Na$^+$ transport is linked to acid excretion and HCO$_3^-$ reclamation. For every Na$^+$ reabsorbed, 1 H$^+$ is excreted. A secreted H$^+$ combines with a filtered HCO$_3^-$ to form H$_2$CO$_3$, which then forms H$_2$O and CO$_2$ (catalysed by carbonic anhydrase in the apical membrane brush border). CO$_2$ can freely diffuse across the apical membrane where the reverse process takes place to allow HCO$_3^-$ to be transported into the peritubular capillary via the Na$^+$ – 3HCO$_3^-$ symporter. Thus for each Na$^+$ reabsorbed, 1 HCO$_3^-$ is reclaimed. The α-intercalated cells in the collecting duct are involved in H$^+$ secretion and HCO$_3^-$ and K$^+$ reabsorption (see Fig. 3.2).

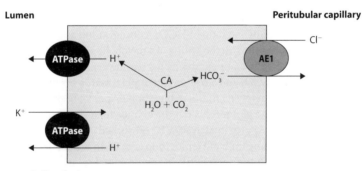

CA = carbolic anhydrase
AE1 = anion exchanger 1

Figure 3.2 The α-intercalated cell in the cortical collecting duct. These cells are primarily concerned with acid excretion (and alkali resorption). H$_2$O and CO$_2$ are dissociated into H$^+$ and HCO$_3^-$ by intracellular carbonic anhydrase. H$^+$ are secreted via a H$^+$-ATPase and via H$^+$,K$^+$-ATPase (in exchange for luminal K$^+$). HCO$_3^-$ is then reabsorbed via a Cl$^-$:HCO$_3^-$ exchanger (anion exchanger 1 or AE1) in the basolateral membrane. H$^+$ excretion is stimulated by acidosis and aldosterone. The activity of the H$^+$,K$^+$-ATPase is increased by hypokalaemia

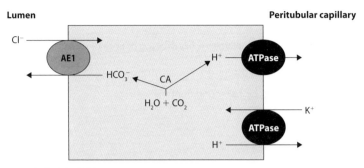

Lumen Peritubular capillary

CA = carbolic anhydrase
AE1 = anion exchanger 1

Figure 3.3 The β-intercalated cell in the cortical collecting duct. In these cells, the arrangement of the transporters in the α-intercalated cells is reversed (i.e. H^+ are secreted into the peritubular capillary by a basolateral H^+-ATPase pump and HCO_3^- anions are secreted into the lumen by an apical anion exchanger, which is probably different from the basolateral Cl^--HCO_3^- exchanger in α-intercalated cells. This allows the loss of HCO_3 into the urine in the presence of an alkaline load

They are primarily concerned with excreting an acid load and defending against acidosis (Answer D incorrect). The excretion of acid by these cells is often inappropriately elevated in conditions of renal alkalosis due to increased delivery of sodium to the collecting duct (which is reabsorbed in exchange for H^+ excretion), elevated aldosterone levels and/or inhibition of the activity of the apical H^+,K^+-ATPase by accompanying hypokalaemia (answer E incorrect). On the other hand, β-intercalated cells in the collecting duct are activated by alkalosis resulting in the excretion of HCO_3^- into the urine in the presence of an alkaline load (see Fig. 3.3). In these cells, the arrangement of the transporters is reversed relative to those in the α-intercalated cells (i.e. H^+ are secreted into the peritubular capillary by a basolateral H^+-ATPase pump and HCO_3^- anions are secreted into the lumen by an apical anion exchanger.

Clinical pearls

- Body defence against metabolic alkalosis includes buffering, hypoventilation, saturation of proximal tubule bicarbonate reabsorption and excretion of HCO_3^- in the collecting duct by β-intercalated cells.
- The Henderson-Hasselbalch equation, $pH = 6.10 + \log(HCO_3/[0.03 \times PaCO_2])$, demonstrates that blood pH is determined by the ratio of HCO_3^- concentration and $PaCO_2$, not by the value of either alone.

Question 3

In this patient, the metabolic alkalosis is likely being maintained by:

(a) hypokalaemia
(b) volume depletion
(c) aldosterone action in the collecting duct
(d) renal acid loss.

Answer

All are correct

Explanation

Hypokalaemia induces a transcellular shift in which potassium leaves the cells, which is counterbalanced by entry of H^+ into cells in order to maintain electro-chemical equilibrium. The movement of hydrogen into the cells increases the plasma bicarbonate concentration (promoting metabolic alkalosis) and lowers the intracellular pH. The intracellular acidosis in renal tubular cells promotes hydrogen secretion and therefore bicarbonate reabsorption and maintenance of a metabolic alkalosis. Hypokalaemia also stimulates the activities of the H^+,K^+-ATPase and H^+-ATPase in the α-intercalated cells in the collecting duct. This leads to increased distal acid excretion and metabolic alkalosis (answers A and D correct).

Volume depletion, as evident in this patient, promotes a metabolic alkalosis via secondary hyperaldosteronism. Aldosterone action in the collecting duct directly enhances urinary acidification by stimulating the activities of the H^+,K^+-ATPase and H^+-ATPase in the α-intercalated cells. Aldosterone also increases the open probability of the epithelial sodium channels (ENaC) in the apical membranes of the adjacent principal cells. This leads to enhanced luminal elec-tronegativity and thus inhibits back-diffusion of secreted H^+ (effectively meaning that increased delivery of sodium to the distal nephron leads to enhanced sodium reabsorption in exchange for H^+ excretion). Chloride depletion also promotes H^+ secretion by α-intercalated cells and inhibits HCO_3^- reabsorption by β-inter-calated cells (answers B, C and D correct). Significant volume depletion may also be accompanied by appreciable urinary losses of bicarbonate-free fluid leading to contraction of the extracellular volume around a relatively constant quantity of extracellular bicarbonate. Such 'volume contraction alkalosis' is commonly seen in disorders characterised by loss of a high chloride, low bicarbonate fluid (e.g. loop diuretics, sweat losses in cystic fibrosis and congenital chloridorrhea).

 Clinical pearl

- Metabolic alkalosis is maintained by one or more of the following factors: hypokalaemia, volume depletion, chloride depletion/hypochloraemia, and aldosterone action.

Question 4

The most important diagnostic test in this patient is:

(a) urinary sodium
(b) urinary chloride
(c) transtubular potassium gradient
(d) urinary-free cortisol
(e) plasma renin/aldosterone ratio.

Answer

B

Explanation

Hypokalaemia often occurs in association with metabolic alkalosis. The first important clinical step is to determine the patient's volume status. If the patient clinically has a normal or increased effective circulating volume, as evidenced by hypertension and/or oedema (not present in this case), one should suspect conditions associated with increased mineralocorticoid effect (e.g. Conn's syndrome, Cushing's syndrome) or external alkali intake (often in the setting of renal failure) (see Fig. 3.4).

In the present case, the patient has a low-normal BP without signs of fluid retention and so is unlikely to have a mineralocorticoid excess state (answers D and E incorrect). Under these circumstances, a urinary chloride test is the most useful investigation to determine whether the cause of the hypokalaemic, metabolic alkalosis is renal or extra-renal. Urinary chloride is more reliable than Na^+ as a guide to volume status in the setting of metabolic alkalosis, as the latter may be misleadingly elevated by the presence of significant bicarbonaturia or excretion of a non-reabsorbable anion (as in some antibiotics such as carbenicillin) (answer A incorrect, answer B correct). In as many as 30% of volume-depleted patients, a difference of 15 mmol/L may be found between the urinary values for Cl^- and Na^+.

A low urinary Cl^- in a volume-depleted patient with metabolic alkalosis suggests vomiting, post-hypercapnia or remote use of diuretics (see Fig. 3.4). Under these circumstances, the kidney is appropriately conserving chloride in order to restore extracellular volume.

A high urinary Cl^- in a volume-depleted patient with metabolic alkalosis suggests renal wasting, as may occur with diuretic use or a hereditary renal tubular disorder (see Fig. 3.4).

The transtubular potassium gradient (TTKG) is calculated as (urine K^+/ plasma K^+) ÷ (urine osmolality/plasma osmolality). This equation estimates the ratio of the potassium concentration at the end of the cortical collecting duct relative to plasma by correcting for the degree of urinary concentration that subsequently takes place in the medullary collecting duct. The TTKG assumes

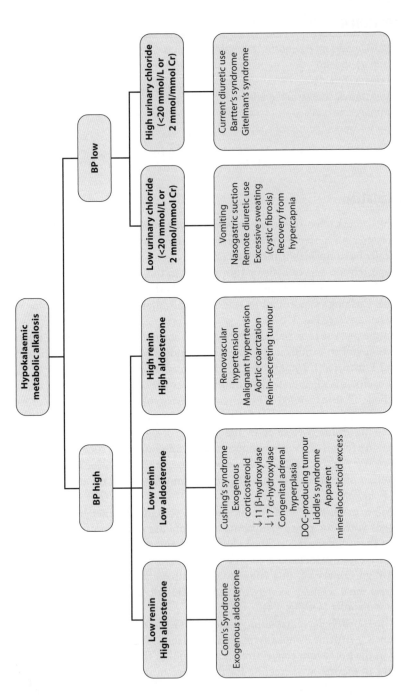

Figure 3.4 The clinical approach to the patient with hypokalaemic metabolic alkalosis

that the osmolality at the end of the cortical collecting duct is similar to that of plasma (since equilibration with the isosmotic interstitium will occur in the presence of antidiuretic hormone) and that there is no appreciable K^+ secretion or absorption in the medullary collecting duct. The formula is relatively accurate provided the urine osmolality exceeds plasma osmolality and the urine sodium concentration exceeds 25 mmol/L (so that sodium delivery is not rate-limiting). An extrarenal cause of hypokalaemia is suggested by a TTKG <2, a urinary K^+ concentration <20 mmol/L or 1.5 mmol/mmol creatinine, or a 24-hour urinary K^+ <15 mmol/day. In hypokalaemia, calculating the TTKG does not usually provide additional useful information beyond that afforded by a spot urinary potassium concentration (answer C incorrect). However, in hyperkalaemia, a TTKG may be very helpful, whereby a value <5 is strongly suggestive of hypoaldosteronism.

 Clinical pearls

- In hypokalaemic metabolic alkalosis, the first clinical step is to assess the patient's BP and volume status.
- If the patient is hypertensive and/or has evidence of hypervolaemia, consideration should be given to a mineralocorticoid or glucocorticoid excess state.
- If the patient clinically has a low extra-cellular fluid volume (the more common scenario), urinary chloride is very useful for narrowing the diagnostic possibilities.
- A low urinary Cl in a volume-depleted patient suggests vomiting, post-hypercapnia or remote use of diuretics (since the kidneys are appropriately conserving chloride in response to volume depletion).
- A high urinary Cl in a volume-depleted patient suggests a hypokalaemic salt-losing tubulopathy (i.e. diuretic use or a genetic tubular transport defect such as Bartter's or Gitelman's syndrome).
- The transtubular potassium gradient (TTKG) is calculated as (urine K^+/plasma K^+) ÷ (urine osmolality/plasma osmolality). In hypokalaemic patients, a value <2 suggests extra-renal K^+ loss, provided the urine osmolality exceeds the plasma osmolality and the urine Na^+ >25 mmol/L.
- Calculating the TTKG is often more helpful in patients with hyperkalaemia, whereby a value <5 is strongly suggestive of hypoaldosteronism.

LEVEL B

Case history continued ...

Additional urinary biochemistry results are obtained on the patient:

K^+	24 mmol/L
Na^+	136 mmol/L
Cl^-	187 mmol/L
Creatinine	6 µmol/L
Osmolality	730 mosm/kg

Question 5

The most likely cause/s of the patient's hypokalaemic, hypochloraemic metabolic alkalosis is/are:

(a) hypokalaemic periodic paralysis

(b) vomiting

(c) renal tubular disorder

(d) diuretic

(e) mineralocorticoid (or glucocorticoid) excess state

(f) diarrhoea.

Answer

C and D

Explanation

The combination of mild volume depletion and inappropriate chloriuresis (urinary chloride >20 mmol/L or >2 mmol/mmol creatinine) in the setting of a hypokalaemic, hypochloraemic metabolic alkalosis strongly suggests a hypo-kalaemic salt-losing tubulopathy (i.e. diuretic administration or hereditary renal tubular disorder) (answers C and D correct). Diuretic administration is gener-ally biochemically indistinguishable from a hereditary salt-losing tubulopathy. However, if a patient stops taking diuretics for a few days prior to urinary testing, their kidneys will appropriately curtail excretion of chloride. On the other hand, in Bartter's and Gitelman's syndromes, inappropriate chloriuresis is a consistent finding. Thus, the finding of even a single low urinary chloride concentration in the urine in a volume-depleted patient with previously documented inappropriate chloriuresis suggests surreptitious diuretic use. Testing the urine for diuretic substances may also be useful if positive.

Clinical situations in which the primary basis for hypokalaemia is a shift of potassium into cells (e.g. familial periodic paralysis, hyperthyroid periodic paralysis, β-agonists, insulin therapy) are usually characterised by a short time course, low urinary potassium excretion (<10 to 15 mmol/day or <1.5 mmol/mmol creatinine or TTKG <2) and the absence of an acid–base disorder. Thus, the basis for the current patient's hypokalaemia is not likely to be primarily explained by a shift of K^+ into cells (e.g. by periodic paralysis) because her urinary potassium concentration is inappropriately high for their degree of hypokalaemia (4 mmol/mmol creatinine) and there is an accompanying metabolic alkalosis (answer A incorrect).

The patient is mildly volume depleted and has a high urinary chloride excretion rate (>20 mmol/L or >2 mmol/mmol creatinine). The inappropriate chloriuresis, together with the high urinary potassium excretion rate, is inconsistent with vomiting (which is characterised by low urinary excretion of both chloride and potassium) (answer B incorrect).

The clinical absence of hypertension and hypervolaemia makes a mineralocorticoid or glucocorticoid excess state unlikely (answer E incorrect).

Diarrhoeal states are associated with a metabolic acidosis (not metabolic alkalosis) due to stool bicarbonate losses (answer F incorrect). The most common causes of hypokalaemia combined with metabolic acidosis are diarrhoea and distal (type 1) or proximal (type 2) renal tubular acidoses.

 Clinical pearls

- The differential diagnosis for hypokalaemia is extensive but can be rationalised by 'concept sorting' with the presence or absence of concurrent acid–base abnormalities.
- Clinical situations in which the primary basis for hypokalaemia is a shift of potassium into cells (e.g. familial periodic paralysis, hyperthyroid periodic paralysis, β-agonists, insulin therapy), are usually characterised by a short time course, low urinary potassium excretion (<10 to 15 mmol/day or <1.5 mmol/mmol creatinine or TTKG <2) and the absence of an acid–base disorder.
- Hypokalaemia in association with metabolic acidosis should prompt consideration of diarrhoea and distal (type 1) or proximal (type 2) renal tubular acidoses.
- Hypokalaemia in association with metabolic alkalosis suggests apparent mineralocorticoid excess states (e.g. Cushing's, Conn's, liquorice, apparent mineralocorticoid excess, Liddle's syndrome), extra-renal chloride losses (e.g. vomiting, sweat) or hypokalaemic salt-losing tubulopathies (diuretics, Bartter's syndrome, Gitelman's syndrome). These can be readily distinguished by measurement of BP, plasma renin and aldosterone (if BP high) and urinary chloride (if BP normal or low).

Question 6

The factors potentially contributing to this patient's hypokalaemia include:

(a) secondary hyperaldosteronism
(b) hypomagnesaemia
(c) metabolic alkalosis
(d) increased sodium delivery to the cortical collecting duct
(e) β-adrenergic stimulation.

Answer

All are correct

Explanation

Metabolic alkalosis is generally accompanied by hypokalaemia. In this patient, the high urinary chloride concentration suggests the presence of a hypokalaemic, salt-losing tubulopathy. Under these circumstances, the ensuing natriuresis leads to mild volume depletion (suggested by the clinical findings), secondary hyperaldosteronism and increased renal K^+ excretion (answer A correct). If volume depletion is sufficiently severe, an ensuing adrenergic response may lead to stimulation of Na^+,K^+-ATPase via β_2-receptors and subsequent intracellular shifting of K^+ (answer E correct).

Hypomagnesaemia is commonly present in hypokalaemic patients. It promotes kaliuresis by uncertain mechanisms, although it is thought that hypomagnesaemia may lead to intracellular ATP depletion thereby releasing luminal potassium channels in the collecting duct and the thick ascending limb of Henle from inhibition. Consequently, loop and collecting duct secretion of potassium is enhanced. This phenomenon is important to recognise as hypokalaemia may be difficult to correct without concurrent treatment of hypomagnesaemia (answer B correct).

Both metabolic and respiratory alkalosis promote hypokalaemia by stimulating intracellular K^+ shifts. H^+ moves out of cells to minimise the rise in extracellular pH. Consequently, K^+ moves into cells to maintain electrochemical neutrality. For each 0.1 unit rise in pH, plasma K^+ may fall by up to 0.4 mmol/L (answer C correct).

Patients with salt-losing tubulopathies have significant natriuresis and kaliuresis by virtue of increased urine output. Moreover, the increased distal delivery of Na^+ results in increased Na^+ reabsorption, which is balanced by increased excretion of K^+ (answer D correct).

 Clinical pearls

- Metabolic alkalosis is frequently accompanied by hypokalaemia due to intracellular K^+ shifts and enhanced urinary potassium excretion (often due to concurrent hyperaldosteronism, increased distal Na^+ delivery, adrenergic stimulation and hypomagnesaemia).

- Hypomagnesaemia is common in hypokalaemic states and exacerbates urinary potassium losses. Under such circumstances, correcting hypokalaemia is often difficult without concurrent magnesium supplementation.

LEVEL C

Case history continued ...

Further tests are ordered on the previous urine specimen:

Ca^{++}	0.3 mmol/L
Mg^{++}	4.2 mmol/L

Question 7

The clinical and biochemical picture would be compatible with which of the following conditions:

(a) Bartter's syndrome
(b) surreptitious thiazide use
(c) surreptitious frusemide use
(d) Gitelman's syndrome
(e) multiple myeloma.

Answer

B and D

Explanation

In the setting of a suspected hypokalaemic, salt-losing tubulopathy (high urinary chloride in a volume-depleted patient), examining the urinary osmolality and calcium excretion helps to determine whether the problem is localised to the loop of Henle (which is responsible for concentrating the urine via the countercurrent mechanism and is an important site for calcium reabsorption) (see Fig 3.5) or the distal tubule (in which Na^+ reabsorption is linked with calcium excretion) (see Fig. 3.6). Consequently, a high or high-normal urinary calcium concentration and isosthenuria (urine osmolality [U_{osm}] 200 to 300 mosm/kg) suggests Bartter's syndrome, loop diuretic therapy or cationic binding of the calcium-sensing receptor on the basolateral membrane of the thick ascending limb of Henle's loop (e.g. by aminoglycosides or myeloma globulins). Conversely, a low urinary calcium and intact urinary concentrating ability suggests Gitelman's syndrome or thiazide diuretic therapy. Since the distal convoluted tubule is the last nephron segment to regulate the excretion of magnesium, hypomagnesaemia is more common with distal convoluted tubule defects than with loop defects.

The current patient has a modestly high urinary osmolality, a low urinary calcium excretion and a low plasma magnesium concentration. This picture best fits a distal convoluted tubule lesion (i.e. thiazide use or Gitelman's syndrome) (answers B and D correct). These conditions are frequently biochemically indistinguishable (as are Bartter's syndrome and loop diuretic use), although useful clues include testing the urine for the presence of diuretics and the intermittent presence of low urinary chloride excretion due to intermittent diuretic cessation.

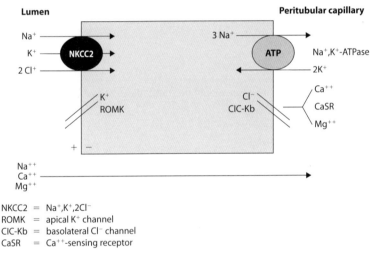

NKCC2 = Na$^+$,K$^+$,2Cl$^-$
ROMK = apical K$^+$ channel
ClC-Kb = basolateral Cl$^-$ channel
CaSR = Ca^{++}-sensing receptor

Figure 3.5 Loop of Henle electrolyte transport processes

Transport processes are actively driven by a basolateral Na$^+$,K$^+$-ATPase, which lowers intracellular Na$^+$ concentration and raises intracellular K$^+$ concentration. The fall in intracellular Na$^+$ concentrations allows lumenal Na$^+$ to enter the cell via the Na$^+$,K$^+$,2Cl$^-$ (NKCC2) co-transporter. K$^+$ is recycled back into the lumen via an apical K$^+$ channel (ROMK). Cl$^-$ is reabsorbed into the peritubular capillaries via a basolateral Cl$^-$ channel (ClC-Kb); this process is controlled by a basolateral membrane Ca^{++}-sensing receptor (CaSR). The net absorption of Cl$^-$ and excretion of K$^+$ creates an electrochemical gradient between the lumen and the peritubular capillary which favours the passive reabsorption of positively charged electrolytes (Na^{++}, Ca^{++}, Mg^{++}) through tight junctions between the cells (paracellular pathway). Since the thick ascending limb of Henle's loop is impermeable to water, the net reabsorption of NaCl without water increases medullary tonicity, which is vital to the effective operation of the countercurrent mechanism (which in turn allows the excretion of highly concentrated urine). Loop diuretics (e.g. frusemide, bumetanide, ethacrynic acid) block the action of NKCC2 resulting in the excretion of a dilute urine and increased urinary excretion of Na^+, K^+, Cl^-, Ca^{++} and Mg^{++}. An identical biochemical picture will also be caused by genetic mutations of NKCC2, ROMK, ClC-Kb or CaSR (which cause Bartter's syndrome). Certain drugs (e.g. aminoglycosides) and abnormal proteins (e.g. myeloma) can also interfere with the action of the CaSR.

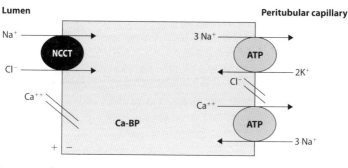

NCCT = Na^+,Cl^--co-transporter
Ca-BP = calcium-binding protein

Figure 3.6 Distal convoluted tubule electrolyte transport processes

Transport processes are actively driven by a basolateral Na^+,K^+-ATPase, which lowers intracellular Na^+ concentration and raises intracellular K^+ concentration. The fall in intracellular Na^+ concentrations allows luminal Na^+ to enter the cell via the apical Na^+,Cl^--co-transporter (NCCT; also know as the thiazide-sensitive co-transporter, TSC). The entry of Na^+ into the cells inhibits the activity of a Ca^{++}-Na^+ antiporter on the basolateral membrane. Consequently, reabsorption of calcium from luminal urine is inhibited, thereby promoting calciuresis. Inhibition of NCCT activity by thiazide diuretics or genetic defects (Gitelman's syndrome) results in increased urinary excretion of Na^+ and Cl^- and reduced urinary excretion of Ca^{++}. Since the loop of Henle transport processes are not affected, the countercurrent mechanism remains intact and so the kidneys can still therefore generate either a dilute or concentrated urine, depending on the hydration status of the individual.

Clinical pearls

- In patients with hypokalaemic, salt-losing tubulopathies (metabolic alkalosis, low extracellular fluid volume, high urinary chloride excretion), urinary concentrating ability and urinary calcium excretion rate are useful for localising the defective nephron segment.
- A high or high-normal urinary calcium and isosthenuria (U_{osm} 200 to 300 mosm/kg) suggests a loop defect (Bartter's syndrome, loop diuretic or cationic binding of the calcium-sensing receptor).
- A low urinary calcium and normal urinary concentration suggests a distal convoluted tubule defect (Gitelman's syndrome or thiazide diuretic).
- Hypomagnesaemia is more common with distal convoluted tubule defects than with loop defects.
- Thiazide use is frequently biochemically indistinguishable from Gitelman's syndrome (as is loop diuretic use from Bartter's syndrome).
- Temporary cessation of a diuretic for a few days will result in a fall in urinary chloride excretion to a low level (cf. urinary chloride excretion is consistently elevated in Bartter's and Gitelman's syndromes).

Question 8

Assuming that the patient is not surreptitiously taking diuretics, which of the following investigation results would be expected in this patient?

(a) Elevated plasma renin and aldosterone concentrations
(b) Increased urinary prostaglandin excretion
(c) A fall in urinary osmolality with frusemide administration
(d) Lack of urinary concentration response to ADH
(e) A mutation in the SLC12A3 gene
(f) Nephrocalcinosis

Answer
A, C and E

Explanation

All of the hypokalaemic, salt-losing tubulopathies are characterised by mild volume depletion and secondary hyperaldosteronism with elevated plasma aldosterone and renin concentrations (answer A correct). Prostaglandin synthesis in the thick ascending limb of Henle's loop is increased in Bartter's syndrome and following loop diuretic administration. In contrast, thiazide diuretics and

Gitelman's syndrome are associated with little or no increase in urinary prostaglandin excretion (answer B incorrect). Since the Na^+-K^+-2 Cl^- co-transporter (NKCC2) in the loop of Henle is intact in Gitelman's syndrome and thiazide diuretic use, such patients will still show a diuretic response to loop diuretics (including a fall in urinary osmolality) (answer C correct). Similarly, the counter-current mechanism is intact in distal convoluted tubule defects, such that ADH will result in appropriate urinary concentration (answer D incorrect). The majority of cases of Gitelman's syndrome identified to date are associated with mutations of the SLC12A3 gene encoding the thiazide-sensitive Na^+-Cl^- co-transporter (NCCT) in the distal convoluted tubule. Medullary nephrocalcinosis is observed in some cases of Bartter's syndrome (reflecting the high urinary calcium excretion rate), but is not seen in Gitelman's syndrome (answer F incorrect).

 Clinical pearl

- Gitelman's syndrome is generally characterised by secondary hyperaldosteronism, normal urinary prostaglandin secretion, intact Henle's loop responses and a mutation of the SLC12A3 gene.

Question 9

Which of the following therapies would be appropriate for this patient?
(a) Indomethacin
(b) Spironolactone
(c) Angiotensin-converting enzyme inhibitor
(d) Potassium supplementation
(e) Magnesium supplementation

Answer
B, C, D and E

Explanation

Non-steroidal anti-inflammatory drugs (NSAIDs) ameliorate the augmented prostaglandin synthesis, hyperreninaemia, hypokalaemia and metabolic alkalosis of Bartter's syndrome. However, NSAIDs have been reported to be of relatively little benefit in Gitelman's syndrome, in which prostaglandin excretion appears to be normal (answer A incorrect). Potassium-sparing diuretics, such as spironolactone and amiloride, promote K^+ and H^+ retention thereby correcting hypokalaemia and alkalosis (answer B correct). One study has found spironolactone to be more effective than amiloride, suggesting that antagonising aldosterone action is more efficacious than blocking ENaC in the collecting duct principal cells. Angiotensin-converting enzyme inhibitors also antagonise the biochemical features of secondary hyperaldosteronism in Gitelman's syndrome, although may exacerbate hypotension in this condition (answer C correct). Despite spironolactone and angiotensin-converting enzyme inhibitor therapy, potassium and magnesium supplementation are still often required in Gitelman's syndrome (answers D and E correct). Hypokalaemia is frequently refractory to treatment unless the magnesium depletion is concurrently addressed.

Question 10

This patient's condition has been linked to a defect of which of the following transporters?

(a) β-subunit of the basolateral chloride channel (ClC-Ka / ClC-Kb) (Barttrin)

(b) Basolateral chloride channel (ClC-Kb)

(c) Na^+-K^+-2 Cl^- co-transporter (NKCC2)

(d) Calcium-sensing receptor (CaSR)

(e) K^+ channel (ROMK)

(f) Na^+-Cl^- co-transporter (TSC or NCCT)

Answer

B and F

Explanation

It has recently been appreciated that Gitelman's syndrome is genetically hetero-geneous and can be caused by mutation of the basolateral chloride channel (ClC -Kb) (Bartter's syndrome type III), as well as of the luminal, thiazide-sensitive Na^+-Cl^- co-transporter (TSC or NCCT) (answers B and F correct) (see Table 3.2). Kindreds with homozygous chloride channel (ClC-Kb) mutations have been reported in which family members variously exhibit Bartter's or Gitelman's phenotypes or start off expressing a Bartter's phenotype and evolve into a Gitelman's phenotype. However, ClC-Kb mutations tend to manifest earlier in life (usually the first 2 years) compared to NCCT mutations, which may not be clinically apparent until adulthood. In addition to genetic heterogeneity, marked variability in the clini-cal phenotype may also be observed among patients with the same mutation.

Clinical pearls

- Significant genetic and phenotypic heterogeneity has been observed among the hereditary, hypokalaemic, salt-losing tubulopathies.
- Gitelman's syndrome is known to be caused by defects of either the luminal, thiazide-sensitive sodium chloride co-transporter (NCCT) in the distal convoluted tubule or the basolateral chloride channel (ClC-Kb) in the distal tubule and the thick ascending limb of Henle's loop.

Table 3.2 Classification of the hereditary, hypokalaemic, salt-losing tubulopathies

Classification	Phenotype	Gene defect	Locus	Transporter defect	Location	Features
BS Type I	Antenatal	SLC12A1	15q15–21	NKCC2	TAL	Nephrocalcinosis
BS Type II	Antenatal	KCNJ1	11q24–25	ROMK	TAL	Nephrocalcinosis Minor K^+ wasting
BS Type III	Classic BS or Gitelman's syndrome	CLCNKB	1p36	ClC-Kb	TAL and/or DCT	Variable Ca^{++} excretion
BS Type IV	BS with deafness	BSND	1p31	Barttrin	TAL/inner ear	Deafness Normocalciuria
Gitelman's	Gitelman's	SLC12A3 or CLCNKB	16q13 or 1p36	NCCT or ClC-Kb	DCT	
Autosomal dominant hypocalcaemia		CASR	3q13.3–q21	Calcium-sensing receptor (CaSR)	TAL/parathyroids	Hypocalcaemia Hypomagnesaemia

Note: BS = Bartter's syndrome, DCT = distal convoluted tubule and TAL = thick ascending limb of Henle's loop

Bibliography

Level A

1. Whittier, W.L. & Rutecki, G.W. (2004) Primer on clinical acid-base problem solving. Dis Mon. 50(3), 122–62.
2. Groeneveld, J.H.M., Sijpkens, Y.W.J., Lin, S.H., Davids, M.R. and Halperin, M.L. (2005) Masterclasses in medicine: an approach to the patient with severe hypokalaemia—the potassium quiz. QJM. 98, 305–16.

Level C

3. Zelikovic, I. (2003) Hypokalaemic salt-losing tubulopathies: an evolving story. Nephrol Dial Transplant. 18, 1696–700.
4. Reinalter, S.C., Jeck, N., Peters, M. & Seyberth, H.W. (2004) Pharmacotyping of hypokalaemic salt-losing tubular disorders. Acta Physiol Scand. 181, 513–21.

Part B
General
nephrology

Case 4
Renal mass

GOPI RANGAN

Case history

A 75-year-old female presents to her general practitioner with mild right-sided flank pain and malaise for 6 months. She has a past history of left-sided nephrectomy for renal cancer at age of 48, hypertension for 10 years, cancer of the left breast with oestrogen receptor-positive nodes treated by radiotherapy and hormone treatment at the age of 72 and hypothyroidism. An abdominal computerised tomography (CT) scan with contrast is performed and reveals a 6.5 cm solid mass (5 Hounsfield units) in the mid-pole of the right kidney.

Question 1

Risk factors for kidney cancer include:
- **(a)** obesity
- **(b)** smoking
- **(c)** end-stage kidney failure
- **(d)** occupational exposure to petrol
- **(e)** von Hippel-Lindau syndrome.

Answer
A, B, C and E

Explanation

Any solid renal mass should be considered malignant until proven otherwise. Renal cell carcinomas account for 95% of all malignant neoplasms arising from the kidney. The male to female ratio is 2:1, and the incidence peaks between the ages of 50 to 70 years. The majority of cancers are sporadic. The strongest environmental factors associated with kidney cancer are cigarette smoking (accounting for 20 to 30% of cases) and obesity. There is no consistent evidence that occupational exposure to petrol is associated with renal cancer. Risk is also increased in those who have tuberous sclerosis and acquired cystic disease associated with end-stage renal failure. Familial cases occur with von-Hippel-Lindau syndrome (VHL), where approximately 35% develop renal cell cancer.

Question 2

True statements about the clinical features of kidney cancer include which of the following?
(a) Flank pain is a common presenting symptom.
(b) A mass is palpable in 25% of patients.
(c) Hypertension occurs in 20% of patients.
(d) Anaemia is less common than erythrocytosis.
(e) More than half of patients have metastatic disease at presentation.

Answer
A, B and C

Explanation

The presenting symptoms and signs of renal cell carcinoma include haematuria, abdominal pain and a flank/abdominal mass. This classic triad occurs in 10 to 20% of patients. The most common presentations are haematuria (40%), flank pain (40%), palpable mass (25%), weight loss (33%), fever (20%), hypertension (20%), anaemia or a varicocele. Anaemia, a sign of advanced disease, is a much more common feature on presentation than erythrocytosis (20% versus 3%). Due to the increasing use of imaging investigations in clinical practice, many cases (up to 50%) of renal cell carcinoma are now diagnosed as an incidental finding. This may, in part, explain the rising incidence of renal cell carcinoma in epidemiological studies and that 50% have localised disease on presentation with 25 to 30% having metastatic disease.

Question 3

Regarding the pathology and molecular genetics of kidney cancers, which of the following statements is/are true?
(a) Clear cell tumours arise from distal tubular epithelial cells.
(b) Papillary tumours arise from proximal tubular epithelial cells.
(c) Mutations of the VHL gene occur in a minority of sporadic cases.
(d) Birt-Hogg-Dube syndrome is associated with chromophobe tumours.

Answer
B and D

Explanation

Kidney cancer is a heterogeneous group of at least five different histological types (Table 4.1). The most frequent histologic type is clear cell, comprising 75% of all renal cancers. The VHL gene is mutated both in hereditary as well as in most cases of sporadic clear cell carcinomas. The former is due to the germ line mutation of one allele and loss of heterozygosity of the other allele, whereas the latter is due to acquired mutations of both alleles. The VHL gene encodes a protein (pVHL) which is important for regulating the tissue response to hypoxia in cancers. The gene whose mutation is responsible for hereditary papillary renal cell carcinoma was found to be the protooncogene c-Met, receptor tyrosine kinase. Renal tumours in the Birt-Hogg-Dube syndrome are associated with cutaneous fibrofolliculoma, pulmonary cysts and pneumothorax.

Table 4.1 Kidney cancer is a heterogeneous group of at least five different histological types

Type	Clear Cell	Papillary	Chromophobic	Oncytoma	CD tumour
Frequency	75%	5–10%	5%	5%	<1%
Cell origin	Proximal tubule	Proximal tubule	Cortical CD	Cortical CD	Medullary CD
Gene mutation	VHL	Met or FH	Birt-Hogg-Dube	Birt-Hogg-Dube	?
Disease	VHL	HPRC or HLRCC	Birt-Hogg-Dube	Birt-Hogg-Dube	

Note: VHL = von Hippel-Lindau, Met = c-Met, FH = fumarate hydratase, HPRC = hereditary papillary renal carcinoma syndrome, HLRCC = hereditary leiomyomatosis renal carcinoma syndrome, CD = collecting duct

Clinical pearl

- More renal cancers are being diagnosed as incidental findings due to the widespread use of imaging procedures in medicine.

LEVEL B

Question 4

Which of the following investigations should be performed to stage kidney cancer?
(a) CT chest
(b) Renal magnetic resonance imaging (MRI)
(c) Urine cytology
(d) Serum calcium
(e) Serum lactic dehydrogenase (LDH)

Answer
A, C and D

Explanation

The standard evaluation of patients with suspected renal cell carcinoma includes a CT scan of the abdomen/pelvis and chest, urine analysis and urine cytology. It is standard also to perform serum electrolytes, liver function tests, calcium and phosphate, and a CT of chest is required if the chest radiograph indicates metastatic disease. Renal MRI is indicated in evaluating the inferior vena cava if its involvement is suspected, as well as in patients for whom contrast cannot be administered due to contraindications or renal dysfunction.

Question 5

Regarding the features of a renal mass on CT, which of the following statements is/are true?
- **(a)** 10-Hounsfield-unit-enhancement with contrast is indicative of malignancy.
- **(b)** Presence of fat is indicative of malignancy.
- **(c)** Calcification is indicative of malignancy.
- **(d)** A cyst with multiple septa is indicative of malignancy.
- **(e)** A fine-needle biopsy should not be performed if an indeterminate mass is greater than 3 cm in size.

Answer
C and D

Explanation

The differential diagnosis of a renal mass includes benign neoplasms (adenoma, angiomyolipoma, oncocytoma), malignant neoplasms (primary, metastatic such as melanoma, Wilms tumour, transitional cell carcinoma of the renal pelvis, sarcoma, lymphoma), cysts or an inflammatory mass (pyelonephritis, abscess). The most important criterion used in differentiating surgical from non-surgical masses is the determination of enhancement. Enhancement of mass with contrast suggests vascularised masses, which may be found with renal cancers. If there is difficulty in assessing enhancement, then this can be determined more objectively by using Hounsfield (HF) units. HF units are a measure of radiodensity, with the radiodensity of distilled water being 0, and muscle and bone, 40 and 100 units respectively. In general, an increase of 10 to 20 HF units suggests malignancy. The differentiation of an angiomyolipoma from a renal carcinoma is important, because, in most cases, the former do not need surgical removal. The diagnosis of an angiomyolipoma is made by demonstrating fat within a solid renal mass. Calcification and multiple septa raise the possibility of malignancy. In the past, there was a theoretical concern that malignant cells could be 'tracked' by the biopsy needle, but improved techniques and imaging of masses have eliminated this potential problem. Therefore, if there is a question as to whether a mass is malignant, biopsy should be considered before surgery, especially in patients with high surgical risk, such as the elderly.

Question 6

Regarding paraneoplastic features associated with renal cell carcinoma, which of the following statements is/are true?
(a) They occur in 5% of patients.
(b) Hypercalcaemia is the most common manifestation.
(c) Serum levels of renin are frequently elevated.
(d) Stauffer's syndrome is due to metastatic hepatic dysfunction.
(e) Secondary amyloidosis is observed in 20% of patients.

Answer
B and C

Explanation

Up to 30% of patients presenting with renal cell carcinoma have evidence of tumour-derived factors with systemic effects. In some cases, paraneoplastic symptoms may be the only manifestation of the disease at the time of presentation. The clinical features of paraneoplastic syndrome associated with renal cell carcinoma include pyrexia (20%); cachexia (33%); and abnormal liver function tests, increased alkaline phosphatase, hypercalcaemia, polycythaemia and neuromyopathy and secondary amyloidosis (2 to 3%). Humoral hypercalcaemia, frequently observed in advanced renal cell carcinoma and due to secretion of tumour-derived parathyroid-like peptide, is associated with a poor prognosis. Renin levels are frequently elevated in patients with renal cell carcinoma and return to normal after surgical resection. This may contribute to the systemic hypertension observed in 20% of patients. Stauffer's syndrome is a reversible syndrome defined as non-metastatic hepatic dysfunction without jaundice that is associated with fever, fatigue and weight loss, and resolves when the tumour is resected.

 Clinical pearls

- Patients with suspected renal cell carcinoma should be staged with a CT scan of the abdomen/pelvis and chest, urine analysis and urine cytology.
- A renal mass that enhances greater than 10 to 20 HF units suggests malignancy.
- Up to 30% of patients presenting with renal cell carcinoma have evidence of tumour-derived factors with systemic effects.

LEVEL C

Question 7

Which of the following statements about the prognosis of kidney cancer is/are true?

(a) Disease confined to the kidney (stage 1) is associated with a greater than 75% five-year survival.

(b) Renal vein involvement is worse than lymph node involvement.

(c) Hypercalcaemia indicates a poor prognosis.

(d) Erythrocytosis is associated with a poor prognosis.

(e) Metastatic disease has a 20% 5-year survival.

Answer
A and C

Explanation

The United States' National Cancer Institute's Surveillance, Epidemiology and Results (SEER) data (www.seer.cancer.gov) indicate that the 5-year survival of patients with localised disease is 89% (Stage 1, which accounts for half of all patients), is 61% with regional disease (defined as extension into the renal capsule or Gerota's fascia [Stage 2] or involvement of the renal vein or inferior vena cava [Stage 3A] or involvement of lymph nodes [Stage 3B]) and only 9% in distant metastatic disease or advanced locally invasive disease (e.g. involving the adrenal gland). Involvement of the lymph nodes has a worse outcome (Stage 3B, 5-year survival 20%) than if there is involvement of the renal vein or inferior vena cava (Stage 3A, 5-year survival 64%). Humoral hypercalcaemia is frequently observed in advanced renal cell carcinoma and is therefore associated with a worse prognosis. Anaemia is a feature of advanced disease and indicative of a poor prognosis.

Question 8

Regarding the surgical management of metastatic renal cell carcinoma, which of the following statements is/are correct?

(a) Nephrectomy is contraindicated in the presence of metastatic disease.

(b) Surgical excision of solitary metastasis to the lung is not effective in prolonging survival.

(c) Nephron-sparing surgery is suitable for treating tumours 5 cm in diameter.

(d) Results achieved with nephron-sparing surgery are similar to those achieved by radical nephrectomy.

(e) Laparoscopic partial nephrectomy is associated with an increased risk of perioperative complications.

Answer

B, D and E

Explanation

Surgical excision is the primary treatment of renal cell carcinoma. Radical nephrectomy, which includes removal of the kidney *en bloc* with Gerota's fascia, the ipsilateral adrenal gland and regional nodes, has been the standard treatment. Nephrectomy may be warranted even in the presence of metastatic disease for alleviation of pain and haemorrhage. The surgical excision of a single metastasis in advanced renal cell carcinoma has not yet been proven to enhance survival. Nephron-sparing surgery may be indicated for localised ipsilateral tumours less than 4 cm in size. Relative indications may also include larger tumours in patients with a single kidney (as in the present case) to reduce the almost certain risk of end-stage renal disease. Decisions determining whether a patient undergoes nephron-sparing surgery or radical nephrectomy depend on the experience of the surgeon, the size and position of the tumour, patient comorbidity and preference. A disadvantage of nephron-sparing surgery is a rate of local recurrence of 3 to 6%. Laparoscopic partial nephrectomy has benefits which include reduced postoperative pain, shorter hospitalisation and quicker patient recovery, but is associated with increased perioperative complications because it is technically more demanding.

Question 9

Regarding the use of chemotherapy and immunomodulatory therapy in renal cell carcinoma, which of the following statements is/are true?

(a) Only 15% of tumours respond to chemotherapy.
(b) Collecting duct carcinomas are more sensitive to chemotherapy than papillary carcinomas.
(c) The combination of interferon-α and nephrectomy has a similar outcome to treatment with interferon-α alone.
(d) High-dose interleukin-2 therapy is more effective than interferon-α.
(e) Immunomodifier agents produce a durable and long term regression of tumour in 10 to 20% of patients.

Answer

D

Explanation

In general, renal cell carcinomas are refractory to cytotoxic agents, have an infrequent and variable response to biological agents, such as immunomodifiers (interferon-α and interleukin-2 [IL-2]) and have a variable clinical course with metastatic disease and the possibility for spontaneous regression. Medical therapies are offered to patients with locally advanced and metastatic disease. Rates of response to chemotherapy are low and generally less than 10%. Drug resistance may be related to the presence of the multidrug resistant transporter in proximal tubule cells which, as discussed earlier, are the cells of origin for clear cell and papillary cell carcinomas. Chemotherapy, therefore, may be more effective in non-clear cell carcinomas, such as the collecting duct type (as shown in case reports) and this hypothesis is being addressed in randomised controlled studies. The aim of immunomodulatory therapy with interferon or IL-2 is to enhance tumour antigenicity and host surveillance. In general, immunomodifiers produce tumour regression in 10 to 20% of patients but rarely produces long term and durable regression. The combination of interferon-α and nephrectomy is superior to interferon-α alone and offers a survival advantage of 3 to 10 months. High-dose IL-2 induces a response in 25% of patients as compared to a response rate of 13% among patients who receive low-dose interferon-α. However, many patients with metastatic disease are unable to tolerate high-dose IL-2 due to the 'capillary leak syndrome'.

Question 10

Regarding the molecular pathogenesis of renal cell carcinoma, true statements include which of the following?

(a) The VHL gene is mutated in more than 75% of clear cell carcinomas.
(b) In normal cells, pVHL is physically associated with hypoxia inducible factor-1 (HIF1).
(c) Inactivation of pVHL directly leads to the transcription of vascular endothelial growth factor.
(d) HIF1α translocates to the nucleus and induces platelet-derived growth factor.
(e) Treatment with vascular endothelial growth factor is effective in reducing progression of renal cell carcinomas.

Answer
A, B and D

Explanation

Although VHL disease accounts for 2% of all cancers, mutations of the VHL gene are present in 80% of sporadic clear cell carcinomas. Renal cell cancer growth requires neoangiogenesis given their parenchymal localisation and, therefore, successful tumours are highly angiogenic. In normal cells, hypoxia induces the activation of the hypoxia inducible factor-1 (HIF1) transcription factor (see Fig. 4.1), which translocates to the nucleus and results in the transcription of several genes whose proteins are important for blood vessel growth and oxygen delivery, such as vascular endothelial growth factor (VEGF), erythropoietin, platelet-derived growth factor and transforming growth factor-α. In normal cells, HIF1α directly interacts with and is complexed with pVHL. This leads to the ubiquitination of HIF and degradation by proteasome-mediated pathways. Therefore, clear cell carcinomas are unable to degrade HIF1α in both normoxic and hypoxic conditions leading to the production of VEGF as well as other angiogenic factors. Consequently, a number of VEGF monoclonal antibodies are currently in phase 3 clinical trials, the results of which are awaited. In addition, inhibitors of intracellular signal transduction pathways, such as tyrosine kinases, mammalian target of rapamycin (sirolimus), HIF inhibitors and cyclin-kinase inhibitors are being tested.

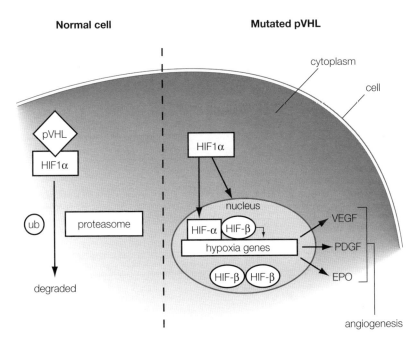

Figure 4.1 Activation of the HIF1 transcription factor

Source: Adapted from Weiss & Lin (2006)

Clinical pearls

- Renal vein involvement has a better prognosis than a patient with lymph node involvement.
- Nephron-sparing surgery is being increasingly performed for the treatment of renal cancer, and the results achieved may be similar to those achieved by radical nephrectomy.

- Renal cell carcinomas are refractory to cytotoxic agents, and have an infrequent and variable response to biological agents, such as immunomodifiers (interferon-α and IL-2).
- Although VHL disease accounts for 2% of all cancers, mutations of the VHL gene are present in 80% of sporadic clear cell carcinomas.

Bibliography

Level A

1. Scher, H.I. & Motzer, R.J. (2001) Bladder and renal cell carcinomas. *Harrison's Principles of Internal Medicine*, 15th edn. Braunweld, E., Fauci, A.S., Kasper, D.L., Hauser, S.L., Longo, D.L. & Jameson, J.L. (eds). New York: McGraw-Hill, 604–8.
2. Lipworth, L., Tarone, R.E. & McLaughlin, J.K. (2006) The epidemiology of renal cell carcinoma. J Urol. 176, 2353–8.

Level B

3. Motzer, R.J., Bander, N.H. & Nanus, D.M. (1996) Renal-cell carcinoma. N Engl J Med. 335, 865–75.
4. Cohen, H.T. & McGovern, F.J. (2005) Renal cell carcinoma. N Engl J Med 353, 2477–90.

Level C

5. Weiss, R.H. & Lin, P.Y. (2006) Kidney cancer: identification of novel targets for therapy. Kidney Int. 69, 224–32.
6. Lineham, W.M., Bates, S.E., Yang, J.C. (2005) Cancer of the kidney. *Cancer: Principles and Practice of Oncology*, 7th edn. DeVita, V.T., Hellman, S. & Rosenberg, S.A. (eds.). Philadelphia: Lippincott Williams & Wilkins, online version.

Case 5
Haematuria

GOPI RANGAN

LEVEL A

Case history

A 56-year-old Caucasian man presents for routine follow-up to a hospital out-patient renal–diabetic clinic. He has had type 2 diabetes mellitus for 8 years (complicated by diabetic nephropathy) and a history of smoking (15 cigarettes per day for the past 25 years). His current medications include perindopril 8 mg/day, metformin 1 g three times a day, atorvastatin 40 mg/day, gliclazide 80 mg three times a day, aspirin 100 mg/day and hydrochlorothiazide 25 mg/day. The supine blood pressure (BP), body weight and urinalysis are checked by the clinic nurse before you see the patient. The supine BP measured using the right brachial pulse is 142/88 mmHg and body weight 82 kg. The urinalysis shows 2+ protein, 2+ red blood cells, a trace of glucose and no ketones. You review the patient's medical file and notice that the microscopic haematuria was not present at previous clinic visits.

Question 1

Regarding asymptomatic microscopic haematuria, which of the following statements is/are true?

(a) It is defined as 2 to 5 RBCs per high power field on urine microscopy.
(b) Exercise is associated with transient microscopic haematuria.
(c) Chronic treatment with clopidogrel is a cause.
(d) It is present in 5% of the Australian population.

Answer

B, C and D

Explanation

Isolated haematuria without proteinuria, urine casts or other cell types indicates bleeding from the urinary tract. Up to 2 million RBCs per day can be excreted in the urine of normal healthy individuals. Microscopic haematuria is defined as 2 to 5 RBCs per high power field, an amount that can also be detected by urine dipstick. Common causes of haematuria include renal stones, cancer of the urinary tract and kidney, infection (cystitis, prostatitis) and trauma. Transient asymptomatic microscopic haematuria is common in the general population and may be due to menstruation, febrile illness, allergy, exercise or trauma. One of the first population-based studies to address the prevalence of asymptomatic microscopic haematuria in Australia was the landmark Australian Diabetes, Obesity and Lifestyle (AusDiab) study. The AusDiab study was a cross-sectional survey of more than 11 000 Australian adults from randomly selected areas throughout the country. A variety of parameters were assessed in this popula-tion-based survey. One of the endpoints, microscopic haematuria (which was defined as $>10 \times 10^6$ RBCs per litre), was present in 4.6% of this cohort. These data are similar to other large screening and population-based studies performed in other countries. Chronic treatment with anticoagulants is not considered to be an independent cause of haematuria, and further investigation to determine a cause is warranted under these circumstances.

Question 2

With regard to assessment of microscopic haematuria by urine dipstick analysis, a positive urine dipstick may also indicate:

(a) rhabdomyolysis
(b) intravascular haemolysis
(c) treatment with diuretics
(d) urinary tract infection
(e) treatment with ascorbic acid.

Answer
A, B and D

Explanation

The most frequently used test to diagnose microscopic haematuria is the urine dipstick. The test is based on a time-dependent colour reaction (yellow to green if positive) due to the oxidation of impregnated substrates on the test strip by peroxide, catalysed by free haemoglobin released when red blood cells lyse on the reagent strip. A limitation of the urine dipstick to assess or haematuria is that the reaction relies on the presence of free haem. Therefore, a positive test can also be caused by myoglobinuria (as in rhabdomyolysis) or haemoglobinuria (as in intravascular haemolysis). False positives (up to 16%) can also be seen in the presence of povidone-iodine and oxidising agents such as hypochlorite or microbial peroxidase activity (such as that associated with a urinary tract infection). False negatives may be due to old (air-exposed) reagent sticks, delayed examination, ingestion of ascorbic acid or presence of dilute urine (e.g. treatment with diuretics). The overall sensitivity and specificity of the urine dipstick in detecting haematuria are approximately 91% and 99% respectively. In addition, certain food dyes, beetroot and drugs (such as rifampicin) may alter the colour of the urine to orange-red, but not signify haematuria and are dipstick negative for blood.

Question 3

The next appropriate step/s in the management of this patient who has new-onset of microscopic hematuria detected on urine dipstick is/are which of the following?

(a) It can be ignored because it is a typical feature of diabetic nephropathy.

(b) A renal ultrasound should be performed as a screening investigation.

(c) A midstream urine should be sent for culture.

(d) Autoimmune serology should be checked as a screening investigation.

(e) The urine dipstick should be rechecked if no specific symptoms are present.

Answer

E

Explanation

Isolated asymptomatic microscopic haematuria may have a number of benign causes and be transient (e.g. exercise, trauma, menstruation). Moreover, as discussed earlier the urine dipstick can be a false-positive result. Therefore, in the absence of specific symptoms, it is important to repeat the urine dipstick on one or two occasions, before undertaking further investigations. Haematuria is an unusual feature of diabetic nephropathy and should alert the clinician to another underlying cause. Autoimmune serology is inappropriate to use as screening test, unless there are additional clinical features to support a diagnosis of autoimmune renal disease, such as systemic lupus erythematosus (SLE) or Wegener's granulomatosis.

 Clinical pearls

- Haematuria is an increase in the number of RBCs excreted in the urine and signifies bleeding from the kidney, ureter, bladder, urethra and/or prostate.
- Microscopic haematuria is a common finding in the general population; it may be transient and have a number of benign causes.
- Urinalysis using a dipstick is a reliable initial test for haematuria but does not distinguish haematuria from haemoglobinuria and myoglobinuria. A cell count of the urine should also be performed.

LEVEL B

Case history continued ...

You advise the patient to return to his general practitioner to repeat the urine dipstick again in one week. The patient ignores your advice. At the next review, four months later, the urinalysis again shows 2+ protein, 2+ RBCs, trace of glucose and no ketones. You are quite concerned about the persistent microscopic haematuria and, on this occasion, immediately organise a urine microscopy and culture, which shows that there are 100×10^6 RBCs per litre. The white cell count is normal ($<10 \times 10^6$ cells per litre) and there is no growth on culture. You also ask the laboratory to perform phase-contrast microscopy of the urine sediment to determine the morphology of the RBCs to help distinguish between a glomerular and a non-glomerular cause for the microscopic haematuria. Approximately 10% of the RBCs are dysmorphic. There are also some hyaline casts.

Question 4

Which of the following statements is/are true regarding phase-contrast microscopy of urinary erythrocytes?

(a) If 10% of the RBCs are dysmorphic then this indicates a glomerular origin for the microscopic haematuria.

(b) If 90% of the RBCs are isomorphic then this indicates a non-glomerular origin for the microscopic haematuria.

(c) If 30% of the RBCs are dysmorphic then this indicates a glomerular origin for the microscopic haematuria.

(d) When performed by an experienced operator and laboratory, this test can predict the site of urinary bleeding in up to 85% of patients with haematuria.

Answer

B and D

Explanation

Examination of the RBC morphology using phase-contrast microscopy can be a very helpful diagnostic tool to differentiate between a glomerular and non-glomerular cause for haematuria. Isomorphic RBCs have regular shapes and contours whereas dysmorphic RBCs have irregular shapes and contours. When isomorphic RBCs predominate (greater than 80% of total RBCs), the haematuria is defined as non-glomerular, whereas when dysmorphic RBCs predominate (greater than 80% of total RBCs), the haematuria is defined as glomerular, particularly when there are accompanying clinical features (hypertension, proteinuria, renal impairment). Therefore, when used early in the evaluation of microscopic haematuria, this test may help avoid unnecessary investigations. However, some important caveats need to be considered. First, the urine should be examined fresh (within 2 hours, otherwise cells may undergo lysis) and second, evaluation of the RBC morphology is subjective with high inter-observer variability.

Question 5

Red blood cell casts in the urine:
- **(a)** are formed in the proximal tubule of the nephron
- **(b)** are often found in patients with focal segmental glomerulosclerosis
- **(c)** are usually present in patients with renal failure due to small-vessel vasculitis
- **(d)** may be present in healthy individuals
- **(e)** contain Tamm-Horsfall protein.

Answer
C and E

Explanation

Urinary casts are cellular or acellular gelatinous fragments that are formed in the lumen of a short segment of a single nephron. Casts cannot form in another distal part of the urinary tract. Therefore, the presence of red blood cell and/or haemoglobin casts in the urine is one of the most convincing pieces of clinical evidence to indicate a glomerular origin for microscopic haematuria. This clinical conclusion is strengthened if there is a high percentage of dysmorphic RBCs and/or proteinuria present in the urine.

Red blood cell and other casts are formed only in the distal convoluted tubule or the collecting duct. The proximal convoluted tubule and loop of Henle are not locations for cast formation. This is because the thick ascending limb of the loop of Henle secretes a mucoprotein called Tamm-Horsfall protein. At a sufficient urine concentration (specific gravity >1.010 g/mL) and acidity (pH <6), Tamm-Horsfall protein mucoprotein transforms into a gelatinous substance that forms a mould of the nephron lumen. Given that the latter can occur in physiological states, the excretion of casts containing only Tamm-Horsfall (called hyaline casts) protein can occur in healthy individuals. In contrast, red cell casts signify glomerular pathology. In the presence of a glomerular disease leading to haematuria, red blood cells will become trapped in the Tamm-Horsfall gel and form a cellular cast which eventually dislodges and is excreted in the urine. Red blood cell casts typically occur in inflammatory glomerulonephritides, such as crescentic glomerulonephritis, which is most often due to small-vessel vasculitis and, to a lesser extent, anti-GBM disease and immune-complex glomerular diseases. Non-inflammatory glomerular diseases, such as focal segmental glomerulosclerosis, diabetic nephropathy and membranous nephropathy are not typically associated with red cell casts in the urine. The presence of red cell casts in the urine of a patient with diabetic nephropathy should raise the possibility of a superimposed inflammatory glomerulonephritis, such as crescentic glomerulonephritis.

Question 6

The indications for renal biopsy in an adult with microscopic haematuria include:
- **(a)** serum creatinine of 160 µmol/L
- **(b)** associated proteinuria greater than 1 gram per day
- **(c)** broad casts in the urine
- **(d)** bipolar renal length of 7 cm on renal ultrasound
- **(e)** red blood cell casts in the urine.

Answer
A, B and E

Explanation

One of the main indications for performing a renal biopsy in patients with microscopic haematuria is if a progressive or inflammatory glomerulonephritis is suspected, where treatment with immunosuppressants may be beneficial in preventing kidney failure. The clinical features supporting this include proteinuria, red cell casts, dysmorphic RBCs, renal impairment, hypertension and presence of clinical features of a systemic autoimmune-mediated disease, such as vasculitis or systemic lupus erythematosus. The presence of small kidneys (less than 8 cm in length) and broad casts indicate advanced scarring of the kidneys. Under these circumstances, renal biopsy is usually not undertaken as the immunosuppressant treatment is unlikely to be beneficial. Broad casts originate in dilated atrophic tubules which are usually present in advanced chronic kidney disease.

Case history continued ...

You organise a renal ultrasound and it reveals that the right kidney measures 12 cm in bipolar length and the left measures 11.5 cm. The renal contour is smooth and the renal cortex appears to be normal. The prostate is normal in size and the post-micturition bladder volume is 30 cc. The patient is referred to a urologist to consider a flexible cystoscopy to exclude a bladder cancer.

Question 7

The risk of bladder cancer is increased by which of the following?
- **(a)** Employment in a tyre factory
- **(b)** Employment in a paint factory
- **(c)** Exposure to asbestos

(d) Previous treatment with cyclophosphamide

(e) Use of artificial sweeteners

Answer

A, B and D

Explanation

Bladder cancer is 2.5 times more common in males than in females. The incidence increases with age and peaks between the 6th and 7th decades of life. Risk factors include smoking (threefold increased risk), analgesic abuse (e.g. phenacetin), previous exposure with cyclophosphamide, and industrial contact with chemicals (aromatic amines, aniline dyes, nitrites and nitrates such as in rubber, textile and paint factories), plastics, coal, tar and asphalt. Chronic irritants such as chronic indwelling catheters, chronic infection with *Schistosoma haematobium* and pelvic irradiation are additional risk factors. Ingestion of coffee, tea and artificial sweeteners has not been shown to be an independent risk factor.

Clinical pearl

- The presence of proteinuria, red cell casts and dysmorphic RBCs indicates a glomerular cause for the haematuria and should prompt referral to a nephrologist to consider a renal biopsy.

LEVEL C

Case history continued ...

The urologist arranges urine cytology performed on three consecutive early mornings; this shows the presence of isolated atypical cells. Renal spiral computerised tomography (CT) scan with contrast shows no abnormalities. A flexible cystoscopy reveals an isolated small pedunculated lesion with no other abnormalities elsewhere in the bladder. A transurethral resection of the lesion is performed and biopsies show a high-grade papillary transitional cell carcinoma with no invasion of the lamina propria and muscular layer.

Question 8

Which of the following statements is/are true regarding superficial bladder cancer?

(a) This is the most common mode of presentation.

(b) Less than 10% of patients develop a recurrence.

(c) Fewer than 5% of patients develop metastatic disease.

(d) Adjuvant intravesical drug treatment with bacille Calmette-Guérin (BCG) should be commenced.

Answer

A and C

Explanation

Bladder cancers are divided into superficial cancers, muscularis propria-invasive cancers and metastatic cancers, according to the depth of invasion and distant spread. Seventy percent of patients with bladder cancer have superficial disease at presentation. Fifty percent of these patients have a recurrence after initial therapy and 15 to 20% also develop more invasive disease. Less than 5% of patients develop metastatic disease. Generally, adjuvant intravesical therapy is not used unless there is significant risk of progressive disease or recurrence. This risk occurs with (1) multi-focal carcinoma *in situ* with or without superficial disease; (2) any tumour that invades the perivascular tissue; (3) multifocal tumours; and/or (4) tumours that recur rapidly after resection.

Case history continued ...

The patient is advised to undergo surveillance cystoscopies every 3 months. Three months later, a recurrent lesion is detected. Following resection of this lesion, the patient receives treatment with weekly intravesical BCG for 6 weeks.

Question 9

Which of the following statements regarding BCG therapy in bladder cancer is/are true?

(a) It may cause abacterial cystitis in 80% of patients.

(b) It may cause fever and joint pain.

(c) It may cause disseminated tuberculosis.

(d) Side effects are common.

(e) Granulomatous prostatitis occurs in 1% of patients.

Answer

All are correct

Explanation

Intravesical BCG has been used by urologists as adjuvant intravesical therapy to treat patients with recurrence of or those at high-risk of developing recurrent bladder cancer following initial detection. The treatment regimen usually consists of once weekly instillation of BCG for 6 weeks. Patients are given a live attenuated BCG in 50 mL of normal saline instilled into the bladder via a urinary catheter. Its widespread use, however, is often limited by the side effects which are common, and include abacterial cystitis (80%), haematuria (40%) and low-grade fever (30%). Granulomatous prostatitis occurs in 1% of patients but granulomas can occur anywhere in the body including the liver, lung and kidneys. Allergic reactions may occur in 1% of patients and include arthralgias and rash. A systemic reaction may occur, and includes fever, pneumonitis, hepatitis and organ dysfunction. The latter can be serious and require admission to the intensive care unit. It is contraindicated in patients with an impaired immune response.

Question 10

The patient develops recurrent invasive bladder carcinoma and requires a radical cystectomy with urinary diversion. True statements regarding urinary diversion include which of the following?

(a) The risk of renal calculi is greater with continent types of diversions than with intestinal conduit types of diversions.
(b) Phenytoin levels may be reduced following urinary diversion.
(c) Osteomalacia may occur if 60 cm of ileum is used for the diversion.
(d) Hyperchloraemic metabolic acidosis may occur when the jejunum is used for the diversion.
(e) Asymptomatic growth of *Proteus* species does not require treatment in patients with a continent type of diversion.

Answer
A

Explanation

Radical cystoprostatectomy and bilateral pelvic node dissection (with or without urethrectomy) is standard surgical treatment for a patient with invasive transitional cell carcinoma of the bladder. The absence of the bladder, therefore, necessitates the surgical creation of a urinary diversion from the distal ureters. Urinary diversions can be divided into continent and non-continent diversions (see Fig. 5.1):

- Non-continent diversions involve the use of a segment of bowel (usually the ileum or colon, and sometimes the jejunum). The distal end is brought to the skin as a stoma and the ureters are implanted into the proximal end. The patient wears a urostomy bag to collect the urine. The advantages of this diversion are the simplicity and the reduced number of immediate and long-term complications (approximately 10% of patients have significant complications).

- Continent diversions consist of a reservoir made of bowel that is fashioned into a pouch-like or bladder-like structure. There are two variations: (1) abdominal continent diversion: a stoma is connected to the urine reservoir (often called a pouch) and the patient usually performs self-catheterisation every 4 to 6 hours; and (2) orthotopic continent diversion: the urethra is connected to the urine reservoir (often called a neobladder), allowing the patient to void by Valsalva. Self-catheterisation is usually necessary in the first six months after surgery and occasionally thereafter.

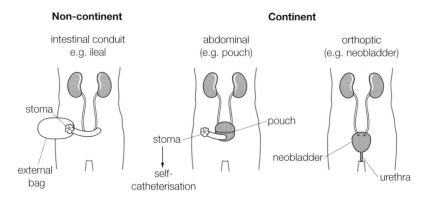

Figure 5.1 Types of urinary diversion

In general, continent diversions are associated with increased long-term postoperative (including metabolic) complications (10 to 30%) but have reduced risk of urine reflux compared to incontinent diversions. The ileal conduit urinary diversion is currently the gold standard, and many of the different approaches require long-term comparisons by clinical trials in the future.

The long-term complications of urinary diversion are listed in Table 5.1. The complications of urinary diversion either arise for mechanical/surgical reasons or are metabolic due to the resection of the bowel and/or effects of urine being in contact with the bowel. With regard to the latter, resection of more than 100 cm of ileum may result in malabsorption of vitamin B12, bile and fat-soluble vitamins (A, D, E and K leading to osteomalacia), and loss of the ileocaecal valve may cause diarrhoea. Oxalate absorption is increased because the unabsorbed fat complexes with calcium, which is no longer available to chelate oxalate. Therefore, serum and urinary oxalate levels are increased, potentially leading to stone formation. The reduced solubility of cholesterol in bile may also lead to gallstones. In addition, exposure of the bowel lumen to urine leads to electrolyte abnormalities. This is because the intestinal wall attempts to maintain iso-osmolality, leading to altered serum sodium and chloride concentrations. Acidosis occurs in up to 50% of patients in the early postoperative period. This may persist if >45 cm of ileal segment has been used to construct a pouch and there is renal dysfunction. Chronic acidosis can lead to a range of long-term complications.

Patients with urinary diversions develop bacteriuria and may suffer from pyelonephritis. At present, there is no evidence that the risk for urinary tract infection is altered by the type of urinary diversion. In general, asymptomatic bacteriuria does not warrant treatment unless there have been recurrent episodes of pyelonephritis or there is infection with urea-splitting organism, such as *Proteus* species, given the potential for stone formation.

Table 5.1 Long-term complications of urinary diversion

Medical	Neuromechanical	Surgical
Electrolyte abnormalities Hyperchloraemic metabolic acidosis, hypocalcaemia and hypomagnesaemia (ileum and colon) Hypokalaemia (colon) Hypochloraemic metabolic acidosis (jejunum) *Renal calculi* (3–4% with conduits compared to 20% in reservoir conduits) *Bacteriuria* Sepsis (10%) *Altered drugs levels* (e.g. increased Dilantin levels, cyclophosphamide) *Loss of >100 cm of ileum* B12 malabsorption, fat and fat-soluble vitamin malabsorption	*Atonic segment* (for continent diversion) Urine retention and hydronephrosis	*Urine leak* *Bowel obstruction or leak* *Pyelonephritis and sepsis* *Renal failure due to obstruction* *Problem with stoma*

Clinical pearls

- The majority of patients with bladder cancer present with superficial disease. Fifty percent of these patients have a recurrence after initial therapy.
- Intravesical BCG has been used by urologists as adjuvant intravesical therapy to treat patients with recurrence or those at high risk of developing recurrent bladder cancer following initial detection.

Bibliography

Level A

1. Horio, M., Orita, Y., Fukunaga, M. (2003) Assessment of renal function. *Comprehensive Clinical Nephrology*, 2nd edn. Johnson, R.J. & Feehally, J. (eds). Philadelphia: Mosby, 27–45.
2. Mathew, T. (2004) What to do when you find microhaematuria? Medical Observer. 33–5. Available at www.kidney.org.au
3. Chadban, S.J., Briganti, E.M., Kerr, P.G., Dunstan, D.W., Welborn, T.A., Zimmet, P.Z. & Atkins, R.C. (2003) Prevalence of kidney damage in Australian adults: the AusDiab kidney study. J Am Soc Nephrol. 14(Suppl 2), S131–8.

Level B

4. Fassett, R.G., Horgan, B.A. & Mathew, T.H. (1982) Detection of glomerular bleeding by phase-contrast microscopy. Lancet. 21, 105–8.

Level C

5. Shipley, W.U., Kaufman, D.S., McDougal, W.S., Dahl, D.M., Michealson, M.D. & Zietman, A.L. (2005) Cancer of the bladder, ureter and pelvis. *Principles and Practice of Oncology*, 7th edn. Philadelphia: Lippincott Williams & Wilkins.
6. Meyer, J.P., Persad, R. & Gillat, D.A. (2002) Use of bacilli Calmette-Guérin in superficial bladder cancer. Postgrad Med J. 78: 449–54.
7. Falagas, M.E. & Vergidis, P.I. (2005) Urinary tract infections in patients with urinary diversion. Am J Kidney Dis. 46, 1030–7.

Case 6
Urinary tract infection

ANNEMARIE HENNESSY

LEVEL A

Case history

A 29-year-old woman presents for assessment of loin pain and fever. Her presenting problem is an episode of fever for 24 hours and right-back pain. She has noted some frequency and painful urination in the last few days and has taken two tablets of cephalothin at the outset of the infection; these antibiotics were left over from treatment for a previous renal tract infection.

There is no other medical or surgical history and no family history of renal disease. She has a history of urinary tract infections since 22 years of age. This has taken the form of 3 to 4 'infections' per year, each often settling with cranberry juice alone. She occasionally had to see a General Practitioner and a course of antibiotics was required. There were occasions when the culture was positive and at one time, bacteriuria was found in a urine test taken for follow-up after resolution of her symptoms.

On examination she looks unwell and is sweating. She has a temperature of 39.0°C, a heart rate of 120 beats/min and blood pressure (BP) of 90/60 mmHg. There is marked tenderness over the right renal angle. Abdominal examination is otherwise normal and there are no enlarged lymph nodes. There are no chest findings and her pre-cordial examination is normal. There are no neurological signs. She weighs 95 kg and her height is 180 cm.

The following blood tests and urine tests are obtained.

Laboratory data

	Result	Reference range
Full blood count		
Haemoglobin	12.9 g/L	(115–145 g/L)
White cell count	20.8×10^9/L	($4–11 \times 10^9$/L)
Platelet count	344×10^9/L	($150–400 \times 10^9$/L)
Differential cell count		
Neutrophil	18.0×10^9/L	($3.5–9.0 \times 10^9$/L)
Lymphocytes	2.0×10^9/L	($0.5–4.0 \times 10^9$/L)

Laboratory data continued

	Result	Reference range
Biochemistry		
Na⁺	135 mmol/L	(136–146)
K⁺	3.5 mmol/L	(3.5–5.5)
Cl⁻	105 mmol/L	(99–109)
HCO₃⁻	25 mmol/L	(22–30)
Urea	4.0 mmol/L	(3.0–8.0)
Creatinine	95 µmol/L	(60–90)
Anion gap	0 mmol/L	

The dipstick urine test shows the following:
- Nitrates: positive
- Leucocytes: Positive
- Protein: +
- Blood: +++

Microscopy results are as follows:
- Leucocytes: 50–100/µL
- Erythrocytes: Nil
- Epithelial: 10–50/µL
- Bacteria: Scanty
- Yeasts: Scanty
- Casts: Nil

The final report states the viable count as <104 colony forming units (CFU) per mL, with no significant growth.

Question 1

The patient's symptoms can be best explained by which of the following?
(a) Partly treated lower tract infection
(b) Right-sided pyelonephritis
(c) Interstitial cystitis
(d) Drug-induced interstitial nephritis
(e) Bladder calculus disease

Answer
B

Explanation

Although her symptoms were initially suggestive of lower urinary tract infection, the presentation with a septic illness and unilateral renal angle pain indicates probable extension beyond the collecting system into the right renal parenchyma (answer B correct). Not all infections are preceded by lower tract infections and generalised symptoms related to sepsis may present first.

Pyelonephritis is a relatively common presentation to general practice and hospital emergency departments and most commonly is caused by *E. coli* and other gram-negative organisms. Only half of infections are acquired from the lower tract and 50% are from haematogenous bacterial spread. Patterns of antimicrobial resistance differ in different communities and depend in part on the rates of antibiotic use in the community.

Differential diagnosis of right-sided abdominal pain and fever can include cholecystitis (pain tends to be more anterior), appendicitis (retrocaecal appendix), or more rarely pancreatitis (generally more central), pelvic inflammatory disease with Fitz-Hugh-Curtis (perihepatic) inflammation or renal infarction. These diagnoses are relatively uncommon in younger women.

Differential diagnosis of ongoing infection in the setting of recent lower urinary tract symptoms could include partially treated infection, but the signs would generally be localised to the lower tract including bilateral renal discomfort (answer A incorrect). Interstitial cystitis is the persistence of lower tract symptoms in the absence of further bacteriuria (answer C incorrect). Drug-induced interstitial nephritis is more likely to present as bilateral renal discomfort or no renal pain and positive urinary findings of red cells, white cells, urinary eosinophils and cellular casts, and perhaps proteinuria, in the absence of bacteriuria (answer D incorrect). Bladder calculus disease is more likely to present with lower tract symptoms (answer E incorrect).

 Clinical pearls

- Urinary tract infection presents as a clinical constellation of symptoms.
- Pyelonephritis is a common infection in younger women.
- Only 50% of infections are associated with lower tract pathology.
- Unilateral symptoms are suggestive of pyelonephritis rather than ureteric extension of cystitis, which is more likely to be bilateral.

Question 2

The conditions which predispose to pyelonephritis in this case include which of the following?

(a) Recurrent urinary tract infection
(b) Obesity
(c) Diabetes
(d) Family history
(e) Childhood history of urinary tract infection

Answer

E

Explanation

The risk profile of women with pyelonephritis is the same as for symptomatic lower urinary tract infection—they are sexually active women. Women with recurrent lower urinary tract infections are no more prone to pyelonephritis than women with infrequent ones (answer A incorrect). Patients with renal calculus disease, pregnancy and delivery, hospitalisation and chronic disease are also at risk. Diabetes and obesity are additional risks factors for all infections. The patient's weight of 95 kg would need to be adjusted for height—weight (kg)/height (m)^2—to assess her body mass index (BMI). A BMI of >30 kg/m^2 defines obesity. If her height was 180 cm, her BMI would be 29.32 kg/m^2 and she would not be obese (answers B and C incorrect).

Family history is relevant because women with certain inherited epithelial surface characteristics (in the urethelium) are particularly prone (Finer & Landau 2004). These tests are not available in everyday clinical practice. The patient had no family history (answer D incorrect).

Childhood infection is important as this could indicate occult ureteric reflux disease which is associated with recurrent urinary tract infection and recurrent pyelonephritis (answer E correct).

In older men the presence of prostate symptoms is an important indicator of the risk of symptomatic urinary tract infection. In older women, senile vaginitis is also a risk factor for urinary tract infection.

 Clinical pearls

- Pyelonephritis often occurs in otherwise well women.
- Natural history profile is recurrent bladder and occasional upper tract infection in sexually active young women.
- Other risk factors include diabetes, hospitalisation, chronic disease, renal calculi, urinary tract obstruction, immunosuppression and pregnancy.
- Prostate disease is a risk factor in older men.

Question 3

The urinary finding of pyuria is relevant because it:
- (a) excludes other pelvic pathology
- (b) confirms bacteriuria
- (c) indicates prognosis and expected rate of recovery
- (d) excludes renal tract obstruction
- (e) strengthens the likelihood of urinary infection.

Answer

E

Explanation

In the presence of sepsis of unknown aetiology, the finding of pyuria on dipstick testing is highly suggestive of urinary tract infection. It does not differentiate upper and lower tract infection. The main confounding diagnosis is that of pelvic inflammatory disease where pyuria is associated in up to 25% of cases.

In this case, the use of recent oral antibiotics makes the likelihood of achieving a positive urine culture less likely. Therefore, reliance on clinical symptoms and signs and the presence of urinary markers of inflammation are important. Dipstick testing is less reliable, whereas the presence on microscopy of white cells has much greater sensitivity and specificity.

 Clinical pearls

- Urinary nitrates and leucocytes have a high post-test probability of indicating infection in women with this history.
- Bladder inflammation as demonstrated by pyuria is supportive in the diagnosis of urinary tract infection.
- Confirmation of infection requires a positive single colony on urine culture but this test can be negative in the presence of recent oral antibiotic use.

Question 4

At this stage the treatment for the patient should include:
(a) continuation of the antibiotics used at home
(b) a different oral antibiotic
(c) parenteral antibiotic therapy
(d) fluid resuscitation alone
(e) imaging of the renal tract.

Answer
C and E

Explanation

Although guidelines exist for the treatment of pyelonephritis, there are limited studies of the various antibiotics and regimens. The goals of treatment are to use the shortest possible course of antibiotics and the lowest dose, and at the same time to limit the occurrence of relapse. Most infections respond very quickly to antibiotic therapy, but to prevent recurrence a longer course is often required.

Empirical therapy (answer A incorrect) in this case would suggest that past inefficient and infrequent use of an antibiotic might allow for antibiotic resistance to emerge and suggest the choice of an alternative agent.

In the case of pyelonephritis, the fever can take up to 5 days to resolve. It is generally prudent to use intravenous antibiotics (answer B incorrect, answer C correct). Even in a patient such as this one, the progression to full-blown septicaemia with multi-organ failure is a possibility. The use of intravenous antibiotics is supported by a need for intravenous fluid resuscitation in view of the high fever, relative hypotension and tachycardia, suggesting a decrease in circulating blood volume of up to 20% due to movement of fluid into extravascular spaces and poor oral intake when unwell. Vomiting occurs in 25% of patients and compromises oral antibiotic strategies. Intravenous antibiotics are generally continued until the patient is non-tender and afebrile.

Renal tract imaging is a contentious issue. In complicated urinary tract infection, there is a high probability of finding abnormalities on either renal tract ultrasound or computerised tomography, but often these abnormalities, which can include perinephric stranding, do not change management. In the rare case of renal tract obstruction or mass lesions such as renal tract carcinoma, management is significantly altered. Patients with renal cysts, duplex systems or ectopic kidneys are at increased risk of future renal tract infection and need frequent screening and early treatment of infection to prevent long-term effects on renal function. The majority of infections are treatable with no long-term effects on renal function.

Clinical pearls

- Where possible, antibiotic therapy should be directed by the microscopy and culture results of urine testing.
- Empirical therapy before culture results are available, or when initially negative, should be based on known resistance patterns of community-acquired bacteriuria.
- Parenteral therapy is indicated when signs of sepsis are present, or there are any concerns about tolerating oral antibiotics.
- The majority of infections are reversible and atypical patterns of infection (rare or multiple types of bacteria) should prompt a search for renal tract obstruction or calculus disease.

LEVEL B

Case history continued ...

The patient has missed two menstrual periods (her cycle is usually 28 days long). She has breast soreness. Her serum β-hCG (human chorionic gonadotrophin) test shows a concentration of 21 000 U/L. An ultrasound of the kidneys, collecting system and pelvis shows she is 8 weeks pregnant. Her renal tract shows mild dilatation of the right collecting system.

Question 5

Which of the following aspects of medical history predispose a patient to pregnancy-related urinary tract sepsis?
(a) Childhood urinary tract infections
(b) Known vesicoureteric reflux nephropathy
(c) Family history of vesicoureteric reflux disease
(d) Bacteriuria in the first trimester of pregnancy only
(e) Pyuria without culture of bacteria

Answer

A and B

Explanation

In pregnancy the rate of bacteriuria is not increased compared to the general population, but the rate of progression to pyelonephritis is increased due to glycosuria, *de novo* vesicoureteric reflux (in 5% of pregnancies), bladder outlet obstruction and sex hormone-dependent difference in urine flow rate and collecting capacity. Perinatal morbidity and mortality are increased due to premature delivery after untreated pyelonephritis.

An increased risk of urinary tract infection in pregnancy occurs in women with a history of childhood infection and ureteric reflux disease (answers A and B correct). Presently, all pregnant women are screened for bacteriuria in the first trimester (its presence in the first trimester is a risk factor for pyelonephritis at any stage of the pregnancy). Pregnant women with asymptomatic bacteriuria (unlike non-pregnant women) should be treated and screened for subsequent infection. The rate of pyelonephritis is the same in all trimesters of pregnancy (answer D incorrect).

The criteria for diagnosis of urinary tract infection are the same in pregnancy as in non-pregnant women. However, white cell excretion rate is increased in normal pregnancy and pyuria without bacteriuria is a common finding. Isolated pyuria has a number of possible causes and atypical bacteria (e.g. mycobacteria, *Chlamydia*) should be considered (Answer E incorrect). The relationship between symptoms and infection in pregnancy is blurred by the presence of bladder symptoms related to pressure from the gravid uterus: frequency and dysuria. Other physiological factors in pregnancy which predispose to infection include *de novo* reflux (3 to 5%), glycosuria (in the absence of gestational diabetes), greater capacity of the collecting system and obstruction to outflow by the gravid uterus.

Clinical pearls

- Pyelonephritis is a more common complication of bacteriuria in pregnancy than outside pregnancy.

- Bacteriuria in pregnancy is common (up to 5%) and should be screened for in the first trimester.
- Pregnant women with asymptomatic bacteriuria should be treated and screened for subsequent infection.
- Physiological factors in pregnancy which predispose to infection include:
  - *de novo* reflux (3 to 5%)
  - glycosuria (in the absence of gestational diabetes)
  - greater capacity of the collecting system
  - obstruction to outflow by the gravid uterus.
- Renal tract dilatation is normal in pregnancy.

Question 6

True statements about antibiotic treatment in pregnancy include which of the following?

(a) Potential fetotoxicity should be considered.

(b) Intravenous therapy has greater potential for crossing the placenta.

(c) Perinatal morbidity is increased in babies born from women with untreated infection.

(d) Maternal morbidity is increased in women with untreated urinary tract infection.

(e) Relief of the right ureteric obstruction is essential for antibiotics to be effective.

Answer

A, C and D

Explanation

The majority of available antibiotics are categorised as safe in pregnancy, *but no antibiotic should be administered without checking the safety classification in pregnancy* (answer A correct). Safety profile is independent of route of administration (answer B incorrect). Category A drugs are considered to be the safest and gain this classification due to extensive used in humans with no known, or theoretical, abnormalities having occurred after human or animal use. Some antibiotics are classified as C (causing reversible effects in babies) and should only be used if there are no safer choices available, if the mother is fully informed and with multidisciplinary discussion involving the obstetrician, midwife and neonatologist.

There is a clear increase in perinatal mortality and morbidity from maternal urinary tract infection A (answer C correct). This justifies the universal screening for bacteriuria in pregnant women. Increased maternal morbidity occurs due to the more severe nature of infections, the delay in diagnosis due to symptoms being masked by the pregnancy, the tenfold increased rate of progression to pyelonephritis and the relative immunosuppression of normal pregnancy (answer D correct). However, the choices of antibiotics (after taking into account potential fetotoxicity) and the prognosis are much the same as for non-pregnant women.

It is essential to assess renal anatomy and function following pyelonephritis, to exclude possible obstruction. Mild hydronephrosis, often more prominent on the right, is normal in pregnancy and with visualisation of ureteric jets (of urine) into the bladder, no further treatment is required (answer E incorrect).

Clinical pearls

- Increased perinatal and maternal morbidity from pyelonephritis are reasons for an increased need in pregnancy to treat asymptomatic bacteriuria and lower urinary tract infection.
- Assessment of renal anatomy and function after pyelonephritis in pregnancy is essential.
- Mild hydronephrosis is normal in pregnancy and no further treatment is required provided ureteric jets are seen, renal function is normal and there is prompt response to antibiotic treatment.
- The safety of antibiotics in pregnancy is outlined in Table 6.1.

Table 6.1 Antibiotic safety in pregnancy

Antibiotic	Category
Penicillins	
Ampicillin, amoxicillin, benzathine penicillin, benzylpenicillin, carbenicillin, cloxacillin, methicillin, phenethicillin phenoxymethylpenicillin, procaine penicillin	A
Amoxycillin with clavulanic acid, flucloxacillin, mezlocillin, piperacillin, piperacillin with tazobactam	B1
Ticarcillin, dicloxacillin	B2
Azlocillin	B3
Cephalosporins	
Cephalexin, cephalothin	A
Ceclor, cefotaxime, cefotetan, cefpodoxime, cefazidime, ceftriaxone, cefamandole, cefazolin	B1
Cefodizime, cefpirome	B2
Tetracyclines	
(After 18 weeks gestation—teeth discoloration)	D
Nitrofurantoin (short-term therapy) (Beware term use: haemolytic anaemia in infants with glucose-6-phosphate dehydrogenase (G6PD) deficiency; crosses the placenta)	A
Macrolide antibiotics	
Clarithromycin	B3
Azithromycin, roxithromycin	B1

Table 6.1 Antibiotic safety in pregnancy continued

Antibiotic	Category
Erythromycin	A
Aminoglycosides	
Gentamicin, amikacin, kanamycin, neomycin, netilmicin, tobramycin (Cross the placenta; unrelated to maternal blood concentrations; possible cranial nerve damage and renal damage)	D
Quinolones	
Ciprofloxacin, enoxacin, fleroxacin, norfloxacin, ofloxacin	B3
Trimethoprim	B3
Sulfonamides	
(Cross the placenta; jaundice and haemolytic anaemia in the newborn)	
Sulfadoxine, sulfadiazine, sulfamethizole, sulfamethoxazole	C
Trimethoprim-sulfonamide combinations	C

Definitions

A   Drugs that have been taken by a large number of pregnant women and women of child-bearing age without any proven increase in the frequency of malformations or other direct or indirect harmful effects on the fetus having been observed.

B1   Drugs that have been taken by only a limited number of pregnant women and women of child-bearing age without an increase in the frequency of malformations or other direct or indirect harmful effects on the human fetus having been observed. Studies in animals have not shown evidence of an increased occurrence of fetal damage.

B2   Drugs that have been taken by only a limited number of pregnant women and women of child-bearing age without an increase in the frequency of malformations or other direct or indirect harmful effects on the human fetus having been observed. Studies in animals are inadequate or may be lacking, but available data show no evidence of an increased occurrence of fetal damage.

B3   Drugs that have been taken by only a limited number of pregnant women and women of child-bearing age without an increase in the frequency of malformations or other direct or indirect harmful effects on the human fetus having been observed. Studies in animals have shown evidence of an increased occurrence of fetal damage, the significance of which is considered uncertain in humans.

C   Drugs that, owing to their pharmacological effects, have caused or may be suspected of causing, harmful effects on the human fetus or neonate without causing malformations. These effects may be reversible.

D   Drugs that have caused, are suspected to have caused or may be expected to cause an increased incidence of human fetal malformations or irreversible damage. These drugs may also have adverse pharmacological effects.

X   Drugs that have such a high risk of causing permanent damage to the fetus that they should not be used in pregnancy or when there is a possibility of pregnancy.

LEVEL C

Case history continued ...

The patient goes on to have a caesarean section for transverse lie position of the fetus at 38 weeks gestation. Her baby has a birth weight of 4.2 kg (above the 95th percentile for a term baby). The patient's blood sugar was elevated at her routine 28-week glucose tolerance test. She was initially treated with dietary restriction of carbohydrates but at 33 weeks gestation insulin injections were required. Her blood sugar level (BSL) was mostly below 6.0 mmol/L but levels of up to 14.0 mmol/L occurred with meals, and her HbA_{1c} was 7.3% (r.r. <6.0 %).

Her post-operative course is complicated on day three by acute abdominal pain, frequency and dysuria. Her BP is 80/50 mmHg and she has a tachycardia of 120 beats/minute. Her temperature is 38.0°C.

The following urine microscopy is reported:

- Leucocytes: >100/µL
- Erythrocytes: >100/µL
- Epithelial: 10–50/µL
- Bacteria: Scanty
- Yeasts: Scanty
- Casts: Nil

The final report is:

- Viable count >10^5 CFU/mL
- *Escherichia coli*
- Antibiotic sensitivities
  — Ampicillin
  — Cephalexin
  — Gentamicin
  — Nitrofurantoin
  — Trimethoprim
- Streptococcus
- Pseudomonas

Question 7

Likely contributors to her urinary tract infection include:

(a) gestational diabetes
(b) bladder instrumentation associated with the procedure
(c) surgical complications of the procedure
(d) use of intra-operative prophylactic antibiotics
(e) fetal macrosomia.

Answer

A, B and C

Explanation

Like all surgical procedures, caesarean section is associated with an increased risk of post-operative sepsis and urinary tract infection (Answer C correct).

In this case, the prior history of urinary tract infection is of importance. There are special risks with delivery by caesarean section, particularly ureteric ablation or suture during the procedure, bladder laceration or bladder disruption from instrumentation. This risk is diminished by catheterisation of the bladder prior to the procedure, and identification of the ureters at the time of surgery. Catheterisation, however, increases the risk of urinary sepsis (answer B correct). Therefore, these are generally placed under sterile conditions and removed as soon as possible after delivery and after the effects of regional anaesthesia (spinal or epidural) have resolved. Prophylactic antibiotics are added at the time of operation to prevent both wound infection and perioperative urinary tract infection (answer D incorrect).

Because urinary tract infections are acquired in hospital, in potentially sick women with antecedent risks, infection is more likely to be complicated by atypical organisms and require more aggressive treatment than community-acquired infections.

Other contributing factors in this case include the neonatal macrosomia, albeit indirectly (answer E partially correct). A birth weight of greater than 4.0 kg is indicative of inadequately treated impaired glucose tolerance or gestational diabetes. Diabetes is a predisposing factor to urinary tract sepsis (answer A correct). Fetal macrosomia is important in that the risk of complications after vaginal delivery is increased. There is an increased risk of malposition as in this case, and malposition requires operative delivery which is a risk factor for urinary sepsis.

Clinical pearls

- Operative delivery is associated with an increased risk of urinary tract infection due to:
  — instrumentation
  — risk of urinary tract damage including ureteric obstruction
  — antecedents to caesarean section such as prolonged labour, malposition, possible ureteric obstruction and gestational diabetes.
- Urinary tract infection is more likely to be complicated by atypical organisms and require more aggressive treatment than community-acquired infections.

Question 8

True statements about renal tract and pelvic imaging in this case include which of the following?

(a) Reduction of physiological right-sided dilatation occurs within days of delivery.

(b) Ureteric obstruction after operative delivery is generally bilateral.

(c) Exclusion of endometritis requires computerised tomography (CT) imaging.
(d) Use of radiocontrast is safe in the immediate post-delivery period.

Answer

A

Explanation

Post-caesarean section ureter obstruction is a rare complication and needs to be excluded by urgent imaging. This is usually unilateral obstruction and of moderate to severe degree (answer B incorrect). It takes 6 weeks for the physiological dilatation to resolve completely, but a reduction would already be expected on day three post-delivery (answer A correct).

Other possible sources of post-caesarean pain and fever can include pelvic thrombophlebitis, wound infection, infected broad ligament haematoma and endometritis.

CT imaging is difficult if contrast is required. Breast milk needs to be discarded for 24 to 48 hours after contrast administration, so there are important implications for a woman attempting to establish breastfeeding. Pelvic and renal ultrasound are generally sufficient, and often better than CT, for excluding pelvic pathology or renal tract obstruction (answer C incorrect). If contrast-enhanced imaging is required, a strong argument needs to be put to the mother about the risks and benefits of such a procedure and the likely strategies to allow the baby to be fed in the absence of the mother.

Clinical pearls

- Ureteric obstruction needs to be excluded after any pelvic surgery if there is a reduction in renal function, unilateral renal pain or urinary tract sepsis.
- Possible sources of post-caesarean pain and fever can include pelvic thrombophlebitis, wound infection, infected broad ligament haematoma and endometritis.
- Management of post-caesarean sepsis (investigations and antibiotic choices) has implications for breastfeeding.
- Physiological dilatation can take up to 6 weeks to resolve completely, but a reduction would already be expected on day three post-delivery.

Question 9

The nature of the culture results suggests which other possibilities?
(a) Mastitis
(b) Perineal infection

(c) Abdominal wound infection
(d) Endometritis
(e) Peritonitis
(f) Cannula site infection

Answer
B, C and D

Explanation

Given the presence of multiple organisms in the urine, the possibility of urine contamination from perineal infection needs to be excluded (answer B correct). However, her presentation is one of sepsis and other potential sources of infection need to be identified. In this case other possibilities include endometriosis and wound infection (answers C and D correct).

The presence of mixed organisms is not uncommon in the setting of urinary tract instrumentation. This patient has signs of septicaemia with hypotension and tachycardia. Progression to multi-organ failure is a real possibility. Given her pre-delivery diabetes, all potential sites needs to be explored (answer A, E and F partially correct). Urgent treatment is required with intravenous fluids and antibiotics (3rd-generation cephalosporin and aminoglycoside and metronidazole); inotropes may be necessary if her BP fails to respond to intravenous fluids. Post-partum women are at particular risk of pulmonary oedema in the setting of excessive fluid resuscitation.

The consequences of treatment, particularly immediately post-delivery, include significant perineal irritation in the form of superimposed fungal infection, passage of fungal infection to the neonate and nipples and interruption of breastfeeding.

Clinical pearls

- Post-caesarean section urinary tract sepsis can complicate other post-operative infections, including wound, perineal and endometrial infection.
- The presence of mixed organisms is not uncommon in the setting of urinary tract instrumentation.
- Urgent broad-spectrum antibiotic treatment and fluid resuscitation are required for septicaemia in the post-partum period.
- Consideration needs to be given to the breastfeeding implications of treatment including candidal superinfection.

Case history continued ...

Following the resolution of the illness with fluid resuscitation and appropriate antibiotics, the patient is discharged from hospital on day 14. At follow-up 6 weeks post-delivery she is complaining of vaginal itchiness and discharge. Her symptoms of frequency and dysuria have never fully resolved and are concerning. She is voiding up to 4 times most nights. Two urinary cultures taken by her general practitioner in the interim have identified *E. coli* resistant to ampicillin, trimethoprim and cephalothin. She has been treated initially with cephalothin 500 mg four times a day and then amoxycillin with clavulanic acid. She has had no treatment for 5 days, but is concerned about ongoing bladder symptoms.

Question 10

Possible consequences of long-term prophylactic antibiotics include:
(a) increased risk of antibiotic adverse reactions
(b) vaginal thrush
(c) neonatal thrush
(d) emergence of microbial resistance
(e) reduced breast-milk production.

Answer
B, C and D

Explanation

Prophylactic treatment for ongoing urinary tract infection is indicated in this case. She has had a severe illness related to urinary tract infection in the post-operative period following an episode of pyelonephritis in early pregnancy. Her ongoing symptoms suggest partially treated infection, interstitial cystitis or recurrent urinary tract infection. Once this infection has been treated with appropriately directed antimicrobial therapy, consideration should be given to 3 to 6 months of antibiotic prophylaxis.

There is no increased risk of idiosyncratic adverse reactions to antibiotics with prolonged use (answer A incorrect). Vaginal candidal infection is a common complication of antibiotic treatment, both acutely and with longer-term use. Transfer to the baby can cause neonatal morbidity and complications with breastfeeding (answers B and C correct). Treatment with neonatal nystatin and maternal topical treatment are required.

The theoretical concern about antimicrobial resistance is important given the >50% penicillin resistance of *E. coli* in most communities. In individual cases, monitoring with repeat urine cultures and adjusting antibiotics where necessary is required, especially if there is re-emergence of urinary tract symptoms (answer D correct).

Reduced breast-milk production is very difficult to diagnose given variations in individual milk production. There is no evidence for an effect of antimicrobial therapy on breast milk production, but this is something that should be discussed to provide maternal reassurance about treatment.

Although many women feel a benefit from cranberry juice and yoghurt treatment, there is limited evidence that this prevents or treats urinary tract infection.

 Clinical pearls

- Antibiotic prophylaxis is indicated for recurrent urinary tract infection.
- In individual cases, monitoring with repeat urine cultures and adjusting antibiotics where necessary is required, especially if there is re-emergence of urinary tract symptoms.
- Vaginal candidal infection is a common complication of antibiotic treatment, both acutely and with longer-term use.
- Although many women feel a benefit from cranberry juice and yoghurt treatment, there is limited evidence that this prevents or treats urinary tract infection.

Bibliography

Level A

1. Albert, X., Huertas, I., Pereiró, I., Sanfélix, J., Gosalbes, V. & Perrota, C. (2004) Antibiotics for preventing recurrent urinary tract infection in non-pregnant women. Cochrane Database Syst Rev. 3.
2. Finer, G. & Landau, D. (2004) Pathogenesis of urinary tract infections with normal female anatomy. Lancet Infect Dis. Oct. 4(10), 631–5.
3. Milo, G., Katchman, E.A., Paul, M., Christiaens, T., Baerheim, A. & Leibovici, L. (2005) Duration of antibacterial treatment for uncomplicated urinary tract infection in women. Cochrane Database Syst Rev. 2.
4. Paul, M., Silbiger, I., Grozinsky, S., Soares-Weiser, K. & Leibovici, L. (2006) Beta lactam antibiotic monotherapy versus beta lactam-aminoglycoside antibiotic combination therapy for sepsis. Cochrane Database Syst Rev. 1.

Level B

5. Smaill, F. & Vazquez, J.C. (2007) Antibiotics for asymptomatic bacteriuria in pregnancy. Cochrane Database Syst Rev. 2.
6. Vazquez, J.C. & Villar, J. (2003) Treatments for symptomatic urinary tract infections during pregnancy. Cochrane Database Syst Rev. 4.

7. Villar, J., Widmer, M., Lydon-Rochelle, M.T., Gülmezoglu, A.M. & Roganti, A. (2000) Duration of treatment for asymptomatic bacteriuria during pregnancy. Cochrane Database Syst Rev. 2.

Level C

8. Jepson, R.G., Mihaljevic, L. & Craig J.C. (1998) Cranberries for treating urinary tract infections. Cochrane Database Syst Rev. 4.
9. Smaill, F. & Hofmeyr, G.J. (2002) Antibiotic prophylaxis for caesarean section. Cochrane Database Syst Rev. 3.

Case 7
Resistant hypertension

PAOLO FERRARI

LEVEL A

Case history

Three months ago a 28-year-old woman was found to have a blood pressure (BP) of 196/114 mmHg, and heart rate 78 beats/min. She was initially started on an angiotensin-converting enzyme (ACE) inhibitor in combination with a diuretic (quinapril 20 mg, hydrochlorothiazide 12.5 mg). Subsequently, a beta-blocker (atenolol 50 mg) and a calcium channel blocker (nifedipine SR 30 mg) were added because of poor response. She was advised to avoid foods high in sodium. Her medical history is uneventful; she is on an oral contraceptive and she takes one to two tablets of paracetamol for headaches every couple of months. She is vegetarian, has never smoked and consumes less then four drinks of alcohol per week. Her grandfather died of a haemorrhagic stroke; her mother and two siblings have hypertension. On examination she appears well; her BP is 174/101 mmHg, heart rate 61 beats/min, her weight is 57 kg, and height 172 cm (body mass index is 19.3 kg/m²). Heart sounds are normal and there is no murmur. There is no rash and no peripheral oedema. The chest is clear, the jugular venous pressure is not elevated and there is no systolic or diastolic epigastric bruit. Peripheral pulses are present and strong. Fundoscopy reveals only moderate narrowing of the arteries, but no cotton-wool exudates, haemorrhages or papilloedema. Her electrocardiogram (ECG) shows left ventricular hypertrophy (LVH).

The following baseline investigations are obtained.

Laboratory data

	Result	Reference range
Na⁺	143 mmol/L	(136–146)
K⁺	3.7 mmol/L	(3.2–5.5)
HCO₃⁻	32 mmol/L	(24–31)
Urea	4.2 mmol/L	(2.5–6.5)
Creatinine	68 µmol/L	(45–90)
Uric acid	0.12 mmol/L	(0.14–0.36)
Glucose	4.7 mmol/L	(3.5–6.0)
Midstream urine	No red blood cells, no white blood cells, no protein	

Question 1

Her resistant hypertension can be explained by which of the following?

(a) Suboptimal therapy
(b) Ingestion of substances that can elevate BP
(c) Secondary hypertension
(d) Pseudohypertension

Answer

B and C

Explanation

Suboptimal therapy is considered the single most common and most correctable cause of resistant hypertension. The major causes of inadequate medical treatment are lack of administration of more effective drugs and failure to prevent volume expansion with adequate diuretic therapy (Table 7.1). This is not the case, as the patient remains hypertensive despite correction of any contributing mechanisms as well as taking several antihypertensive drugs, including a thiazide diuretic (answer A incorrect). A variety of prescription and recreational drugs can increase the BP and, in some cases, reduce the efficacy of antihypertensive agents (Table 7.2). These include cocaine, sympathomimetic drugs (including amphetamines), anabolic steroids, cyclosporine, antidepressants, non-steroidal anti-inflammatory drugs, liquorice and oestrogen-containing oral contraceptives (answer B correct). Patients with resistant hypertension are much more likely to have some form of secondary hypertension, most often due to intrinsic renal disease, renal artery stenosis or primary aldosteronism (answer C correct). Some older patients have thickened, calcified arteries. Thus, with a sphygmomanometer a cuff pressure greater than that present within the artery is required to compress the brachial artery. The net effect, called pseudohypertension, is that the systolic and diastolic pressures estimated from the sphygmomanometer may be considerably higher than the directly measured intra-arterial pressure. Pseudohypertension is very unlikely in this patient due to the presence of end-organ damage (left ventricular hypertrophy [LVH] on ECG) and her young age (answer D incorrect).

Other causes of resistant hypertension are: relative or absolute volume expansion, which is often at least partially responsible for an inability to control the systemic BP; poor compliance with medical or dietary therapy, office or 'white coat' hypertension (see Table 7.1).

Table 7.1 Reasons for lack of responsiveness to hypertension therapy

- Inadequate therapy
  - Doses too low
  - Inappropriate combinations (ACE-inhibitor and ARB)
  - No diuretic
  - Drug interactions   *(continued)*

Table 7.1 Reasons for lack of responsiveness to hypertension therapy *continued*

- Volume overload
  — Inadequate diuretic therapy
  — Excess sodium intake
  — Fluid retention from reduction of blood pressure
- Non-adherence to therapy
  — Cost of medication and related care
  — Instructions not clear and/or not given to the patient in writing
  — Failure of physician to increase or change therapy to achieve blood pressure goals
  — Inadequate or no patient education
  — Lack of involvement of the patient in the treatment plan
  — Side-effects of medication
  — Organic brain syndrome (e.g. memory deficit)
  — Inconvenient dosing schedule
- White coat hypertension
- Pseudohypertension
- Secondary hypertension
  — Renal (renal parenchymal disease or renovascular disease)
  — Endocrine (primary aldosteronism, overproduction of other mineralocorticoids, congenital adrenal hyperplasia, Cushing's syndrome, phaeochromocytoma)
  — Pregnancy-induced hypertension
  — Sleep apnoea
  — Coarctation of the aorta
  — Neurologic disorders (dysautonomia, increased intracranial pressure, lead poisoning)
- Drug-related causes
  — (See Table 7.2)
- Associated conditions
  — Increasing obesity
  — Excessive alcohol intake
  — Sedentary lifestyle

Table 7.2 Commonly used medications and other substances that may interfere with blood pressure control

- Non-steroidal anti-inflammatory drugs
- Over-the-counter nasal sprays, oral decongestants
- Appetite suppressants containing vasoactive compounds (phenylpropanolamine hydrochloride, ephedrine, pseudoephedrine used for long periods, oxymetazoline hydrochloride)
- Anabolic steroids, corticosteroids
- Oral contraceptives containing oestrogen
- Cholestyramine (decreases absorption of diuretics)
- Rifampicin (increases clearance of propranolol)
- Tyramine and monoamine oxidase (MAO) inhibitors
- Phenothiazines
- Cyclosporine
- Erythropoietin
- Recreational drugs or illicit substances
  — Amphetamines
  — Cocaine
  — Alcohol (consumption of more than 28 mL of ethanol [680 mL of beer, 225 mL of wine or 57 mL of liquor] has a direct pressor effect that may lessen benefit of antihypertensive agent)

Clinical pearls

- Some patients have hypertension that is apparently resistant to conventional medical therapy.
- Resistance is defined as a BP above goal despite adherence to appropriate treatment.
- Appropriate antihypertensive therapy is considered a three-drug regimen including a diuretic.
- BP target is ≤140/90 mmHg in most patients and ≤130/80 mmHg in those with diabetes or renal disease.

Question 2

The plasma uric acid in this case is consistent with:

(a) vegetarian diet

(b) volume expansion

(c) treatment with a thiazide diuretic

(d) treatment with an ACE inhibitor.

Answer

B

Explanation

The connection of gout and hyperuricaemia with gluttony, obesity and over-indulgence in food and alcohol dates from ancient times. Uric acid (urate) is the end product of purine degradation. Although eating foods rich in purines contributes to the total pool of uric acid, most uric acid is derived from the metabolism of endogenous purine (answer A incorrect). Uric acid plasma concentration depends largely on its renal clearance. The renal handling of urate involves complete glomerular filtration followed by reabsorption and secretion mainly in the proximal renal tubule. The amount of urate excreted depends on the extracellular fluid volume. Expansion of extracellular fluid volume increases (answer B correct) and contraction of extracellular fluid volume decreases the clearance of urate. In the syndrome of inappropriate secretion of antidiuretic hormone, there is volume expansion associated with low uric acid. A comparable situation is observed whenever exaggerated amounts of free water are consumed. Similarly, hypouricaemia and a tendency to low serum sodium (Na^+) concentrations are observed in normal pregnancy, a state with volume expansion, and in mineralocorticoid hypertension, which is associated with Na^+ and water retention. On the other hand, when contraction of extracellular fluid volume is present, as is often the case when thiazides or loop-diuretics are administered, increased serum uric acid concentrations are observed (answer C incorrect). Although the ACE inhibitors captopril, enalapril and ramipril have been found to increase uricosuria (probably by lowering the net reabsorption of uric acid in the proximal tubule), the effect is too mild to be of clinical relevance (answer D incorrect).

Clinical pearls

- Plasma uric acid concentration is a useful marker of extracellular fluid volume.
- A low uric acid level is usually found with expansion of the extracellular fluid volume, while extracellular fluid volume contraction increases plasma uric acid level.
- Hypouricaemia is observed in normal pregnancy, a state with volume expansion. Hyperuricaemia, and volume contraction, occur in pre-eclampsia.
- Hypouricaemia is also observed in forms of mineralocorticoid hypertension.

Case history continued ...

The patient is asked to discontinue her oral contraceptive. Two months later her BP still remains high and her latest reading is 172/97 mmHg.

Question 3

The most likely cause of this woman's resistant hypertension is:

(a) renovascular disease
(b) mineralocorticoid hypertension
(c) Cushing's syndrome
(d) coarctation of the aorta.

Answer

B

Explanation

Renovascular disease due to renal artery stenosis is caused either by fibromuscular dysplasia or atherosclerosis. The former predominates in young women while atherosclerosis is usually encountered in older individuals. The most common clinical manifestation of fibromuscular dysplasia is hypertension, which can frequently be cured or significantly improved with percutaneous balloon dilation. BP usually responds well to treatment with an inhibitor of the renin–angiotensin system, even if BP can't be normalised. Thus, even if fibromuscular dysplasia could be a likely cause of this patient's hypertension, the poor BP response to quinapril argues against this aetiology (answer A incorrect).

Clinical findings other than resistant hypertension may be of little help in identifying mineralocorticoid hypertension. Primary aldosteronism is the most common form of mineralocorticoid hypertension. Hypokalaemia, whether spontaneous or provoked, provides the best clue to the presence of primary aldosteronism, but it is found in <20% of cases. As with any form of mineralo-corticoid hypertension, the most important mechanism for the increase in BP is renal Na^+ retention producing volume expansion. Moreover, activation of the mineralocorticoid receptor leads to increased renal excretion of potassium (K^+) and hydrogen ions. This patient had low plasma uric acid and high bicarbonate, with low normal serum K^+ (answer B correct). A history of considerable weight gain and recent change in facial appearance together with characteristic physical (e.g. truncal obesity, moon face, plethora, purplish skin striae) and biochemical (hyperglycaemia) features are indicative of Cushing's syndrome. None of these signs is present in this patient (answer C incorrect). Coarctation of the aorta is often asymptomatic in adults. Absent or reduced pulses in the legs, together with lower blood pressure in the legs than in the arms, are a valuable clue to diagnosis. Upper extremity systolic blood pressure is elevated disproportionately to diastolic blood pressure, resulting in a wide pulse pressure and bounding pulses (answer D incorrect).

Clinical pearls

- Hypertension with metabolic alkalosis, with or without hypokalaemia, in association with hypouricaemia, is suggestive of mineralocorticoid hypertension.
- In most cases of mineralocorticoid hypertension, activation of the mineralocorticoid receptor leads to renal Na^+ reabsorption and increases excretion of K^+ and hydrogen ions.
- Resistant hypertension is often the only relevant clinical finding in primary aldosteronism, the most common form of mineralocorticoid hypertension.

Question 4

The possible explanation of the mild retinal target-organ damage is:

(a) hypertension of short duration
(b) beta-blocker-associated decrease in eye pressure

(c) primary aldosteronism

(d) white coat hypertension.

Answer

C

Explanation

Hypertensive retinal changes are usually dependent on the severity of hypertension and the underlying mechanism for the increase in BP, rather than the duration of hypertension. In hypertensive disorders where vasoconstriction is primarily involved, such as with high circulating renin (renal artery stenoses) or catecholamines (phaeochromocytoma), severe retinopathy is more common; in states of fluid retention with or without vasodilation, hypertensive retinopathy is usually mild. Severe retinopathy can be observed in previously normotensive women with short duration of pregnancy-related hypertension and pre-eclampsia (answer A incorrect).

Topical beta-blockers are commonly used agents in the treatment of raised intraocular pressure and can lower the eye pressure by 4 to 6 mmHg (20 to 35%). Oral atenolol causes a moderate, non-significant fall in intraocular pressure of approximately 10 to 15%. However, glaucomatous retinal changes are distinct from hypertensive retinal changes, and systemic beta-blockers are unable to reverse hypertensive retinopathy beyond their blood pressure lowering effect (answer B incorrect). The severity of hypertensive retinopathy in primary aldosteronism is subclinical and similar to that observed in essential hypertension without LVH, but significantly milder than in essential hypertension with LVH (answer C correct). However, in primary aldosteronism LVH can be pronounced, even in patients with mild retinopathy. White coat hypertension should be suspected in patients who remain resistant to therapy in the absence of target organ damage (retinopathy, renal insufficiency, LVH), who manifest symptoms of overmedication (orthostatic symptoms, persistent fatigue) and/or who report home blood pressure values significantly lower than values measured in the office. This patient has demonstrated LVH (answer D incorrect).

 Clinical pearls

- Fundoscopic examination of the retina is an often-neglected clinical examination that provides important clues to the relevance of measured BP.
- White coat hypertension should be suspected in patients without retinopathy despite increased office BP.
- Patients with primary aldosteronism tend to have subclinical hypertensive retinopathy.

LEVEL B

Case history continued ...

The ACE-inhibitor, diuretic and beta-blocker are ceased and after a week the following results are obtained on this patient.

Laboratory data

	Result	Reference range
Plasma		
Na^+	142 mmol/L	(136–146)
K^+	3.4 mmol/L	(3.2–5.5)
Osmolality	288 mosmol/kg	(275–295)
Urine		
Volume	1240 mL/d	
Na^+	79 mmol/L	
K^+	76 mmol/L	
Osmolality	739 mosmol/kg	(40–1200)

Question 5

These additional results indicate which of the following?

(a) Excessive salt consumption

(b) Excessive renal K^+ loss

(c) Inadequate renal H_2O retention

(d) Excessive Na^+ retention

Answer

B

Explanation

A Na^+ excretion of 97 mmol/d (= 79 mmol/L × 1.24 L/d) corresponds to a salt intake of 5.6 g NaCl daily, which is low for a western-type diet (answer A incorrect). Secretion of K^+ in the distal nephron accounts for the vast majority of K^+ excreted in the urine and is mainly influenced by aldosterone. The degree of aldosterone activity can in theory be estimated by measuring the tubular fluid K^+ concentration at the end of the cortical collecting tubule, the site responsible for most of K^+ secretion. This measurement can be estimated clinically from calculation of the transtubular potassium gradient (TTKG) using osmolality and K^+ in plasma and urine, and is an index of the gradient of K^+ achieved at K^+ secretory sites, independent of urine flow rate:

$$\text{TTKG} = (\text{urine } K^+ \div [\text{urine osmolality/plasma osmolality}]) \div \text{plasma } K^+$$

Use of the TTKG assumes that negligible amounts of K^+ are secreted or reabsorbed distal to these sites and that the final urinary K^+ concentration then depends on water reabsorption in the medullary collecting ducts.

This formula is accurate as long as the urine osmolality exceeds that of the plasma (so that the K^+ concentration of the cortical collecting tubule can be estimated) and the urine Na^+ concentration is >25 mmol/L (so that Na^+ delivery is not limiting). An inadequately high renal K^+ loss is present when TTKG >2 for plasma K^+ <3.5 mmol/L or TTKG >6 for plasma K^+ 3.5 to 4.0 mmol/L. In this case, TTKG = $(76 \div [739/288]) \div 3.4 = 8.7$. This high value is consistent with hyperaldosteronism (answer B correct). While the urine osmolality of 739 mosmol/kg suggests stimulated ADH secretion, the resulting water retention cannot be considered inadequate in view of the normal plasma Na^+ concentration (answer C incorrect). In states of chronic mineralocorticoid excess there appears to be no excessive Na^+ retention. This phenomenon has been called aldosterone escape. The escape phenomenon appears to be due to decreased Na^+ reabsorption in some other nephron segment, perhaps the loop of Henle or the papillary collecting tubule. It does not represent aldosterone resistance, since urinary K^+ loss continues and the cortical collecting tubule remains responsive to aldosterone (answer D incorrect).

 Clinical pearls

- Secretion of K^+ in the distal nephron accounts for the vast majority of K^+ excreted in the urine and is mainly influenced by aldosterone.
- Calculation of the transtubular potassium gradient (TTKG)—using plasma and urine osmolality and K^+—provides an index of the gradient of K^+ achieved in the distal nephron under the influence of aldosterone.

Case history continued ...

Based on the patient's history and clinical and laboratory findings, a strong suspicion of primary (rather then secondary) aldosteronism is raised.

Question 6

Which investigations would you request to confirm the possible diagnosis of primary aldosteronism (PA)?

(a) Abdominal computed tomographic (CT) scan

(b) Plasma renin

(c) Plasma aldosterone/renin ratio

(d) Fludrocortisone suppression test

Answer

C

Explanation

Adrenal CT imaging can detect most, but not all, aldosteronomas, since a unilateral excess of aldosterone secretion in the absence of adenoma or hyperplasia may be caused by an adrenal microadenoma not detectable by radiologic imaging. In the most common form of PA, idiopathic hyperaldosteronism, the adrenals appear normal on CT scan. Conversely, the appearance of a non-functional incidentally discovered adrenal nodule on CT imaging occasionally causes confusion regarding its functional significance. Thus, biochemical diagnosis of aldosteronism needs to be established before determining the subtype of the disorder (answer A incorrect).

Although spontaneous hypokalaemia in a patient with hypertension is a strong indicator of classic PA, most patients with this condition have normal serum K^+ levels. Plasma renin activity is suppressed in almost all patients with untreated PA. However, many patients with essential hypertension may present with low-renin hypertension. Thus, neither measurements of serum K^+ nor measurements of plasma renin are suitable or reliable methods of screening for PA (answer B incorrect). Determining the aldosterone/renin ratio (ARR) in patients with untreated hypertension seems to be the most appropriate screening method for distinguishing patients with PA from those with essential hypertension. In the presence of severe or symptomatic hypertension, patients should take only antihypertensive medications that are least likely to affect measurements of renin and aldosterone (answer C correct).

The fludrocortisone suppression test (FST) is not a screening test for PA and is used to further characterise the condition once its biochemical diagnosis has been established, to prove autonomous production of aldosterone, independent of angiotensin II. With the FST the diagnosis of PA is based on failure of aldosterone to be suppressed to <180 pmol/L after 4 days of fludrocortisone 0.1 mg every 6 hours. The major drawback of this test is that it has to be carried out with the patient in hospital for 4 days under a strict regimen of Na^+ intake and K^+ substitution (answer D incorrect).

 Clinical pearls

- The biochemical diagnosis of aldosteronism needs to be established before determining the subtype of the disorder by more specific tests and imaging.

- Most patients with primary aldosteronism have normal serum K⁺ levels.
- Determining the ARR in patients with untreated hypertension seems to be the most appropriate screening method for distinguishing patients with primary aldosteronism from those with essential hypertension.

Question 7

Which antihypertensive drugs are best avoided to adequately interpret plasma aldosterone and renin studies?

(a) Calcium channel blockers
(b) ACE-inhibitors/angiotensin receptor blockers
(c) Beta-blockers
(d) Alpha-blockers

Answer

B and C

Explanation

The ARR is best measured in patients with untreated hypertension. In the presence of severe or symptomatic hypertension, patients should take only anti-hypertensive medications that are least likely to affect measurements of renin and aldosterone, such as calcium channel blockers or alpha-blockers (answer A and D incorrect). ACE-inhibitors and angiotensin receptor blockers may 'falsely elevate' plasma renin in patients with primary aldosteronism and, therefore, in patients treated with these agents a low ARR does not exclude primary aldosteronism (answer B correct). Conversely, beta-blockers may 'falsely reduce' plasma renin in subjects with essential hypertension and therefore produce a false-positive raised ARR (answer C correct), while diuretics increase both plasma renin and aldosterone.

 Clinical pearls

- Antihypertensive drugs least likely to affect measurements of renin and aldosterone include calcium channel blockers and alpha-blockers.
- Diuretics, ACE-inhibitors and angiotensin receptor blockers may 'falsely elevate' and beta-blocker may 'falsely reduce' plasma renin.
- It is impossible to interpret data obtained from patients treated with aldosterone receptor antagonists.

LEVEL C

Case history continued ...

Her plasma aldosterone and renin studies yield the following results.

Immunoreactive renin	3.5 mU/L	(4–29)
Aldosterone	680 pmol/L	(56–730)
ARR	194 pmol/mU	(<100)

Question 8

Given the patient's history, what is the likely cause of her primary aldosteronism?

(a) Idiopathic aldosteronism

(b) Adrenal adenoma

(c) Glucocorticold-remediable aldosteronism

(d) Adrenal carcinoma

Answer

C

Explanation

The ARR is clearly increased and plasma renin is suppressed, but aldosterone is within the normal range. Although plasma aldosterone is not elevated, an increased ARR in the presence of plasma aldosterone levels >650 pmol/L suggest primary aldosteronism (PA). The term PA is used to describe a heterogeneous group of conditions characterised by an overproduction of aldosterone by the adrenal gland. Known causes of PA are unilateral or bilateral micro- or macronodular adrenal hyperplasia (idiopathic aldosteronism, ~70%), adrenocortical adenoma (~30%) and adrenal carcinoma (<1%). These subtypes of PA are sporadic and a strong family history of hypertension is usually absent (answers A, B and D incorrect).

This patient has a strong family history. One form of PA with a strong family history, and thus also known as familial hyperaldosteronism type I, has been recently characterised and called glucocorticoid-remediable aldosteronism (GRA). GRA is a rare, autosomal dominant form of familial hypertension with suppressed plasma renin and variable aldosteronism (aldosterone may be elevated or within normal limits) that is sometimes (but not always) associated with hypokalaemia. GRA should be suspected in patients with early onset of severe hypertension, a history of severe hypertension in first-degree relatives, or a family history of early haemorrhagic stroke (answer C correct). Under normal conditions, the renin–angiotensin system and K^+ balance regulate aldosterone production. In GRA, adrenocorticotrophic hormone (ACTH), and not angiotensin II, regulates aldosterone secretion and the renin–angiotensin system is suppressed. Because a hormone that is not sensitive to Na^+ balance stimulates aldosterone secretion, aldosterone production is autonomous, resulting in a chronic mineralocorticoid excess state. Suppression of ACTH with glucocorticoids decreases aldosterone secretion and cures the hypertension.

Clinical pearls

- The term primary aldosteronism is used to describe a heterogeneous group of conditions, which include idiopathic aldosteronism, adrenal adenoma and carcinoma, and a genetic form called glucocorticoid-remediable aldosteronism (GRA).
- In GRA, aldosterone secretion is regulated by ACTH; suppression of ACTH with glucocorticoids decreases aldosterone secretion and cures the hypertension.
- Family history of hypertension and early haemorrhagic stroke in patients with suppressed plasma renin and high aldosterone are suggestive of GRA.

Question 9

What is the molecular basis of glucocorticoid-remediable aldosteronism?

(a) Mutations in the 11β-hydroxysteroid dehydrogenase type 2 gene
(b) Mutations in the WNK4 gene
(c) Chimeric duplication of the aldosterone synthase and 11β-hydroxylase genes
(d) Mutations in the subunit of the epithelial sodium channel

Answer
C

Explanation

Mutations in the 11β-hydroxysteroid dehydrogenase type 2 (11βHSD2) gene are the cause of apparent mineralocorticoid excess (AME) syndrome. In AME cortisol acts as the mineralocorticoid receptor (MR) agonist. This disease is characterised by hypokalaemic hypertension, with suppressed circulating renin and aldosterone. Cortisol and aldosterone bind with equal affinity to the MR. Plasma concentrations of cortisol are 1000-fold higher than those of aldosterone, but in MR-target cells the enzyme 11βHSD2 converts cortisol to the receptor-inactive form cortisone, protecting the MR from occupation by cortisol (answer A incorrect).

WNK4 is a serine–threonine kinase containing a cysteine instead of the usual lysine at a key position in the active site of serine–threonine kinases. WNK4 gene mutants are the cause of some forms of pseudohypoaldosteronism type II, an autosomal dominant disorder characterised by hypertension, hyperkalaemia and renal tubular acidosis. Wild-type WNK4 inhibits the renal thiazide-sensitive NaCl co-transporter NCCT; mutations that cause type II pseudohypoaldosteronism relieve this inhibition allowing unrestricted Na^+ reabsorption by the distal convoluted tubule (answer B incorrect).

GRA is caused by a chimeric gene duplication arising from unequal crossing-over, such that the coding sequences of aldosterone synthase come under the control of the regulatory sequences of steroid 11β-hydroxylase. The adrenal cortex in GRA produces large quantities of 18-oxygenated cortisol compounds, 18-oxocortisol (18-oxo-F), and 18-hydroxycortisol (18-OH-F). Elevated levels of these compounds in a timed 24-hour urine collection provide a highly sensitive and specific test to diagnose GRA (answer C correct). Mutations in the C-terminus of the β- or γ-subunits of the epithelial sodium channel (ENaC) are the cause of another hereditary monogenic form of hypertension, also known as Liddle syndrome. Liddle syndrome is characterised by hypoaldosteronism, hypokalaemia and decreased renin and angiotensin. Thus, in this syndrome the hypertension is not due to hyperaldosteronism but rather to a renal tubular defect (Answer D incorrect).

 ## Clinical pearls

- All currently known monogenetic mutations altering BP regulation involve disturbances of Na^+ reabsorption in the renal tubule.
- Most genetic hypertensive disorders involve the mineralocorticoid axis and are characterised by low plasma renin, metabolic alkalosis and hypokalaemia.
- Monogenic forms of low renin hypertension can be identified in the following well-characterised disorders: 11β-hydroxylase and steroid 17-hydroxylase deficiencies (congenital adrenal hyperplasia), glucocorticoid-remediable hyperaldosteronism, apparent mineralocorticoid excess, activating mutations of the mineralocorticoid receptor, Liddle syndrome and familial pseudohypoaldosteronism type II.
- Genetic analysis in patients with glucocorticoid-remediable hyperaldosteronism demonstrates the presence of a hybrid gene for 11β-hydroxylase and aldosterone synthase.

Bibliography

Level A

1. Erdine, S. & Arat-Özkan, A. (2003) Resistant hypertension. *European Society of Hypertension Scientific Newsletter: Update on hypertension management.* 4(15), www.eshonline.org/education/newsletter/2003_15.pdf
2. Chobanian, A.V., Bakris, G.L., Black, H.R., Cushman, W.C., Green, L.A., Izzo, J.L. Jr., Jones, D.W., Materson, B.J., Oparil, S., Wright, J.T. Jr. & Roccella, E.J. (2003) Seventh report of the Joint National Committee on Prevention, Detection, Evaluation, and Treatment of High Blood Pressure. Hypertension. 42, 1206–52.
3. Kaplan, N.M. (2005) Treatment of hypertension: drug therapy. *Clinical Hypertension*, 9th edn. Kaplan, N.M. (ed.). Baltimore: Lippincott Williams & Wilkins.
4. Jorgensen, H. & Sundsfjord, J.A. (1974) The relation of plasma renin activity to left ventricular hypertrophy and retinopathy in patients with arterial hypertension. Acta Med Scand. 196, 307–13.
5. Weinman, E.J., Eknoyan, G. & Suki, W.N. (1975) The influence of the extracellular fluid volume on the tubular reabsorption of uric acid. J Clin Invest. 55, 283–91.
6. Muxfeldt, E.S., Bloch, K.V., Nogueira, Ada R. & Salles, G.F. (2005) True resistant hypertension: is it possible to be recognised in the office? Am J Hypertens. 18, 1534–40.

Level B

7. Ethier, J.H., Kamel, K.S., Magner, P.O., Lemann, J. & Halperin, M.L. (1990) The transtubular potassium concentration in patients with hypokalemia and hyperkalemia. Am J Kidney Dis. 15, 309–15.
8. Ferrari, P., Shaw, S.G., Nicod, J., Saner, E. & Nussberger, J. (2004) Active renin versus plasma renin activity to define aldosterone-to-renin ratio for primary aldosteronism. J Hypertens. 22, 377–81.
9. Ferrari, P. & Bonny, O. (2003) Forms of mineralocorticoid hypertension. Vitam Horm. 66, 113–56.

Level C

10. Lifton, R.P., Gharavi, A.G. & Geller, D.S. (2001) Molecular mechanisms of human hypertension. Cell. 23(104), 545–56.
11. Ferrari, P. & Bonny, O. (2003) Forms of mineralocorticoid hypertension. Vitam Horm. 66, 113–56.

Case 8
Hypertension in pregnancy

GEORGE MANGOS AND MARK BROWN

LEVEL A

Case history

A 28-year-old female presents for assessment of hypertension. There is a four-year history of stage 1 hypertension. A non-pharmacological approach was undertaken initially and the patient, who had originally weighed 82 kg, lost 20 kg over the 12-month period prior to presentation. There is no other past medical history. She is asymptomatic. There is no history of hypertension in her first-degree relatives. She smoked occasionally and prior to her pregnancy consumed alcohol on weekends with up to 120 g of alcohol consumed over the two-day period.

At the first consultation the patient announces that she is 10 weeks' gestation in her first pregnancy. Her weight is 62.5 kg. Her blood pressure (BP) is 152/88 mmHg and her pulse is 72 in sinus rhythm. The peripheral pulses are normal. There is no radio-femoral delay. The remainder of the cardiac and respiratory examinations is normal. The abdominal examination reveals no tenderness, no organomegaly and a very soft bruit in the epigastrium. The urinalysis shows a pH of 5 and is negative for blood, protein, leucocytes and glucose.

Results of blood analyses include serum creatinine 54 μmol/L, potassium 3.8 mmol/L, bicarbonate 20 mmol/L and urate 0.3 mmol/L. Thyroid function is normal.

A 24-hour ambulatory BP study is abnormal with an average BP of 135/84 mmHg (normal <130/80 mmHg). The systolic loads are 58% and diastolic loads 54%. Office BP is remeasured at 172/100 mmHg and the patient is managed with oral oxprenolol and subsequently the addition of oral hydralazine. The BP remains elevated and hydralazine is not tolerated; subsequently this drug is suspended and replaced by methyldopa. Methyldopa and oxprenolol provided good BP control until 29 weeks gestation when prazosin is added. During this time there is no clinical evidence of pre-eclampsia and fetal growth is satisfactory.

At 33 weeks gestation the patient develops moderate hypertension with office BP measured at 154/100 mmHg despite three antihypertensive agents. Proteinuria develops, initially detected by positive dipstick urinalysis and confirmed by quantitation (spot protein/creatinine ratio 69 mg/mmol). The patient is admitted to hospital and betamethasone administered intramuscularly to enhance fetal maturation. Severe hypertension develops, with BP measured up to 220/120 mmHg. This is managed with oral nifedipine and intravenous hydralazine.

Labour is induced at 33.5 weeks gestation. The patient has severe hypertension during labour, treated with hydralazine infusion. Fortunately vaginal delivery is successful and a premature female infant weighing 1650 g is delivered.

Question 1

How should hypertension in early pregnancy be managed?

(a) Pharmacologic therapy should be commenced at the first visit.

(b) Hypertension should be managed as an emergency when severe (BP >170/110 mmHg) during pregnancy.

(c) Mild hypertension (BP 140–159/90–99 mmHg) does not require treatment.

(d) Atenolol is a useful beta-blocker in this circumstance.

Answer

B

Explanation

Severe hypertension in early pregnancy is associated with an increased risk of growth restriction, pre-eclampsia and fetal demise (answer B correct). It is more likely that severe hypertension will develop later in pregnancy if early pregnancy BP control is poor. There is a little controversy about the management of severe hypertension in early pregnancy; pharmacological therapy is indicated. For mild to moderate hypertension, there continues to be controversy. Twenty per cent of women who present before 20 weeks gestation with hypertension will have white coat hypertension. Ambulatory BP monitoring is useful to diagnose this condition which generally will not require treatment with medication (answer A incorrect). Antihypertensives used in early pregnancy for mild to moderate hypertension are generally safe, well tolerated and proven outside of pregnancy to be of long-term cardiovascular benefit. Treatment of hypertension needs to be weighed against the risks of exposing the fetus to pharmacological agents (answer C incorrect). There is some concern that atenolol used from early pregnancy is associated with fetal growth restriction (see Question 2) (answer D incorrect).

 Clinical pearl

- White coat or office hypertension should be considered when BP is elevated in the first half of pregnancy.

Question 2

Which of the following statements about the use of antihypertensive medication in early pregnancy is/are incorrect?

(a) Antihypertensive medication for chronic hypertension reduces the risk of the development of pre-eclampsia.

(b) Antihypertensive medication is generally safe in pregnancy.

(c) Angiotensin-converting enzyme inhibitors are contraindicated in pregnancy.

(d) Antihypertensive agents reduce the risk of cerebral haemorrhage.

Answer

A

Explanation

Unfortunately, no useful treatment has been proven to reduce the risk of pre-eclampsia, except for a small benefit for aspirin in high-risk women (Duley et al. 2003). Ketanserin (a serotonin receptor antagonist) has been shown to reduce pre-eclampsia but safety concerns limit its use (Steyn & Odendall 1997). Antihypertensive medication has not been shown to reduce the development of superimposed pre-eclampsia in women with chronic hypertension (answer A). Generally, however, there is widespread experience with antihypertensive medication in pregnancy in several thousands of women in published clinical trials. Beta-blockers (except atenolol), hydralazine, clonidine, methyldopa, prazosin and many calcium channel blockers have all been used with safety in pregnancy (answer B correct). Atenolol, however, has been associated with growth restriction in hypertensive pregnancy women (Bayliss et al. 2002). ACE inhibitors (and therefore angiotensin receptor blockers [ARBs]) should be avoided in pregnancy in view of the potential risks of oligohydramnios, renal agenesis, growth restriction and neonatal renal failure as well as congenital heart or neurological abnormalities and ossification defects (Cooper et al. 2006) (answer C correct). Similarly, diuretics are generally avoided in view of the potential effect of reducing intravascular volume in women who are already predisposed to volume contraction. The primary benefit of antihypertensive medication in pregnancy is to lower BP to a safe range; indeed, antihypertensives do prevent cerebral haemorrhage (answer D correct).

 Clinical pearls

- Atenolol, ACE inhibitors, ARBs and diuretics are best avoided during pregnancy.
- No treatment is proven to reliably prevent pre-eclampsia.

Question 3

The presence of an epigastric bruit:

(a) is highly sensitive and specific for renal artery stenosis
(b) is neither sensitive nor specific for renal artery stenosis
(c) is not sensitive but highly specific for renal artery stenosis
(d) is abnormal
(e) will correlate with the need for angiographic diagnosis.

Answer

B

Explanation

Epigastric bruits in pregnancy may be due to increased blood flow associated with a hyperdynamic circulation due to plasma volume expansion and tachycardia (answers A and D incorrect). The splenic artery may be responsible for an epigastric bruit (answer C incorrect). The presence of an epigastric bruit is therefore neither sensitive (i.e. relying on a bruit will miss true renal artery stenosis) nor specific (i.e. there are many false positive causes of a bruit) for renal artery stenosis (answer B correct). Radiologic interventions during pregnancy should be avoided in view of the potential risk of ionising radiation exposure to the fetus; hence, an angiogram should be delayed until the post-partum period (answer E incorrect).

 Clinical pearl

- Epigastric bruits are common, not necessarily pathological, but should raise suspicion of renal artery stenosis.

Question 4

The diagnosis of pre-eclampsia can be established by the presence of:

(a) severe hypertension
(b) hypertension and proteinuria
(c) hypertension and evidence of target organ involvement
(d) hypertension and ankle oedema.

Answer

B and C

Explanation

Pre-eclampsia can be defined as a condition where *de novo* hypertension in pregnancy occurs in the presence of target organ involvement (answer B correct—some definitions of pre-eclampsia *require* proteinuria). Commonly this includes proteinuria, but pre-eclampsia may be hypertension associated with new onset abnormal liver function, thrombocytopenia, reduced glomerular filtration rate or central nervous system symptoms and signs (answer C correct). Table 8.1 gives the classification of the hypertensive disorders of pregnancy. Severe hypertension alone does not constitute a diagnosis of pre-eclampsia (answer A incorrect). Proteinuria should be diagnosed by 24-hour urine collection or spot protein/creatinine ratio; urinalysis cannot be relied upon for diagnosis of pre-eclampsia or for timing of delivery. Ankle oedema is a weak predictor of pre-eclampsia, and is a common phenomenon in normal pregnancy (answer D incorrect). However, the rapid development of oedema in a pregnant woman should indicate a need for monitoring for the signs and symptoms of pre-eclampsia as oedema often precedes the clinical development of pre-eclampsia (see Table 8.2).

Table 8.1 Classification of the hypertensive disorders of pregnancy

- Pre-eclampsia-eclampsia: *de novo* hypertension after 20 weeks' gestation with proteinuria properly documented (by 24-hour urine collection or midstream urine protein/creatinine ratio)
- Gestational hypertension: *de novo* hypertension alone after 20 weeks' gestation
- Chronic hypertension: hypertension that antedates pregnancy or identified before 20 weeks' gestation
- Pre-eclampsia superimposed on chronic hypertension

Source: Brown 2001

Table 8.2 Clinical features of pre-eclampsia

- Systolic BP >140 mmHg and/or diastolic BP >90 mmHg
- Urinary protein excretion >300 mg/day or spot protein/creatinine ratio >30 mg/mmol
- Increased plasma uric acid (this is common but not always present)
- Increased aminotransferases and epigastric pain
- Cerebral involvement (headaches, blurred vision, visual scotomata)
- Thrombocytopenia
- Reduced GFR, acute renal failure
- Pulmonary oedema
- Coagulopathy (rarely)

 Clinical pearls

- Pre-eclampsia is a systemic disorder, affecting multiple vascular beds.
- Proteinuria should be diagnosed by 24-hour urine or spot protein/creatinine ratio; urinalysis should be considered a screening test only.
- The presence or absence of proteinuria stratifies maternal and fetal risk, not the amount of proteinuria, unless at exceptionally high levels (≈9 g/day).

Question 5

Delivery of the fetus at 33.5 weeks gestation was indicated because:

(a) severe hypertension carried significant maternal risk
(b) the fetus was at risk in view of the maternal proteinuric pre-eclamptic syndrome
(c) the administration of intramuscular glucocorticoids to the mother reduced risk to the fetus.
(d) all of the above.

Answer
D

Explanation

The most common cause of death in pre-eclamptic disease is cerebral haemorrhage, and this is associated with severe hypertension. Therefore, severe hypertension in pregnancy should be managed as an emergency and certainly in hospital. If pharmacological control fails, delivery is usually indicated (answer A correct). The fetus was at risk in view of proteinuric pre-eclampsia. The presence of maternal pre-eclampsia increases perinatal mortality risk by approximately three-fold. Proteinuria frequently associates with reduced or diminishing fetal growth. Fetal distress, growth restriction, abruption and fetal demise may occur in this situation (answer B correct). Where delivery is considered to be likely within days, the administration of intra-muscular betamethasone has been shown to reduce the risk of neonatal respiratory distress syndrome, necrotising enterocolitis and neonatal cerebral leukoencephalopathy/haemorrhage (answer A correct).

 Clinical pearls

- The timing of delivery in early-onset pre-eclampsia is not necessarily an easy decision, and depends on both maternal and fetal wellbeing.
- Intramuscular betamethasone administered to the mother improves the outcomes for premature infants.

LEVEL B

Case history continued ...

An ultrasound of the kidneys in the first trimester showed a right kidney 11.8 cm in length and a left kidney 13.3 cm in length. Cortical thickness was normal bilaterally. There were Doppler features of a high-grade renal artery stenosis on the right side, estimated 60 to 99%.

Because of labile, severe hypertension at the time of delivery, a screen for phaeochromocytoma was sent. Fasting plasma metanephrines were normal (0.2 nmol/L – NR <0.4 nmol/L) but plasma normetanephrines were markedly elevated (12.9 nmol/L, normal range <0.7).

Early in the post-partum period a non-contrast computerised tomography (CT) scan of the abdomen identifies a suspicious nodule in the right adrenal gland. After alpha-blockade, a further CT scan with intravenous contrast confirmed the presence of an enhancing lesion measuring 3.5 cm in diameter, displacing the IVC anteriorly in the region of the right adrenal gland (see Fig. 8.1). The whole body I-123 MIBG (Iodine-123-meta-iodobenzylguanidine) scintiscan identified a focus of tracer uptake in the region of the right adrenal gland. Repeat normetanephrine analysis in the plasma was again markedly elevated. The above results were consistent with a right functioning phaeochromocytoma.

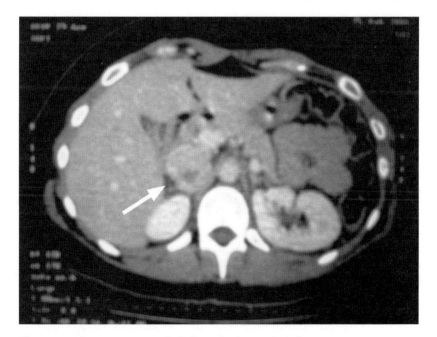

Figure 8.1 Mass anterior to right kidney, displacing the inferior vena cava inferomedially. There is a peripheral enhancing region and a central hypodense area suggestive of necrosis or cystic formation

Question 6

Which of the following statements regarding the management of severe hypertension (BP greater than or equal to 170 mmHg systolic or 110 mmHg diastolic) in pregnancy is/are correct?

(a) Management can be safely undertaken as an outpatient using oral antihypertensive agents.

(b) This level of hypertension is diagnostic of pre-eclampsia.

(c) If confirmed, overnight rest in bed is an acceptable management strategy.

(d) Severe hypertension is most likely to be due to an underlying secondary cause.

(e) None of the above.

Answer

E

Explanation

Severe hypertension should be considered an emergency and managed in hospital using parenteral agents (answer A incorrect). At this level of BP, there is an increased risk of acute maternal compromise, specifically cerebral haemorrhage and placental abruption. Severe hypertension may occur with gestational hypertension (i.e. non-proteinuric hypertension) or with proteinuric pre-eclampsia but it is not a diagnostic criterion for pre-eclampsia (answer B incorrect). Nevertheless, it indicates a severe form of gestational hypertension at least, and 25% of women with gestational hypertension will subsequently develop pre-eclampsia.

For the reasons above, answer C is incorrect. When using parenteral agents to control hypertension, continuous monitoring of fetal heart rate is indicated, and the authors also use plasma expansion of 500 mL/4 hrs (which equates approximately to the estimated intravascular deficit in pre-eclampsia). In the second half of pregnancy, it is more common for a woman to develop severe hypertension as a consequence of gestational hypertension or pre-eclampsia than from an underlying secondary cause.

 Clinical pearls

- Control of hypertension during pregnancy reduces maternal risk of serious intracerebral bleeding.
- When BP cannot be controlled, delivery should be strongly considered.

Question 7

Appropriate management of proteinuric pre-eclampsia at 33 weeks' gestation includes:
- **(a)** the administration of intramuscular betamethasone to the mother
- **(b)** immediate delivery
- **(c)** bed rest and reduction in sodium intake
- **(d)** assessment of fetal wellbeing
- **(e)** further assessment of maternal wellbeing.

Answer

A, D and E

Explanation

Intramuscular betamethasone reduces the risk of neonatal hyaline membrane disease and is indicated in women where premature delivery is likely to occur, particularly where caesarean section seems likely (answer A correct). Forty-eight hours are generally required to allow the effects of glucocorticoids to be maximised (answer B incorrect). The appropriate management of proteinuric pre-eclampsia is delivery. However, expectant management is appropriate up to 34 weeks gestation to allow fetal maturation (Churchill & Duley 2002). After 37 weeks proteinuric pre-eclampsia should usually be managed by delivery. Between 34 and 37 weeks' gestation expectant management is appropriate, only if maternal and fetal condition is stable and there is ongoing careful attention given to both maternal and fetal wellbeing, usually in hospital.

Reduction in sodium intake has not been shown to be beneficial in pre-eclamptic women (whose intravascular volume may be contracted) (answer C incorrect) (Duley, Henderson & Meher 2005). Antihypertensive agents are useful to control BP and reduce the risk of severe hypertension and its sequelae. Bed rest has not been shown to be of benefit. Answers D and E are correct, focusing on target organ involvement in pre-eclampsia (i.e. central nervous system involvement, liver involvement, coagulation system abnormality and renal function).

 Clinical pearl

- Expectant management of pre-eclampsia should occur in hospital and with careful attention to both fetal and maternal wellbeing.

Question 8

At what stage in pregnancy is it safe to perform a renal angiogram?
- **(a)** After 30 weeks' gestation.
- **(b)** After 20 weeks' gestation.

(c) After 14 weeks' gestation.
(d) It is safe at any time during pregnancy.
(e) None of the above.

Answer

E

Explanation

While there are case reports of successful renal angioplasty during pregnancy, the indications to intervene with radioactive contrast are few, if any (answer E correct). Hypertension can generally be controlled with medication. The effects of the contrast and the ionising radiation diminish as the pregnancy proceeds; however, a procedure such as renal angiogram should never be considered 'safe' in any stage of pregnancy (Lowe 2004).

 Clinical pearl

- Ionising radiation should be avoided during pregnancy.

Question 9

Which of the following statements regarding the diagnosis of renal artery stenosis is/are true?

(a) Doppler examination of the renal arteries offers high sensitivity and specificity.
(b) The diagnostic test of choice is a digital subtraction angiogram of the renal arteries.
(c) CT angiography has replaced angiography as the investigation of choice.
(d) Magnetic resonance imaging (MRI) of the renal arteries is the investigation of choice, particularly in pregnancy.

Answer

B

Explanation

Renal artery Doppler studies are presently characterised by both poor sensitivity and specificity, unless carried out frequently by one operator in a referral unit which does a high volume of such cases. The examination is a particularly difficult study to interpret in the presence of abdominal obesity and pregnancy (answer A incorrect). The gold standard remains digital subtraction angiography of the renal arteries (answer B correct). CT angiography, however, is progressing as a new technique and as the number of 'slices' increases, so does resolution (answer C incorrect). The safety of magnetic resonance imaging in pregnancy at this stage is debated (answer D incorrect).

Clinical pearls

- The digital subtraction angiogram has not yet been surpassed as the investigation of choice for renal artery stenosis.
- The safety of abdominal MRI in pregnancy has not been proven.
- In pregnant women, such investigations can usually be deferred until the post-partum period.

LEVEL C

Case history continued ...

In the early post-partum period, the patient undergoes a laparoscopic resection of an extra adrenal phaeochromocytoma (see Fig. 8.2). All antihypertensive agents are suspended after surgery and at follow-up, a 24-hour ambulatory BP monitoring study average is 101/63 mmHg with 0% systolic and 0% diastolic BP loads. The abnormal renal artery Doppler study initially performed was assumed to be a consequence of the large, vascular phaeochromocytoma adjacent to the right kidney. As the patient was no longer hypertensive, a renal angiogram was not performed.

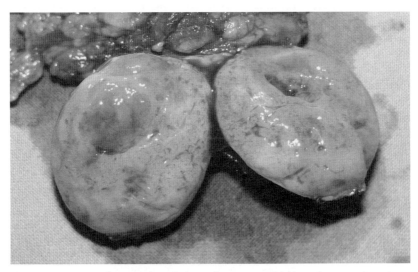

Figure 8.2 Resected extra-adrenal phaeochromocytoma. Note the central cystic structure

Source: We are grateful to Dr Peter Campbell for the photograph of the tumour. Permission was obtained from the patient for publication of this picture.

Question 10

Which of the following statements regarding screening for phaeochromocytoma is/are true?

(a) Fasting plasma metanephrines/normetanephrines are the most useful test presently available for screening.

(b) A CT scan with contrast is a useful screening tool.

(c) Scanning with the radionuclide MIBG is unnecessary and unreliable.

(d) The most appropriate test is 24-hour urinary catecholamine excretion.

Answer

A

Explanation

Fasting plasma free metanephrines carry a high sensitivity (97 to 99%) at the expense of specificity (82%) (Lenders et al. 2002) (answer A correct). False positive tests can occur with certain medications and in non-fasting patients. Twenty-four hour urinary fractionated metanephrines are similarly highly sensitive (96%) but more specific (98%) (Sawka et al. 2003) but require the collection of urine over 24 hours. False positives can be excluded by following up fasting plasma free metanephrine studies with 24-hour urinary fraction-ated metanephrines. The appropriate screening test may be dictated by local availability. A rare disease requires a screening test with high sensitivity, hence plasma catecholamines (sensitivity 69 to 92%), urinary catecholamines (sensitivity 79 to 91%), urinary total metanephrines (sensitivity 60 to 88%) and urinary VMA (sensitivity 46 to 77%) are less useful tests for screening (Lenders et al. 2002) (answer D incorrect). CT scanning is useful after bio-chemical tests are suggestive, not beforehand, because small adrenal nodules (so called incidentalomas) are common (answer B incorrect). Intravenous contrast should be avoided in patients with suspected phaeochromocytoma. The administration of radionuclide MIBG is useful to exclude multiple lesions in a patient suspected of having phaeochromocytoma with positive screening study (answer C incorrect).

 Clinical pearls

- The screening test for phaeochromocytoma will depend on local availability.
- Generally, patients find a blood sample easier than a 24-hour urine collection.

Question 11

Which of the following statements about a patient with phaeochromocytoma is/are true?
(a) It is unlikely to be a familial condition.
(b) It is prudent to screen for multiple endocrine neoplasia (MEN) syndromes.
(c) The patient is cured of her condition.
(d) The patient should be followed up because of the risk of malignancy/or recurrence.

Answer
A, B and D

Explanation

Most phaeochromocytomas are sporadic (answer A correct), though familial phaeochromocytomas are more common than previously thought, with germ line mutations present in about 25% of patients with apparently sporadic tumours (Neumann et al. 2002). It is appropriate to screen for the multiple endocrine neoplasia (MEN) syndromes by measuring calcitonin (for MEN 2A and B) and parathyroid hormone (PTH) (for MEN2A) (answer B correct). Familial Von-Hippel Lindau Syndrome can cause phaeochromocytomas (and can be screened for by determining the presence of the VHL polymorphism). The succinate dehydrogenase subunits B and D predispose carriers to phaeochromocytomas, and screening for these polymorphisms will probably become increasingly important. Recurrence rate at 5 years is about 10%, so a cure cannot be claimed until considerable disease-free follow-up has been achieved. Malignancy is not always apparent histologically, further emphasising the importance of long-term follow-up (answer D correct).

 Clinical pearl

- Familial genetic disorders causing phaeochromocytoma are more common than previously thought, accounting for about 25% of tumours.

Question 12

The pre-operative management of phaeochromocytoma includes:
(a) restricting fluid in view of the risk of pulmonary oedema
(b) alpha-blockade
(c) beta-blockade alone
(d) none of the above.

Answer
B

Explanation

Affected patients are usually volume-contracted and have reduced sympathetic responses, and hence are prone to hypotension and shock during surgery. Haematocrit may be elevated. Volume expansion is required pre-operatively, often 3 to 5 L of saline to lower haematocrit (answer A incorrect). Alpha-blockade should be initiated once the diagnosis is established; phenoxybenzamine provides long lasting alpha-blockade (answer B correct). Selective alpha-1 agonists are useful during the work-up phase in a patient suspected of phaeochromocytoma. Beta-blockade should only be initiated once alpha-blockade is complete in view of the paradoxical increase in BP which may occur due to antagonism of beta-mediated skeletal muscle vasodilatation (answer C incorrect).

 Clinical pearl

- Patients must be adequately alpha- and beta-blocked prior to surgery for phaeochromocytoma.

Question 13

Which of the following statements about the long-term outcome for women with proteinuric pre-eclampsia is/are true?

(a) Pre-eclampsia is a condition confined to pregnancy and confers no long-term cardiovascular risk.
(b) The development of pre-eclampsia is associated with increased future risk for cardiovascular disease.
(c) The risk factors for cardiovascular disease (hypertension, obesity, dyslipidaemia) are also risk factors for the development of pre-eclampsia.
(d) Women who have had pre-eclampsia should be managed with lifelong antihypertensive medication.

Answer

B and C

Explanation

Evidence is accumulating for worse long-term cardiovascular outcomes in women who have had a hypertensive disorder of pregnancy, both gestational hypertension and pre-eclampsia, compared with those who have had previous normal pregnancies (answer A incorrect). Pregnancy can therefore be considered a 'stress test' for future cardiovascular disease. Whether the pre-eclamptic pregnancy actually increases the risk, or whether women who develop hypertension in pregnancy are at increased risk for cardiovascular disease because of existing risk factors has not yet been clarified (Mangos 2006) (answer B correct). It is now well known that the risk factors for cardiovascular disease later in life are the same as those predisposing to pre-eclampsia (obesity, family history, diabetes, dyslipidaemia) (answer C correct). Accumulating evidence favours the hypothesis that women who develop hypertension in pregnancy have existing risk factors for future cardiovascular disease, but the development of pre-eclampsia remains an excellent 'alerting' condition for future cardiovascular events. Almost all women who have developed *de novo* hypertension during pregnancy will have normal BP by 3 months post-partum. Hence life-long antihypertensive medication is not usually required (answer D incorrect). These women should be counselled about their potential future cardiovascular risk and the importance of healthy eating, physical activity, smoking cessation, weight control and moderation of alcohol intake.

Clinical pearls

- Women with a previous hypertensive disorder of pregnancy are at higher risk of future cardiovascular disease.
- It is prudent to advise such women on the benefits of a healthy lifestyle.

Bibliography

Level A

1. Duley, L., Henderson-Smart, D.J., Knight, M. & King, J.F. (2003) Antiplatelet agents for preventing pre-eclampsia and its complications. Cochrane Database Syst Rev. 4.
2. Steyn, D.W. & Odendaal, H.J. (1997) Randomised controlled trial of ketanserin and aspirin in prevention of pre-eclampsia. Lancet. Nov. 1, 350 (9087), 1267–71.
3. Bayliss, H., Churchill, D., Beevers, M., Beevers, D.G. (2002) Anti-hypertensive drugs in pregnancy and fetal growth: evidence for 'pharmacological programming' in the first trimester? Hypertens Pregnancy. 21(2), 16–74.
4. Cooper, W.O., Hernandez-Diaz, S., Arbogast, P.G., Dudley, J.A., Dyer, S., Gideon, P.S., Hall, K. & Ray, W.A. (2006) Major congenital malformations after first-trimester exposure to ACE inhibitors. N Engl J Med. 354(23), 2443–51.
5. Brown, M.A., Lindheimer, M.D., De Swiet, M., Van Assche, A. & Moutquin, J.M. (2001) The classification and diagnosis of the hypertensive disorders of pregnancy: statement from the International Society for the Study of Hypertension in Pregnancy (ISSHP). Hypertens Pregnancy. 20(1), IX–XIV.

Level B

6. Churchill, D. & Duley, L. (2002) Interventionist versus expectant care for severe pre-eclampsia before term. Cochrane Database Syst Rev. 3.
7. Duley, L., Henderson, S.D., Meher, S. (2005) Altered dietary salt for preventing pre-eclampsia, and its complications. Cochrane Database Syst Rev. 4.
8. Lowe, S.A. (2004) Diagnostic radiography in pregnancy: risks and reality. Aust N Z J Obstet Gynaecol. 44(3), June, 1991–6.

Level C

9. Lenders, J.W., Pacak, K., Walther, M.M., Linehan, W.M., Mannelli, M., Friberg, P., Keiser, H.R., Goldstein, D.S. & Eisenhofer, G. (2002) Biochemical diagnosis of pheochromocytoma: which test is best? JAMA. 287(11), 1427–34.

10. Sawka, A.M., Jaeschke, R., Singh, R.J. & Young, W.F. Jr. (2003) A comparison of biochemical tests for pheochromocytoma: measurement of fractionated plasma metanephrines compared with the combination of 24-hour urinary metanephrines and catecholamines. J Clin Endocrinol Metab. 88(2), 553–8.

11. Neumann, H.P.H., Bausch, B., McWhinney, S.R., Bender, B.U., Gimm, O., Franke, G., Schipper J, Klisch J, Altehoefer, C., Zerres, K., Januszewicz, A., Eng, C., Smith, W.M., Munk, R., Manz, T., Glaesker, S., Apel, T.W., Treier, M., Reineke, M., Walz, M.K., Hoang-Vu, C., Brauckhoff, M., Klein-Franke, A., Klose, P., Schmidt, H., Maier-Woelfle, M., Peçzkowska, M. & Szmigielski, C.; Freiburg-Warsaw-Columbus Pheochromocytoma Study Group. (2002) Germ-Line Mutations in Nonsyndromic Pheochromocytoma. N Engl J Med. 346(19), 1459–66.

12. Mangos, G.J. (2006) Cardiovascular disease following pre-eclampsia: understanding the mechanisms. J Hypertens. 24(4), 639–41.

Case 9
Proteinuria

CAROL POLLOCK

Case history

A 58-year-old Caucasian female presents for a routine cervical Pap smear. She has a long history of mild well-controlled asthma, but no known additional medical problems and is symptomatically well. Her last medical review was two years earlier when she had previously presented for her cervical Pap smear, which was normal. Her blood pressure (BP) was checked at the time and found to be 135/90 mmHg. No urine analysis was undertaken. On this occasion her BP is 150/95 mmHg and her urine analysis demonstrates blood 3+ and protein 2+.

LEVEL A

Question 1

The most appropriate way to determine the degree of proteinuria is the following:
(a) Urinary albumin/creatinine ratio
(b) Urinary protein concentration
(c) Urinary protein/creatinine ratio
(d) Urinary electrophoresis (urinary EPG)
(e) Serum albumin and serum cholesterol

Answer
C

Explanation

Urinary albumin/creatinine ratio is measured in the assessment for microalbuminuria. It is not generally done in the setting where macroproteinuria is present (i.e. when there is protein 2+ on urine analysis). Microalbuminuria is assessed in patients with diabetes mellitus where it is an early marker of nephropathy and increasingly in patients who are considered to have a high risk of vascular pathology. The presence of any degree of proteinuria (including microalbuminuria) is considered a significant risk factor for vascular disease. The urinary protein concentration will vary depending on the urinary volume. A 24-hour urine collection is the most accurate way to determine urinary protein excretion.

However, because of inaccuracies in collection and the inconvenience, the urinary protein/creatinine ratio is the most clinically useful method to determine and monitor urinary protein excretion. Variations in the concentration of the urine can be accounted for by determining the ratio. Urinary EPG (and generally an immunoelectrophoretogram) is done in patients in whom a paraprotein is considered to account for the proteinuria. Although light chains can be quantified by this method, it is not accepted as a method to quantify proteinuria. Serum albumin is low and cholesterol elevated in patients with nephrotic syndrome, but their measurement does not reflect the degree of proteinuria.

Question 2

Given the following possibilities, which is the most likely diagnosis?
- **(a)** Urinary tract infection
- **(b)** IgA nephropathy
- **(c)** Focal sclerosing glomerulonephritis
- **(d)** Reflux nephropathy
- **(e)** Renal artery stenosis

Answer
B

Explanation

IgA nephropathy is the most likely diagnosis. The presence of haematuria, proteinuria and hypertension is suggestive of a glomerular abnormality. A urinary tract infection is more likely to be symptomatic and unlikely to be associated with hypertension unless concurrent renal parenchymal pathology exists. Focal sclerosing glomerulonephritis is less likely to have haematuria as a prominent feature. Renal artery stenosis is unlikely to cause haematuria and only results in proteinuria if longstanding and severe and complicated by secondary focal sclerosis (due to ischaemia).

Question 3

The presence of proteinuria increases the risk of:
- **(a)** progressive renal failure
- **(b)** tubulointerstitial disease
- **(c)** myocardial infarction
- **(d)** progressive osteoporosis
- **(e)** a familial form of glomerulonephritis.

Answer
A, B and C

Explanation

The presence and degree of proteinuria are well known to correlate with progressive renal disease in both diabetic and non-diabetic renal disease. Reducing proteinuria, predominantly achieved by blockade of the renin-angiotensin system, has been shown to slow the progression of renal disease. An increase in filtered proteins increases tubulointerstitial disease as when the renal tubules are exposed to albumin, an enhanced expression of fibrogenic and inflammatory cytokines (including transforming growth factor $\beta 1$, monocyte chemattractant protein, tumour necrosis factor and interleukin-8). Population-based studies, as well as studies in patients with hypertension and/or diabetes mellitus, have demonstrated the increased cardiovascular risk in patients with any degree of proteinuria. Although proteinuria is associated with increased excretion of Vitamin D-binding protein, osteoporosis is described more when corticosteroids are used to treat various types of glomerular disease. Although proteinuria can occur in familial forms of nephritis, its presence in an individual does not increase the likelihood of this diagnosis.

Question 4

Relevant laboratory tests, in addition to an estimation of urinary protein excretion, include:

(a) serum IgA level
(b) urinary electrolytes
(d) serum urea, electrolytes and creatinine
(e) serum complement levels
(f) urine microscopy.

Answer
C and E

Explanation

Urine microscopy confirms the presence of glomerular pathology by demonstrating cast formation. The presence of red cell casts would suggest active glomerular pathology. Granular casts are likely to be present in both active and more quiescent phases of the disease. Urinary electrolytes are not of value in the evaluation of glomerular disease. They are more likely to be of value in the presence of primary electrolyte or acid–base disturbances. An assessment of renal function and detection of any serum electrolyte abnormality is required if glomerular pathology is suspected. An elevation in serum IgA may be seen in up to half of the patients with IgA nephropathy, but it has no diagnostic or prognostic value. Serum complement levels are normal in patients with IgA nephropathy and hence are not measured.

Case history continued ...

Initial investigations yield the following results.

Haemoglobin	131 g/L	(115–145g/L)
White cell count	4.2 × 10⁹/L	(4–11 × 10⁹/L)
Platelets	238 × 10⁹/L	(150–400)
Sodium	138 mmol/L	(136–146)
Potassium	4.2 mmol/L	(3.5–5.5)
Urea	6.1 mmol/L	(3.5–7.5)
Creatinine	82 µmol/l (resulting in an estimated glomerular filtration rate of 90 mL/min/1.73m²)	(40–120)
Serum cholesterol	5.6 mmol/L	
Urinary protein excretion	900 mg/24 hours.	

Question 5

Which one of the following investigations should be undertaken next?
(a) Renal ultrasound
(b) Multislice computerised tomography (CT) scan
(c) MAG-3 Renal scan
(d) Duplex scanning of the renal vessels
(e) Renal biopsy

Answer

A

Explanation

Delineation of the renal anatomy is required in patients presenting with glomerular pathology, particularly if a renal biopsy is to be subsequently considered. An ultrasound provides sufficient information with minimal radiation exposure. Increased echogenicity of the cortex and lack of definition of the corticomedullary junction is suggestive of more severe glomerular pathology. A CT scan is not routinely indicated in glomerular disease. A MAG-3 renal scan is primarily used to assess differential function, with patterns of renal blood flow and excretion of the tracer also providing information on renal artery stenosis and ureteric obstruction. This test is unlikely to be useful in glomerular disease. Duplex scanning of arteries is undertaken to look for renal artery stenosis and of veins for venous occlusion, hence not indicated. A renal biopsy should not be undertaken prior to imaging of the kidneys. In the presence of relatively preserved renal function and less than

1 g proteinuria per day, many clinicians would adopt a 'wait and watch' approach rather than confirming the diagnosis with renal biopsy.

Question 6

Treatment options include which of the following?

(a) Prednisone at 1 mg/kg/day
(b) Aspirin 100 mg/day
(c) Fish oil 3 g/day
(d) Angiotensin-converting enzyme (ACE) inhibitor or angiotensin receptor blocker
(e) Vitamin E

Answer

D

Explanation

Antihypertensive treatment is indicated and in the presence of glomerular disease an agent that interrupts the renin-angiotensin system is appropriate. The target BP is in the order of 120/75 mmHg. At present the data are more persuasive for ACE inhibitors (ACEi) than for angiotensin receptor blockers (ARB). If the urinary protein was greater than 1 g per day that would also be an indication for the use of these agents, independent of the BP, because of their antiproteinuric and renoprotective properties. Steroids, aspirin, fish oil and antioxidants have not been shown to be beneficial.

LEVEL B

Case history continued ...

She was commenced on perindopril at 4 mg/day and returns in 6 months for review. Her BP is 130/90 mmHg. Her results show the following:

Proteinuria	2.3 g	
Na^+	138 mmol/L	(136–146)
K^+	4.9 mmol/L	(3.5–5.5)
Creatinine	150 µmol/L with eGFR 42 mL/min/1.73m²	(40–120)
Total cholesterol	6.1 mmol/L	(3.9–5.5)
LDL cholesterol	4.1 mmol/L	

The dose of perindopril had been increased to 8 mg per day some 8 weeks ago by her general practitioner because of inadequate BP control at the time.

Question 7

Further investigations at this time should include:

(a) renal biopsy
(b) CT scan to exclude renal vein thrombosis
(c) 24-hour BP monitor
(d) cardiac echo
(e) plasma renin and aldosterone.

Answer

A

Explanation

The renal function has significantly declined in a relatively short period of time and histological assessment is required to guide management and determine prognosis. The other tests listed have no specific relevance to this case.

Question 8

Based on evidence, treatment should now include:

(a) a calcium channel blocker
(b) a diuretic
(c) cyclosporin A
(d) a statin
(e) an angiotensin receptor blocker.

Answer

E

Explanation

The renal function is deteriorating, proteinuria is increasing and the BP is not optimal. Hence additional treatment is warranted. The COOPERATE study demonstrated a benefit of the combination of ACEi and ARB in slowing progression of renal failure. The main problem with the combination is hyperkalaemia, but with a baseline potassium of 4.9 mmol/L, the addition of an ARB would not be contraindicated. Serum potassium should be measured serially in a patient with renal impairment on the combination of ACEi and ARB. Other forms of BP control and treatment directed to cholesterol lowering have not been uniformly shown to be effective in reducing morbidity.

The patient enquires as to the genetic implications of the diagnosis IgA nephropathy.

Question 9

Which of the following statements is/are true?
- **(a)** Fertility is impaired when the serum creatinine is greater than 150 μmol/L.
- **(b)** Transplanted kidneys derived from living related donors are more likely to develop IgA nephropathy.
- **(c)** Prenatal genetic testing for IgA nephropathy is available to detect affected fetuses.
- **(d)** Treatment with blockade of the renin-angiotensin system is more beneficial in patients with the DD genotype.
- **(e)** Familial IgA nephropathy is likely to be less severe in successive generations.

Answer

A

Explanation

An increase in serum creatinine above 150 μmol/L is associated with impaired fertility, independent of the cause. Recurrence of IgA deposits may occur in renal grafts of recipients whose primary diagnosis was IgA nephropathy. Many genetic polymorphisms have been associated with the development or progression of IgA nephropathy, but the associations are weak and of uncertain significance. Initial studies suggested a difference in the responsiveness of patients with a DD versus II genotype. However, these differences have not been substantiated. A small number of patients have a form of familial IgA nephropathy which is more likely to be associated with renal failure, but there is no evidence for successive generations to have more severe disease.

LEVEL C

Question 10

Tubular reabsorption of albumin:
- **(a)** occurs in both proximal and distal tubules
- **(b)** largely occurs via paracellular transport
- **(c)** largely occurs via receptor mediated endocytosis
- **(d)** is inhibited by statin therapy
- **(e)** is reduced in glomerular disease.

Answer

C and D

Explanation

Tubular reabsorption of albumin occurs primarily in the early segments of the proximal tubule through receptor-mediated endocytosis. The best described endocytic receptors are megalin and cubulin. Although a paracellular pathway has been proposed, it is generally considered that tight junctions prevent paracellular transport of most proteins. The endocytosis of the megalin–albumin or cubulin–albumin complex requires signalling by prenylated G-proteins. As prenylation of proteins may be inhibited by statins, tubular protein reabsorption may be limited by statins. The more potent statins such as rosuvastatin are more likely to cause tubular proteinuria, but this has not been associated with increased renal dysfunction. Tubular reabsorption of albumin is increased when there is increased filtration of proteins.

Case history continued ...

A renal biopsy is planned for one month later, now some 7 months after initial presentation. Her BP is now 180/100 mmHg and her serum creatinine is now 260 μmol/L with 3.32 g urinary protein per day. Renal biopsy shows 50% of glomeruli affected by segmental cellular crescents with vascular thickening, approximately 20% of tubules atrophic and extracellular matrix replacing approximately 30% of the tubulointerstitium.

Question 11

Which of the following statements is/are true?

(a) Immunosuppression is likely to be of short-term benefit.
(b) Dihydropyridine antihypertensives should be avoided.
(c) Plasma exchange is of demonstrated benefit in the presence of crescentic IgA nephropathy and should be instituted.
(d) Anticoagulation with heparin or clexane should be instituted within 24 hours of renal biopsy.
(e) A vasculitic screen should be undertaken as a superimposed vasculitic renal disease is likely.

Answer

A

Explanation

Immunosuppression in IgA nephropathy is still hotly debated. It is generally agreed that in the presence of vasculitic disease, immunosuppression is likely to be of at least short-term benefit. The long-term efficacy is unknown. Control of BP is paramount and in the presence of concurrent agents that block the reticular activating system (RAS), treatment with a dihydropyridine Ca channel blocker is appropriate to reduce BP. Plasma exchange is not indicated and a vasculitic screen is unlikely to yield additional pathology.

Question 12

The pathogenesis and progression of IgA nephropathy has been linked to:

(a) aberrant O-linked galactosylation of the IgA hinge region

(b) the lack of a tonsillectomy as a child

(c) the absence of CD10 positive podocytes

(d) an aggressive exercise regimen

(e) platelet-derived growth factor stimulating glomerular proliferation.

Answer

A, C and E

Explanation

Both the presence of abnormally galactosylated IgA1 and the size of the polymeric IgA1 influence binding in the glomeruli. The tonsils are an important source of hypogalactosylated IgA1. However, tonsillectomy has not been shown to alter the disease progression. Podocyte abnormalities are prominent in progressive disease and have been demonstrated pathogenetically to link to the progression of IgA nephropathy. Exercise was originally considered to worsen progression of IgA nephropathy, but more recent data suggest this is not the case. Proliferative components of IgA nephropathy has been linked to synthesis of platelet-derived growth factor (PDGF) isoforms, and inhibition of the PDGF–PDGF-receptor interaction has been shown to slow the progression of IgA nephropathy.

Bibliography

Level A

1. Barratt, J. & Feehally, J. (2006) Treatment of IgA nephropathy. Kidney Int. 69, 1934–8.
2. Barratt, J. & Feehally, J. (2005) IgA nephropathy. J Am Soc Nephrol. 16, 2088–97.
3. D'Amico, G. & Bazzi, C. (2003) Pathophysiology of proteinuria. Kidney Int. 63, 809–25.
4. Lambers Heerspink, H.J., Brinkman, J.W., Bakker, S.J., Gansevoort, R.T. & de Zeeuw, D. (2006) Update on microalbuminuria as a biomarker in renal and cardiovascular disease. Curr Opin Nephrol Hypertens. Nov.; 15(6), 631–6.
5. Chiurchiu C., Remuzzi G. & Ruggenenti P. (2005) Angiotensin-converting enzyme inhibition and renal protection in nondiabetic patients: the data of the meta-analyses. J Am Soc Nephrol. Mar.; 16, supplement 1, S58–63.
6. de Zeeuw, D., Remuzzi, G., Parving, H.H., Keane, W.F., Zhang, Z., Shahinfar, S., Snapinn, S., Cooper, M.E., Mitch, W.E. & Brenner, B.M. (2004) Proteinuria, a target for renoprotection in patients with type 2 diabetic nephropathy: lessons from RENAAL. Kidney Int. June; 65(6), 2309–20.

Level B

7. Barratt, J., Feehally, J. & Smith, A.C. (2004) Pathogenesis of IgA nephropathy. Semin Nephrol. 24, 197–217.
8. Locatelli, F., Vecchio, L.D. & Pozzi, C. (2006) IgA glomerulonephritis: beyond angiotensin converting enzyme inhibitors. Nat Clin Pract Nephrol. 2, 24–31.
9. Wakai, K., Kawamura, T., Endoh, M., Kojima, M., Tomino, Y., Tamakoshi, A., Ohno, Y., Inaba, Y. & Sakai, H. (2006) A scoring system to predict renal outcomes in IgA nephropathy from a nationwide prospective study. Nephrol Dial Transplant. 10, 2800–8.

Level C

10. Coppo, R. & Amore, A. (2004) Aberrant glycosylation in IgA nephropathy. Kidney Int. 65, 1544–7.
11. Moura, I.C., Arcos-Fajardo, M., Sadaka, C., Leroy, V., Benhamou, M., Novak, J., Vrtovsnik, F. Haddad, E., Chintalacharuvu, K.R. & Monteiro, R.C. (2004) Glycosylation and size of IgA1 are essential for interaction with mesangial transferrin receptor in IgA nephropathy. J Am Soc Nephrol. 15, 622–34.
12. Horie, A., Hiki, Y., Odani, H., Yasuda, Y., Takahashi, M., Kato, M., Iwase, H., Kobayashi, Y., Nakashima, I. & Maeda, K. (2003) IgA1 molecules produced by tonsillar lymphocytes are under-O-glycoslyated in IgA nephropathy. Am J Kidney Dis. Sept.; 42(3), 486–96.
13. Floege, J. (2006) Is mycophenolate mofetil an effective treatment for persistent proteinuria in patients with IgA nephropathy? Nat Clin Pract Nephrol. 2, 16–17.
14. Chihara Y., Ono, H., Ishimitsu, T., Ono, Y., Ishikawa, K., Rakugi, H., Ogihara, T. & Matsuoka, H. (2006) Roles of TGFB1 and apoptosis in the progression of glomerulosclerosis in Human IgA nephropathy. Clin Nephrol. 65, 385–92.
15. Birn, H. & Christensen, E. (2006) Renal albumin absorption in physiology and pathology. Kidney Int. 69, 440–9.
16. Tonelli, M. (2006) Do statins protect the kidney by reducing proteinuria? Ann Intern Med. 145, 147–9.

Case 10
Oedema and nephrotic syndrome

VINCENT LEE

A 50-year-old woman presents to her general practitioner with a 1-month history of bilateral leg oedema. On examination she has pitting oedema in both legs extending up to the knees. Her blood pressure (BP) is 110/70, her pulse rate is 70 beats/min and regular, her temperature is 36.5°C, and her peripheries well perfused. On examination of her chest, the apex beat is not displaced and is normal in character; there are no abnormal heaves and there are dual normal heart sounds with no added murmurs. The jugular venous pressure is not elevated. Abdominal examination is normal. Her urinalysis is positive for protein (4+) but negative for blood.

LEVEL A

Question 1

What pathophysiological factors are likely to contribute to this woman's oedema?
- **(a)** Decreased intravascular oncotic pressure
- **(b)** Increased capillary permeability
- **(c)** Increased venous hydrostatic pressure
- **(d)** Increased arterial hydrostatic pressure
- **(e)** Increased renal salt and water retention

Answer
A and E

Explanation

Oedema is the swelling of an organ or tissues due to an increase in interstitial fluid. The presence of oedema in the dependent peripheries, associated with proteinuria in a euvolaemic individual suggests that the woman has nephrotic syndrome. In nephrotic syndrome, oedema is caused by an imbalance in Starling forces at the capillary–interstitial compartment interface (see Table 10.1) as well as a total body increase in sodium and water due to renal reabsorption (answer E correct). This woman is likely to have hypoalbuminaemia due to abnormal urinary protein losses, leading to decreased intravascular oncotic pressure (answer A correct). This woman does not have symptoms or signs consistent with right heart failure (jugular venous pressure not elevated and cardiac examination normal) or lymphoedema (which causes non-pitting oedema) (answer C incorrect), sepsis (which would cause fever, tachycardia and cold peripheries) (answer B incorrect) or significant arterial hypertension (answer D incorrect).

Table 10.1 Common causes of peripheral oedema

Pathophysiology	Clinical manifestation
• Decreased oncotic pressure	• Hypoalbuminaemia — Cirrhosis — Nephrotic syndrome — Malnutrition — Systemic illness
• Increased venous hydrostatic pressure	• Right heart failure • Venous thrombosis or obstruction
• Decreased lymphatic flow leading to increased interstitial pressure	• Lymphatic obstruction — Idiopathic — Cancer • Parasitic
• Increased arterial hydrostatic pressure	• Severe arterial hypertension
• Increased capillary permeability	• Sepsis • Burns • Allergy
• Increased salt retention	• Kidney disease • Cirrhosis

Question 2

Which of the following is/are likely to be found in this woman?
(a) Hypoalbuminaemia
(b) Hypercholesterolaemia
(c) Red cell casts
(d) Oval fat bodies in the urine

Answer
A, B and D

Explanation

Given the history of heavy proteinuria and oedema, nephrotic syndrome is the most likely diagnosis in this woman. Hypoalbuminaemia is definitive of and hyperlipidaemia is commonly associated with the nephrotic syndrome (answers A and B correct). It must be pointed out that some patients with 'nephrotic range' proteinuria in fact have 'normal' levels of serum albumin. In nephrotic syndrome, levels of low-density lipoprotein (LDL) cholesterol and occasionally triglycerides are markedly elevated. Hypercholesterolaemia and hypertriglyceridaemia are due to diminished catabolism of LDL cholesterol and triglycerides respectively. Additionally, there is enhanced liver production of triglycerides due to stimulation of hepatocytes by decreased oncotic pressure. In contrast, the nephritic syndrome is a constellation of oedema, proteinuria (usually not in the nephrotic range), glomerular haematuria (with red cell casts), reduced glomerular filtration rate and hypertension. Red cell casts are unlikely to be found in this woman because her urinalysis is negative for blood (answer C incorrect) and her BP is normal. Oval fat bodies are cells with birefringent fat droplets within their cytoplasm which typically creates a Maltese cross appearance, and is usually found when the urine is rich in lipid such as in nephrotic syndrome (answer D correct).

Clinical pearl

- Nephrotic syndrome is defined by the presence of heavy proteinuria, oedema and hypoalbuminaemia, and is frequently accompanied by hyperlipidaemia.

Question 3

Which of the following are possible causes of this clinical presentation?
(a) Minimal change glomerulopathy
(b) Focal segmental glomerulosclerosis
(c) Penicillamine
(d) Anti-glomerular basement membrane (anti-GBM) disease
(e) Membranous glomerulonephritis

Answer
A, B, C and E

Explanation

There are many causes of nephrotic syndrome, including certain types of glomerulonephritis (GN), amyloidosis, type 2 diabetes, drugs (see Table 10.2) and infections (HIV and hepatitis B and C). To narrow the differential diagnosis, one must consider the age of the patient. Older patients such as this woman (over the age of 40) are likely to have focal segmental glomerulosclerosis (FSGS), membranous glomerulonephritis, diabetic nephropathy, IgA nephropathy, drug-induced glomerulonephritis (see Table 10.2) or amyloidosis (answers B, C and E correct). While this woman is not known to be diabetic, type 2 diabetes is often undiagnosed until end-organ damage has already occurred. Children (under the age of 15) are most likely to have minimal change glomerulopathy. Although less common, adults over the age of 40 may develop minimal change glomerulopathy (answer A correct). Individuals aged between 15 and 40 are likely to have

FSGS, minimal change glomerulopathy and membranous glomerulonephritis. Anti-GBM disease (including Goodpasture's disease) is associated with rapidly progressive GN, with haematuria, proteinuria and acute renal failure (answer D incorrect).

 Clinical pearl

• Nephrotic syndrome has many causes, the most common of which are primary GN and diabetes. Narrowing the differential diagnosis involves consideration of the individual's background medical history and age.

Table 10.2 Some drugs that can cause nephrotic syndrome, listed by the type of GN most commonly associated

Type of glomerulonephritis (GN)	Drugs that can cause GN
Membranous GN	Antirheumatic agents: penicillamine, gold Non-steroidal anti-inflammatory drugs: diclofenac Anticytokine agents: infliximab High dose captopril Tiopronin (used for treating cystinuria) Sirolimus
Minimal change GN	Non-steroidal anti-inflammatory drugs Gold Lithium Tiopronin Pamidronate
Focal segmental glomerulosclerosis	Heroin Lithium

Source: Rose 2006

Question 4

Which of the following investigations may be useful in diagnosing the cause of this woman's disease?
(a) Spot urine protein/creatinine ratio
(b) Antinuclear antibody
(c) Hepatitis B and C serology
(d) Serum and urine electrophoresis

Answer
B, C and D

Explanation

The first aim in investigation of the nephrotic syndrome is to identify any associated systemic diseases such as systemic lupus erythematosus (SLE) (over 90% of SLE patients are positive for antinuclear antibody), diabetes mellitus, hepatitis B and C, myeloma and amyloidosis (usually characterised by serum and urine paraproteinaemia) (answers B, C and D correct). A spot urine protein/creatinine ratio is useful in quantifying proteinuria and as a baseline to monitor therapy, but by itself is not helpful in diagnosis (answer A incorrect). A spot urine protein/creatinine ratio estimation gives a reliable estimate of proteinuria without the inaccuracies associated with a 24-hour urine collection for proteinuria. The urinary creatinine is important to correct for total urinary concentration.

Recommendations such as the Caring for Australasians with Renal Impairment (CARI) guidelines in fact suggest the use of timed collections when significant proteinuria is present. A protein/creatinine ratio (or albumin/creatinine ratio) may help in determining the significance of small amounts of dipstick proteinuria but may be highly variable in the setting of large amounts as is often present in the nephrotic syndrome.

 Clinical pearls

- Initial serological testing in cases of nephrotic syndrome should be directed at the common causes (e.g. antinuclear antibody is present in the majority of patients with lupus nephritis).
- Urine protein/creatinine ratio is easier to obtain than a 24-hour urine protein for quantitating proteinuria.

Question 5

Which of the following are likely to be beneficial in treating this patient?
(a) Angiotensin converting enzyme (ACE) inhibitor
(b) 3-hydroxy-3-methylglutaryl coenzyme A reductase inhibitor (HMG-CoA reductase inhibitor or 'statin')
(c) Protein restriction to less than 0.7 g/kg body weight/day
(d) Frusemide

Answer
A, B and D

Explanation

There is convincing evidence that pharmacological blockade of the renin–angiotensin–aldosterone system, either with ACE inhibition and/or angiotensin receptor blockade, is indicated in all patients with diabetic and non-diabetic chronic kidney disease, and that the benefit in reducing progression of disease is greatest in those individuals with heavy proteinuria (answer A correct). HMG-CoA reductase inhibitors are beneficial in lowering both LDL cholesterol and triglyceride levels in individuals with nephrotic syndrome. There are limited data that suggest that statins may possibly also reduce progression of kidney disease by ameliorating glomerular injury (answer B correct). This woman is at high risk of vascular disease due to her age and her heavy proteinuria. However, while statins confer protection against vascular disease in the general population, it is uncertain if this is also the case in patients with nephrotic syndrome or chronic kidney disease in general. Protein restriction to 0.7 g/kg of body weight/ day has been shown to reduce progression of chronic kidney disease (Klahr et al. 1994). However, restricting protein intake in this woman who is already losing heavy amounts of protein through her urine may lead to protein caloric malnutrition. According to current Australasian (CARI) guidelines, patients with chronic kidney disease should have a minimum protein intake of 1.0 g/kg of body weight/day. Nephrotic individuals should have at least this amount of dietary protein intake (answer C incorrect). Diuretics are useful in treating the symptoms of leg oedema (answer D correct).

Clinical pearl

- Inhibitors of the renin–angiotensin–aldosterone axis and cholesterol-lowering drugs form the cornerstones of therapy for all causes of nephrotic syndrome.

LEVEL B

Case history continued ...

This 50-year-old woman who is otherwise well has nephrotic syndrome. The following investigations are performed:

- Serum creatinine 70 µmol/L (50–110)
- Fasting blood glucose 5.0 mmol/L (3.6–6.0)
- Antinuclear antibody negative
- No evidence of serum or urinary paraprotein
- Hepatitis B, C and HIV serology negative
- Twenty-four-hour urine protein 7.9 grams
- Urine microscopy: granular casts, no red cell casts, no white cells.

Question 6

A renal biopsy is performed on the patient. Which one of the following is the most likely pathological diagnosis?

(a) Thin membrane nephropathy
(b) Membranous GN
(c) Minimal change nephropathy
(d) IgA nephropathy

Answer

B

Explanation

Membranous GN (or membranous nephropathy, MN) is the most common primary renal cause of nephrotic syndrome in adults (Rivera, Lopez-Gomez & Perez-Garcia 2004) (answer B correct), closely followed by FSGS and membranoproliferative GN. Minimal change nephropathy is the most common cause of nephrotic syndrome in children (90% of children under 10 years of age and over 50% of older children) but is less frequent in adults (10 to 15%) (answer C incorrect). IgA nephropathy usually presents with haematuria and proteinuria but may occasionally present with acute nephritis or nephrotic syndrome (answer D incorrect). Individuals with 'thin membrane nephropathy' present with asymptomatic haematuria with normal renal function and no significant proteinuria. Electron microscopy of renal biopsies of these patients shows thinner than normal glomerular basement membranes (answer A incorrect).

 Clinical pearl

- Membranous GN is the most common cause of primary renal disease causing nephrotic syndrome in adults.

Question 7

This patient was found to have membranous glomerulonephritis on renal biopsy. What condition/s may be associated with her condition?

(a) Renal vein thrombosis
(b) Malignancy
(c) Cirrhosis
(d) Cryoglobulinaemia
(e) Elevated lipoprotein (a) levels

Answer

A, B and E

Explanation

Membranous nephropathy is associated with an increased risk of venous and arterial thrombosis (answer A correct). Proposed mechanisms include alterations in endogenous anticoagulants such as protein C, protein S and antithrombin 3 (increased urinary loss, increased catabolism or decreased functionally active protein), enhanced platelet reactivity and increased whole blood viscosity. About 10% of middle- to older-aged people with membranous nephropathy will have an underlying malignancy. Careful but limited screening of common cancers (such as breast cancer in women, prostate cancer in men, lung cancer in both), or other cancers as suggested by symptoms and signs, is indicated for this patient (answer B correct). Screening tests that are definitely indicated in this woman include mammography, cervical examination and smear, and testing for faecal occult blood. In men, cirrhosis is most commonly associated with IgA nephropathy (answer C incorrect). Cryoglobulinaemia is associated with membranoproliferative GN (answer D incorrect). As with other causes of nephrotic syndrome, membranous nephropathy is associated with elevated LDL, lipoprotein (a) and triglyceride levels (answer E correct), as well as normal to low HDL levels.

 Clinical pearls

- Membranous GN may be associated with malignancy.
- Nephrosis may be associated with thrombosis.

Question 8

Which of the following would be associated with a worse prognosis in this patient (assuming the disease is idiopathic)?
(a) Variable proteinuria between 4 and 7 g/24 hours
(b) Presence of moderate interstitial fibrosis at the time of biopsy
(c) Reduced glomerular filtration rate
(d) Development of hypertension on follow-up

Answer
B, C and D

Explanation

Indicators of a poor prognosis in membranous nephropathy are male gender, older age (over 60 years), heavy proteinuria (particularly persistent proteinuria over 8 g/day for longer than 6 months) (answer A incorrect), reduced or declining glomerular filtration rate (answer C correct), presence of hypertension (the patient's BP was 110/70 mmHg) (answer D incorrect), tubulointerstitial fibrosis (answer B correct) and crescents on renal biopsy.

Clinical pearl

- As with most types of GN, the predictors of prognosis are the extent of functional and histopathological (especially tubulointerstitial) renal damage and the presence/absence of hypertension.

Question 9

This 50-year-old woman with nephrotic syndrome is likely, based on clinical presentation, to have membranous nephropathy. What histological features are likely to be present on renal biopsy in this woman?

(a) Increased mesangial cellularity

(b) Electron dense deposits within the subepithelial space across the glomerular basement membrane ('spikes')

(c) 'Hump-shaped' subepithelial electron dense deposits on top of the glomerular basement membrane

(d) Thinned basement membrane

(e) Lymphocyte and eosinophil infiltration within the tubulointerstitium

Answer

B

Explanation

Membranous nephropathy is characterised on light microscopy by thickened glomerular capillary loops. Glomerular cellularity is normal. In the early stages of disease, light microscopy shows diffuse thickening of the glomerular capillaries with 'spikes'—these represent projections of glomerular basement membrane interspersed between deposits of immune complex formation in the basement membrane (answer B correct). With advanced disease, these GBM projections completely surround the immune deposits. In membranous nephropathy, immunofluorescence staining demonstrates granular IgG and complement C3 staining along the capillary walls. The presence of IgM, IgA, C1q and C4 is less common, and if present suggests that the membranous nephropathy is due to SLE (so-called type V lupus nephritis). Electron microscopy reveals electron-dense deposits along the glomerular basement membrane in the subepithelial space, along with localised podocyte foot process effacement (in contrast to subepithelial deposits with a 'hump' appearance typical of post-infectious glomerulonephritis—answer C incorrect).

In individuals with early disease, glomeruli may appear normal and the only changes of membranous nephropathy are seen on immunofluorescence and electron microscopy. An increase in mesangial cellularity is not usually found in membranous nephropathy (a notable exception is membranous nephropathy due to systemic disease such as SLE or hepatitis B) but is typically found in cases of IgA nephropathy (answer A incorrect). Eosinophilic infiltration is not seen in individuals with membranous glomerulonephritis but has been reported in some with superimposed interstitial nephritis due to celecoxib (answer E incorrect). Leukocyte infiltration is a common accompaniment of tubulointerstitial injury associated with progression of most types of kidney disease. The presence of tubulointerstitial or vascular injury signifies a poorer prognosis. Basement membrane thinning is found in thin basement membrane disease (answer D incorrect).

 Clinical pearls

- Differentiation of membranous nephropathy from other types of glomerulonephritis can be difficult. In early disease, glomeruli appear normal and the light microscopic appearance is indistinguishable from that of minimal change nephropathy (MCD), whereas immunofluorescence shows granular IgG and C3 staining (opposed to no or minimal staining in MCD) and EM shows subepithelial immune deposits (compared with podocyte foot process effacement in MCD).
- In intermediate stages of membranous nephropathy are seen the typical changes on LM of thickened glomerular capillary loops.
- In advanced stages of membranous nephropathy the glomerular capillary loops are sclerosed and difficult to distinguish from those of other causes of glomerulosclerosis such as FSGS.

LEVEL C

Question 10

Which of the following are possible factors in the pathogenesis of this woman's disease?

(a) Anti-neutral endopeptidase
(b) Complement regulatory proteins
(c) C5b-9 membrane attack complex
(d) IgM

Answer

A, B and C

Explanation

Membranous nephropathy is characterised by glomerular basement membrane thickening with little or no cellular proliferation or infiltration. Electron microscopy shows immune complex deposition within the basement membrane. It is thought that this disease arises by the development of circulating antibodies against glomerular self-antigens. Much of what we know today of the pathophysiology of membranous nephropathy comes from studies using a rat model of membranous nephropathy called Heymann nephritis. In this model, an antibody against a tissue antigen fraction derived from proximal tubular brush border (anti-Fx1A) is administered directly ('passive model') or induced by immunisation with Fx1A ('active model'), and leads to the development of subepithelial glomerular deposits closely resembling human membranous nephropathy. The nature of the putative antigen against which the antibody was directed was identified as a combination of megalin and a receptor-associated protein known as the Heymann nephritis antigenic complex, a protein found on the rat podocyte membrane and tubular brush border. However, the Heymann nephritis antigenic complex is not found constitutively in human glomerular podocytes (Ronco & Debiec 2006). In 2002, Debiec and colleagues described the presence of circulating antibodies against neutral endopeptidase as the cause of a case of antenatal membranous nephropathy (answer A correct) (Debiec et al. 2002). This discovery may, in the near future, lead to identification of the causative antibody or antibodies in adult membranous nephropathy (Couser 2005).

Studies in Heymann nephritis have helped unravel the mechanisms of renal injury induced in membranous nephropathy. In this disease, the autoantibodies formed are IgG—the type of IgG is predominantly IgG1 and 2 in malignancy-associated MN, and IgG 2 and 3 in lupus-associated MN (answer D incorrect). *In situ* formation of immune deposits in the glomerular subepithelial space produces glomerular injury by damaging and/or activating podocytes through complement-dependent processes. C5b-9 formation and insertion into podocyte cell membranes causes glomerular injury in MN (answer C correct) (Nangaku, Shankland & Couser 2005). Defending the podocytes against complement and antibody-mediated attack are cell surface bound complement regulatory proteins (CRP). The role of CRP in membranous nephropathy was demonstrated when the antibody used to induce proteinuria in Heymann nephritis was found to contain antibodies against a CRP called Crry—when this antibody was depleted, anti-Fx1A was no longer able to induce proteinuria (answer B correct) (Schiller et al. 1998).

 Clinical pearl

- The cause of membranous nephropathy is at present unknown. However, work using the Heymann nephritis model, along with the discovery of neutral endopeptidase as a causative antigen in antenatal membranous nephropathy, may eventually lead to precise identification of the pathogenic antibody or antibodies in adult-onset membranous nephropathy and thus a specific treatment for this condition.

Question 11

The patient's renal biopsy shows thickened glomerular capillary loops, with silver stain positive for spike formation. There is minimal interstitial fibrosis and tubular atrophy. Immunofluorescence shows granular linear staining within glomeruli that is strong for IgG and weak for C3. Which of the following therapeutic regimens has been shown to increase renal survival?

(a) Cytotoxic agent and steroids
(b) Cyclosporin alone
(c) Steroids alone
(d) Mycophenolate alone

Answer

A

Explanation

The decision of whether or not to use immunosuppressive agents in the treatment of membranous nephropathy is highly controversial. A recent meta-analysis (Schieppati et al. 2004) found that there was no strong evidence that adults with nephrotic syndrome have a long-term benefit from treatment with immunosuppressive agents. However, selected patients at high risk of developing end-stage renal failure may benefit from immunosuppressive agents.

Ponticelli et al. (1995) performed a ten-year follow-up of eighty-one patients with idiopathic membranous nephropathy and nephrotic syndrome who received a 6-month course of alternating cycles of chlorambucil and prednisone. He found that the group on chlorambucil and prednisone had significantly greater renal survival than the control (no immunosuppression) group (92% versus 60%). However, the same group (Ponticelli et al. 1998) compared a regimen of 6 months of alternate monthly cycles of steroids combined with either oral chlorambucil or oral cyclophosphamide. After at least 1 year of follow-up, there were equivalent rates of remission (83% versus 92%) but significantly more side effects in the chlorambucil group. However, this regimen is not widely used. Therapies with single agents such as cyclosporin, steroids and mycophenolate have all been shown to induce remission (i.e. reduction of proteinuria) but have not been demonstrated to improve renal survival (answers B, C and D incorrect). In contrast, the combination of cyclosporin and prednisone may improve renal survival. Several groups advocate the use of immunosuppressive agents (especially cyclophosphamide, which is better tolerated than chlorambucil) in selected patients with a high risk of progression to end-stage renal failure (answer A correct).

Clinical pearl

- The choice of treatment of membranous nephropathy is highly controversial. A combination of cytotoxic agent and steroids has been shown to improve renal survival compared to steroids or no immunosuppressive agents, but is associated with toxic side effects.

Question 12

Treatment is commenced with an ACE inhibitor, HMG-CoA reductase inhibitor and advice on salt restriction. You see her 6 months later. In which of the following scenarios should you commence immunosuppressive therapy?

(a) Serum creatinine 70 μmol/L, BP 110/70 mmHG, proteinuria 2 g/day
(b) Serum creatinine 70 μmol/L, BP 160/90 mmHG, proteinuria 6 g/day
(c) Serum creatinine 140 μmol/L, BP 110/70 mmHg, proteinuria 10 g/day
(d) Serum creatinine 140 μmol/L, BP 160/90 mmHg, proteinuria 10 g/day

Answer

C

Explanation

The natural history of membranous nephropathy is difficult to define (Cattran 2005). Earlier studies were performed prior to the current (and mandated) use of antihypertensive agents (in particular, antagonists of the renin–angiotensin–aldosterone axis) and lipid-lowering therapy. Up to 30% of patients will undergo spontaneous remission. Predicting which patients will progress (and therefore require early intervention) is one of the dilemmas of treatment of membranous nephropathy. Up to 20% of patients with membranous nephropathy will have an underlying secondary cause such as neoplasia, infection, SLE or drug therapy. Treatment of the underlying disease may induce renal remission and should be tried first along with other supportive therapy. In any case, immunosuppression may worsen underlying malignancy or infection.

The majority of cases of membranous nephropathy have no known cause (idiopathic). These patients can be classified based on their clinical characteristics over a 6-month observation period: low, medium and high risk. Low-risk patients (such as in scenario A) have normal renal function and proteinuria <4 g/day, have less than a 5% risk of progression over 5 years of observation and should be treated conservatively (answer A incorrect). Medium-risk patients are defined as those with normal renal function and medium-range persistent proteinuria (4 to 8 g/day) despite optimum BP control. The patients in scenarios B and D need to have their BP optimised by maximising the dose of ACE inhibitor and angiotensin receptor blocker, and the addition of other antihypertensive agents as necessary (answers B and D incorrect).

If she has persistent proteinuria despite optimum BP control, then the choice of therapy for this patient is debatable. Immunosuppression—either cyclophosphamide and steroids, or cyclosporine and steroids—has been shown to induce remission (i.e. reduce proteinuria to non-nephrotic levels) and prolong renal survival. Steroids alone are not effective at prolonging renal survival. However, side-effects are substantial (66%) and relapse rate is high (30%). Many physicians elect to carefully monitor these patients, as a large proportion of them will spontaneously improve (Schieppati et al. 1993). High-risk patients have deteriorating renal function and/or persistent high-grade proteinuria >8 g/day despite optimum supportive therapy, and should be treated with immunosuppression (answer C correct). This approach has been validated prospectively (Cattran et al. 1997). Current guidelines (Canada, Australia) agree that immunosuppression is indicated in poor-prognosis individuals such as in scenario C.

Two other points are worth mentioning. First, if a patient develops rapidly worsening renal function (such as in scenario C), it is important to consider complications such as renal vein thrombosis, interstitial nephritis or superimposed crescentic glomerulonephritis. Second, treatment of relapsed patients is, at present, not evidence-based as there are no randomised controlled trials addressing this question.

 Clinical pearls

- Of patients with membranous nephropathy, those with the worst prognosis (declining renal function and persistent proteinuria over a 6-month observation period) are likely to benefit the most from immunosuppressive therapy.
- Patients with normal renal function and non-nephrotic range proteinuria should not receive immunosuppression.
- Individuals that fall between these two extremes should be watched carefully and immunosuppressive therapy instituted if proteinuria or renal function worsens despite optimum supportive therapy.

Bibliography

Level A
1. Rose, B.D. (2006) Causes of membranous nephropathy. UpToDate, Rose, B.D. (ed.). Waltham, MA: UpToDate.

2. Klahr, S., Levey, A.S., Beck, G.J., Caggiula, A.W., Hunsicker, L., Kusek, J.W. & Striker, G. (1994) The effects of dietary protein restriction and blood-pressure control on the progression of chronic renal disease. Modification of Diet in Renal Disease Study Group. N Engl J Med. 330, 877–84.

Level B

3. Rivera, F., Lopez-Gomez, J.M. & Perez-Garcia, R. (2004) Clinicopathologic correlations of renal pathology in Spain. Kidney Int. 66, 898–904.

Level C

4. Ronco, P. & Debiec, H. (2006) Molecular dissection of target antigens and nephritogenic antibodies in membranous nephropathy: towards epitope-driven therapies. J Am Soc Nephrol. 17, 1772–4.
5. Debiec, H., Guigonis, V., Mougenot B., Decobert, F., Haymann, J.P., Bensman, A., Deschênes, G. & Ronco, P.M. (2002) Antenatal membranous glomerulonephritis due to anti-neutral endopeptidase antibodies. N Engl J Med. 346, 2053–60.
6. Couser, W.G. (2005) Membranous nephropathy: a long road but well traveled. J Am Soc Nephrol. 16, 1184–7.
7. Nangaku, M., Shankland, S.J., Couser, W.G. (2005) Cellular response to injury in membranous nephropathy. J Am Soc Nephrol. 16, 1195–204.
8. Schiller, B., He, C., Salant, D.J., Lim, A., Alexander, J.J. & Quigg, R.J. (1998) Inhibition of complement regulation is key to the pathogenesis of active Heymann nephritis. J Exp Med. 188, 1353–8.
9. Schieppati, A., Perna, A., Zamora, J., Giuliano, G.A., Braun, N. & Remuzzi, G. (2004) Immunosuppressive treatment for idiopathic membranous nephropathy in adults with nephrotic syndrome. Cochrane Database Syst Rev.
10. Ponticelli, C., Zucchelli, P., Passerini, P., Cesana, B., Locatelli, F., Pasquali, S., Sasdelli, M., Redaelli, B., Grassi, C., Pozzi, C., Bizzarri, D. & Banfi, G. (1995) A 10-year follow-up of a randomized study with methylprednisolone and chlorambucil in membranous nephropathy. Kidney Int. 48, 1600–4.
11. Ponticelli, C., Altieri, P., Scolari, F., Passerini, P., Roccatello, D., Cesana, B., Melis, P., Valzorio, B., Sasdelli, M., Pasquali, S., Pozzi, C., Piccoli, G., Lupo, A., Segagni, S., Antonucci, F., Dugo, M., Minari, M., Scalia, A., Pedrini, L., Pisano, G., Grassi, C., Farina M. & Bellazzi, R. (1998) A randomized study comparing methylprednisolone plus chlorambucil versus methylprednisolone plus cyclophosphamide in idiopathic membranous nephropathy. J Am Soc Nephrol. 9, 444–50.
12. Cattran, D. (2005) Management of membranous nephropathy: when and what for treatment. J Am Soc Nephrol. 16, 1188–94.
13. Schieppati, A., Mosconi, L., Perna, A., Mecca, G., Bertani, T., Garattini, S. & Remuzzi, G. (1993) Prognosis of untreated patients with idiopathic membranous nephropathy. N Engl J Med. 329, 85–9.
14. Cattran, D.C., Pei, Y., Greenwood, C.M., Ponticelli, C., Passerini, P. & Honkanen, E. (1997) Validation of a predictive model of idiopathic membranous nephropathy: its clinical and research implications. Kidney Int. 51, 901–7.

Case 11
Progressive chronic renal disease

ROB MACGINLEY

LEVEL A

Case history

A 50-year-old male with type 2 diabetes mellitus for 5 years is referred for renal assessment as his general practitioner is concerned that he may have developed kidney disease. Initially his diabetes was difficult to control with oral medications alone for a period of a few years but recently he has had good control with a combination of long- and short-acting insulin. He monitors his own blood glucose levels with good pre-meal values of 5 to 7 mmol/L and '2 hrs post-prandial' glucose concentrations of less than 10 mmol/L. His most recent HbA_{1c} values vary between 6.5 and 7.5%. He denies any symptoms of peripheral neuropathy and has not required any laser therapy for retinopathy. He has hypertension that is difficult to control and the presence of albuminuria.

Question 1

In large epidemiological surveys for diabetes and chronic kidney disease, which of the following statements is/are correct?

(a) About 1 in 20 people have abnormalities on urinalysis.
(b) About 8% of the general population have evidence of diabetes mellitus.
(c) About 1 in 10 type-2 diabetics have evidence of diabetic nephropathy.
(d) Those with diabetes are at risk of end-stage kidney failure.

Answer
B and D

Explanation

AusDiab, a recent large community screening study of a representative sample of the general population, demonstrated the prevalence of chronic kidney disease (CKD) to be in as high as one in seven individuals. CKD was defined by the presence of blood or protein on urinalysis, and/or a serum creatinine >150 µmol/L. The same study showed that approximately 8% of those surveyed were diabetic (of whom half were unaware of the diagnosis) and 30% were hypertensive (again, half of these were not known previously to be hypertensive).

Type-2 diabetics have a significant chance of developing diabetic nephropathy, with one in three patients developing evidence of kidney disease during their lifetime. Diabetic nephropathy is now the most common cause of end-stage kidney failure in both developed and developing nations. There is a disproportionately high incidence of diabetic nephropathy in indigenous populations around the world.

Risk factors for CKD include hypertension, diabetes, family history of kidney disease, age (more than 50 to 60 years), ethnicity (Aboriginal and Torres Strait Islanders [ATSI]), smoking and obesity.

 Clinical pearls

- CKD is common, with a prevalence as high as one in seven of the general population in Australia.
- Diabetes is now the major cause of end-stage kidney disease in developed and developing countries.
- Risk factors for CKD include hypertension, diabetes, family history of kidney disease, age (>50 to 60 years), ethnicity (ATSI), smoking and obesity.

Question 2

Which one of the following is the most appropriate investigation when screening for CKD (including diabetic nephropathy)?

(a) Twenty-four hour urinary protein excretion
(b) Twenty-four hour urinary albumin excretion
(c) Urinary protein/creatinine ratio on a spot or timed urine sample
(d) Urinary albumin/creatinine ratio on a spot or timed urine sample
(e) Midstream urine with dipstick urinalysis, spot urinary albumin/creatinine ratio, microscopy and (if appropriate) culture

Answer
E

Explanation

Guidelines from Caring for Australasians with Renal Impairment (CARI) and Kidney Health Australia's Kidney Check Australia Taskforce (KCAT) have reviewed existing evidence for the role of urine tests in screening for renal disease. The ideal screening is a combination of a midstream urine (MSU) and spot urine protein/creatinine ratio, blood pressure (BP) and serum creatinine, from which the glomerular filtration rate (GFR) is estimated (eGFR), on a yearly basis in high-risk groups. In the higher risk groups of diabetics and ATSIs, albumin/creatinine ratio may be preferable as it allows earlier detection and treatment of nephropathy. The MSU should be done to exclude infection and to quantify, and if possible characterise, urinary red blood cells. In an asymptomatic patient it is arguably not worthwhile to perform an MSU solely to exclude infection as a cause of proteinuria. (See Case 5 for a more detailed discussion of haematuria.) The use of a single dipstick analysis for either proteinuria or albuminuria alone is associated with an at least 10% false positive rate and 10% false negative rate. However, the reliability of dipstick analysis is substantially greater with repeat testing. A 24-hour urine collection is less favoured for screening as it is inconvenient and may be unreliable due to inaccurate timing.

 Clinical pearls

- A single urine dipstick analysis for protein has limitations as the sole method of screening for CKD due to its false positive and negative rate.
- Kidney function should be measured at least yearly in those at increased risk of CKD.
- Screening should include measurement of BP, serum creatinine assay (and from that eGFR) and an MSU for dipstick urinalysis, microscopy and a protein/creatinine ratio (probably albumin/creatinine ratio in diabetics and ATSIs).

Question 3

Which of the following is/are true statements concerning tests for assessing CKD?

(a) Serum creatinine is an accurate measure of renal function and if <120 µmol/L excludes nephropathy.

(b) GFR estimated from a formula (such as MDRD) is an accurate measure of renal function.

(c) A deterioration in eGFR (estimated GFR) of more than 15% over a period of months is a sign of acute renal failure.

(d) An eGFR of more than 20 mL/min/1.73m² excludes clinically relevant renal disease.

Answer

B

Explanation

Serum creatinine may not be above the normal reference range until over 50% of GFR is lost. Serum creatinine is also dependent on age, weight, gender and muscle mass. People who are small (low muscle mass), elderly or female (or the combination of all three), may have significant renal impairment despite a serum creatinine within the normal reference range. GFR can be assessed by creatinine clearance derived from a timed (usually 24 hours) urinary collection. GFR also can be estimated from serum creatinine from formulae such as the Modification of Diet in Renal Disease (MDRD) equations. To increase the identification of individuals with CKD, eGFR (based on a modified version of the MDRD formula) is now reported universally in Australia along with serum creatinine. eGFR falls detectably over hours to days or weeks with acute renal failure, and over weeks to months or even years with CKD.

eGFR is also used to stage CKD which provides a useful guide to its expected clinical manifestations (see Table 11.1).

Table 11.1 Classification of chronic kidney disease

Stage	GFR mL/min/ 1.73m²	Expected clinical manifestations [+]
1. Normal GFR	>90*	None, or of the primary disease process
2. Early	60–89*	None; hyperparathyroidism, increased risk of cardiovascular disease
3. Moderate	30–59	Nocturia, abnormal extracellular fluid volume, anaemia, raised serum creatinine level, low 1,25-dihydroxycholecalciferol level, dyslipidaemia
4. Severe	15–29	Uraemic symptoms, abnormalities of serum electrolyte levels
5. End-stage kidney disease	<15	Severe uraemic symptoms, dialysis

Notes: * associated with urinary abnormalities, + plus manifestations of earlier stages of CKD

 Clinical pearls

- eGFR is useful (in conjunction with assessment of BP and urinalysis) as a screening tool for CKD.
- eGFR is also used to stage CKD, which provides a useful guide to expected clinical manifestations.

LEVEL B

Case history continued ...

Over the next 12 months the patient's renal disease progresses, with serum creatinine rising to 312 μmol/l (see Table 11.2). Risk factors for cardiovascular disease remain poorly controlled despite the commencement of appropriate therapy. Systolic BP is persistently 145 to 155 mmHg in the setting of four-drug therapy—an angiotensin-converting enzyme inhibitor (ACEi), calcium channel blocker, beta-blocker and frusemide. He is hyperlipidaemic despite simvastatin (40 mg) with recent total cholesterol of 5.8 mmol/L. His urine protein excretion rate increases from 475 mg to 800 mg/24 hours, despite the use of an ACEi.

Table 11.2 Serial blood tests in this patient

	Feb 2006	June 2006	Oct 2006	Jan 2007	May 2007
K⁺ mmol/L	5.2	5.4	5.6	5.8	5.9
Creatinine μmol/L	137	170	220	290	312
Urea mmol/L	12	16	23	27	29
Haemoglobin g/L	130	117	112	107	103

Question 4

In slowing the progression of renal disease and avoiding the development of malnutrition in CKD patients with an eGFR 15 to 30 mL/min/1.73 m^2, which of the following statements is/are correct?

(a) Nephrotic patients need a high-protein diet.

(b) Reducing proteinuria to less than 1 g/24 hrs is associated with a reduction in rate of decline of renal function.

(c) Proteinuria is a good measure of renal dysfunction.

(d) Heavy proteinuria (>3 g/24 hrs) predicts the response to ACEi.

Answer

B and D

Explanation

Multiple randomised controlled trials (RCTs), as well as a meta-analysis of these RCTs, have not demonstrated convincingly that protein restriction slows the rate of decline in GFR of CKD patients to a clinically useful degree. Because of this, and the risk of malnutrition associated with excessive dietary restriction, current Australasian guidelines (CARI) have advised against excessive protein restriction for slowing renal functional decline. Conversely, the use of high-protein diets in patients with severe proteinuria (a state of high malnutrition risk) does little to correct the malnourished state and potentially could accelerate the decline in renal function.

Control of BP alone can significantly reduce proteinuria. However, greater reductions of proteinuria can be achieved with certain antihypertensives, including ACEi, angiotensin receptor blockers (ARB) and aldosterone antagonists, especially when used in combination. This antiproteinuric effect is to some extent independent of the antihypertensive effect of these agents. The Ramipril in non-diabetic renal failure (REIN) study (Ruggenenti, Perna & Remuzzi 1997) demonstrated that the greater the level of proteinuria, the greater the impact of ACEi in preventing decline in renal function in patients with CKD. Moreover, the protective effect was greatest in those with the largest reduction in proteinuria.

 Clinical pearls

- Low-protein diets may slow the progression of renal dysfunction in CKD, but only to a small extent and at the risk of malnutrition.
- High-protein diets are not effective in treating the malnutrition associated with the nephrotic syndrome and may accelerate the rate of decline of renal function.
- Lowering BP reduces proteinuria.
- The degree of preservation of renal function achieved with antihypertensive agents may be directly proportional to the reduction of proteinuria.
- ACEi and/or ARB appear to slow renal functional decline to an extent greater than is explained by their antihypertensive effect alone.

Question 5

When an individual with type-2 diabetes mellitus is assessed for diabetic nephropathy, which of the following statements is/are correct?

(a) The absence of proteinuria excludes diabetic nephropathy.

(b) Hypertension usually indicates the presence of concomitant macrovascular (e.g. renal arterial) disease.

(c) The severity of diabetic nephropathy is related to the severity of hypertension.

(d) The absence of diabetic retinopathy excludes diabetic nephropathy.

(e) Kimmelstiel-Wilson lesions must be present to diagnose diabetic nephropathy.

Answer

B and C

Explanation

Up to one-third of the type 2 diabetic individuals with a creatinine >150 μmol/L in the NHANES III survey had no evidence of proteinuria. This is because nephropathy of type 2 diabetics may be characterised more by a vasculopathy (particularly microvascular) than by the classic histological changes of glomerular basement membrane thickening and mesangial expansion. The vasculopathy is almost invariably associated with hypertension and may not be associated with proteinuria. As with the classic diabetic histologic features, this vasculopathy leads to progressive renal function decline which may be accelerated by poor diabetic control and poor BP control. The classic histological changes are accompanied by proteinuria, and in a minority may progress to nodular Kimmelstiel-Wilson lesions. Although commonly found together, not all patients with diabetic nephropathy have concomitant diabetic retinopathy.

If hypertension is resistant to therapy, then the possibility of renal arterial stenosis needs to be considered. (See Case 14 for a discussion of renal arterial disease.)

Clinical pearls

- Not all type-2 diabetics with reduced kidney function have proteinuria.
- Hypertension is common in diabetic nephropathy and may be associated with worse renal functional impairment.
- Consider renal artery stenosis (macrovascular disease) as a cause of difficult-to-control hypertension in patients with diabetes.
- Diabetic retinopathy and nephropathy are commonly but not invariably found together.

Question 6

Which of the following statements is/are true regarding treatment aimed at slowing the progression of CKD and at preventing cardiovascular events such as myocardial infarction and cerebrovascular accidents?

(a) The target BP to slow progression of renal functional decline in CKD is ≤ 140/90 mmHg.

(b) Of antihypertensive agents, only ACEi and ARB slow progression of CKD.

(c) In large studies, ACEi have been demonstrated to improve overall survival in diabetics with large and small vessel vasculopathy.

(d) The presence of renovascular disease is a contraindication to the use of ACEi and/or ARB.

Answer

C

Explanation

To slow the progression of non-diabetic kidney disease, recent studies have demonstrated that the target BP should be ≤130/80 mmHg. In diabetic and non-diabetic kidney disease with proteinuria greater than 1 g/24 hours (and in the absence of contraindications such as critical arterial stenosis) target BP is ≤120/75 mmHg, especially in younger patients.

BP reduction alone, irrespective of the agent used, is successful in slowing the progression of CKD. However, of the various antihypertensive classes, ACEi and ARB have the greatest efficacy in slowing the progression of renal disease.

Large secondary prevention studies (HOPE and PROGRESS) have shown that ACE inhibition in high-risk populations reduces the risk of cardiovascular events.

The presence of atherosclerotic renovascular disease with evidence of renal artery stenosis is not an absolute contraindication to the use of ACEi or ARB. However, caution and close monitoring is required to ensure that possible associated acute increases in serum creatinine and potassium are small and not sustained.

Clinical pearls

- Target BPs to slow the progression of non-diabetic CKD:
  — If proteinuria < 1 g/24 hr, target BP ≤ 130/80 mmHg.
  — If proteinuria ≥ 1 g/24 hr, target BP ≤ 120/75 mmHg.
- For diabetic CKD, target BP is ≤ 120/75 mmHg, especially in younger patients.
- ACEi and ARB are the preferred antihypertensive agents in the setting of CKD. However, effective BP control regardless of the agent used is of paramount importance.
- Atherosclerotic vascular disease is not an absolute contraindication to the use of ACEi or ARB.

Question 7

In general, which of the following results in someone of this patient's age (50 years) indicate the need for referral to a nephrologist?

(a) A diabetic with eGFR <60 mL/min/1.73 m² and poorly controlled hypertension.

(b) A non-diabetic with an eGFR 30 to 60 mL/min/1.73 m², proteinuria <0.5 g/d, controlled BP.

(c) Proteinuria >1 g/24 hours with normal eGFR.

(d) Unexplained decline in kidney function (>15% drop in GFR over 3 months).

Answer

A, C and D

Explanation

Because late referral to a nephrologist has been shown to be accompanied by greater impact of associated morbidity, both for those approaching the need for renal replacement therapy and for those receiving conservative care, recommendations have been developed for specialist referral. These guidelines are somewhat controversial and the decision to refer should always be individualised. A period of observation before referral is frequently useful. Patient age is an important consideration; it may not be appropriate to refer an elderly patient even with moderate or severe CKD, whereas in younger patients the threshold for referral should be lower.

In general, stable patients with eGFR >30 mL/min/1.73 m² do not require referral. However, a significant proportion of the patients with diabetes may benefit from early referral (e.g. eGFR <60 mL/min/1.73m²) to allow earlier and more aggressive intervention to slow the progression of their CKD, timely management of the secondary complications of their renal failure including disordered mineral metabolism and anaemia and attention to cardiovascular risk reduction. Individuals with non-diabetic stage 3 CKD with controlled BP (<130/80 mmHg) and controlled proteinuria on ACEi/ARB in general do not require referral. They require 3- to 6-monthly monitoring by their general practitioner and referral if treatment targets (cardiovascular risk, BP, proteinuria) are not met or if there is a significant decline in renal function.

Individuals with unexplained proteinuria >1 g/24 hours on a timed urine collection usually need referral to a nephrologist to establish a renal diagnosis. They will usually require a renal biopsy. Similarly, patients with unexplained rapid deterioration of renal function (>15% reduction in eGFR over weeks to months) need referral to a nephrologist for diagnosis and management.

 Clinical pearl

- Indications of referral to a nephrologist include:
  — proteinuria >1 g/24 hours
  — eGFR <30 mL/min/1.73m² in non-diabetics
  — eGFR <60 mL/min/1.73m² in diabetics
  — unexplained decline in kidney function (>15% drop in eGFR over weeks to months)
  — glomerular haematuria with proteinuria
  — CKD with difficult-to-control hypertension
  — otherwise unexplained anaemia (<100 g/L) with eGFR <60 mL/min/1.73 m².

Question 8

The patient's haemoglobin level fell further to 90 g/L, and treatment with erythropoietin was commenced. With respect to the investigation of iron stores and haemoglobin levels in the management of renal anaemia, which of the following statements is/are correct?

(a) The most common cause for anaemia in a CKD patient with eGFR <60 mL/min/1.73 m^2 is bleeding from the upper gastrointestinal tract.

(b) In patients on erythropoietin, iron therapy is not required if serum ferritin is >100 µg/L.

(c) Treating the anaemia of CKD is not required until haemoglobin (Hb) falls below 100 g/L.

(d) Oral iron is usually adequate for correcting anaemia of CKD in patients on erythropoietin.

(e) The anaemia occurs earlier in the course of CKD in diabetic than non-diabetic patients.

Answer

C and E

Explanation

It has long been thought that there is an increased risk of gastrointestinal haemorrhage in CKD patients; however, the literature consists of small contradictory cohort studies without high-level evidence. The anaemia of CKD is due to relative erythropoietin deficiency, becomes manifest during stage 3 disease and tends to be more severe in diabetic than non-diabetic CKD patients.

Prior to the availability of erythropoietin, iron deficiency was not common in the dialysis population because of the widespread use of blood transfusion to treat severe anaemia. With the advent of treatment with recombinant erythropoietin, iron deficiency has become common because of the increased requirements for haemoglobin (Hb) synthesis. In Australia, erythropoietin may be prescribed for patients once their Hb has fallen below 100 g/L, and accepted target levels are in the range of 115 to 120 g/L. Recent large RCTs (CHOIR, CREATE) have demonstrated the possibility of a worse outcome in patients for whom Hb is raised to higher levels than these. Renal anaemia, whether treated with erythropoietin or not, is frequently iron-responsive. Because of impaired gastro-intestinal absorption of iron in the face of increased requirements for iron, patients on erythropoietin frequently need to receive iron parenterally. It is common practice to aim for a serum ferritin of >100 µg/L in patients prior to use of erythropoietin and 200 to 500 µg/L once erythropoietin is started; and transferrin saturation of >20% prior to and 30 to 40% with erythropoietin therapy, to ensure adequate iron stores and optimal response to erythropoietin. Iron deficiency is the commonest cause of hyporesponsiveness to erythropoietin; other causes include infection, recent surgery, severe hyperparathyroidism, vitamin deficiency, aluminium toxicity and other causes of anaemia.

Clinical pearls

- Impaired absorption of oral iron and the increased utilisation of iron with erythropoietin therapy have contributed to the development of iron deficiency as a common occurrence in CKD patients.
- To optimise responsiveness to erythropoietin, commonly accepted target values for ferritin are 200 to 500 µg/L and for transferrin saturation 30 to 40%.

LEVEL C

Case history continued ...

Within a few months the patient's CKD progresses to the point that he needs dialysis. The patient's general practitioner questions whether other therapies may have prevented such a rapid progression to end-stage kidney disease.

Question 9

For which of the following therapies is there Level 1 evidence for efficacy in the CKD population?

(a) Cholesterol lowering with statins both to slow progressive decline of renal function and to reduce the increased cardiovascular risk associated with CKD.

(b) Uric acid reduction to slow progression of CKD.

(c) Exercise and weight loss to improve insulin resistance and slow progression of CKD.

(d) An additive effect of aldosterone blockade to slow progression of CKD in patients treated with ACEi.

(e) An additive effect of ARB to slow progression of CKD in patients treated with ACEi.

Answer

E

Explanation

There is some evidence that the reduction of plasma uric acid, cessation of smoking and weight loss may slow the progression of CKD, but for each the evidence is from small uncontrolled and non-randomised studies and case series.

Post-hoc analyses of the large statin studies identified a small cohort of patients with mild CKD and demonstrated that cholesterol-lowering therapy reduced cardiovascular events and slowed the progression of renal disease.

However, these conclusions need to be viewed with caution, because the numbers were small and there were no patients with stage 4 or 5 CKD included in the analyses. The 4D study failed to demonstrate any benefit of lipid-lowering therapy in a high-risk group of diabetic patients already on haemodialysis, more than 30% of whom had previous cardiovascular events. The results of the SHARP study (Study of Heart And Renal Protection—a randomised placebo-controlled study of simvastatin and ezetimibe in 9000 CKD patients, including 6000 predialysis patients) should be available in 2010. Thus, to date there is no RCT evidence to support the role of lipid-lowering therapy in CKD, either to slow the progression of renal disease or to reduce the risk of cardiovascular events.

The additive effect of ACEi and ARB in reducing proteinuria and slowing the progression of CKD is established (COOPERATE). Although aldosterone antagonists have been shown to add to the antiproteinuric effect of ACEi (probably to a greater extent than ARB), an additive effect on slowing CKD progression is yet to be proven.

 Clinical pearls

- Allopurinol, cessation of smoking, weight loss and exercise may slow the progression of CKD but to date there is no level 1 evidence to support their use.
- The possible beneficial effect of lipid lowering on CKD progression and cardiovascular risk is yet to be proven.
- Both ARB and aldosterone antagonists add to the antiproteinuric effect of ACEi, but to date only ARB have been proven to add to the effect of ACEi in slowing CKD progression.

Question 10

In type 2 diabetes, ACEi or ARB have been shown to slow the development or progression of nephropathy in patients who are:
(a) normoalbuminuric and normotensive
(b) normoalbuminuric and hypertensive
(c) microalbuminuric and hypertensive
(d) macroalbuminuric and hypertensive.

Answer
B, C and D

Explanation

There are now a number of large RCTs which have examined the efficacy of ACEi or ARB at different stages of diabetic renal disease. The Bergamo Nephrologic

Diabetes Complication Trial (BENEDICT study) showed that the ACEi tran-dolapril was able to reduce the risk of microalbuminuria in type 2 diabetics with hypertension but normal urinary albumin excretion. To date, a similar effect for normotensive normoalbuminuric diabetics has not been shown. The Irbesartan Microalbuminuria in Hypertensive Patients with Type 2 Diabetes (IRMA2) trial showed that an ARB could reduce the risk of macroalbuminuria in microalbuminuric, hypertensive patients with early type 2 diabetic renal disease. The Irbesartan Diabetic Nephropathy Trial (IDNT) showed that an ARB reduced the risk of doubling of serum creatinine, end-stage kidney disease or death in type 2 diabetics with hypertension and macroalbuminuria. The Reduction of Endpoints in NIDMM with the AII Antagonist Losartan (RENAAL) study demonstrated a similar result using another ARB.

 Clinical pearl

- ARB or ACEi have been proven in hypertensive type 2 diabetics to slow the development of microalbuminuria, macroalbuminuria, renal impairment and end-stage kidney failure.

Bibliography

Level A

1. Chadban, S.J., Briganti, E.M., Kerr, P.G., Dunstan, D.W., Welborn, T.A., Zimmet, P.Z. & Atkins, R.C. (2003) Prevalence of kidney damage in Australian adults: the AusDiab Kidney Study. J Am Soc Nephrol. 14, S131–8.
2. Caring for Australians with Renal Impairment (CARI) Guidelines. http://www.cari.org.au
3. KCAT online learning modules: http://www.kidney.primed.com.au
4. Caring for Australians with Renal Impairment (CARI) Guidelines. (2004) Urine protein as a diagnostic test: performance characteristics of tests used in the initial evaluation of patients at risk of renal disease. J Nephrology (Carlton). 3, S8–14.

Level B

5. Wolf, G. & Ritz, E. (2005) Combination therapy with ACE inhibitors and angiotensin II receptor blockers to halt the progression of chronic renal disease: pathophysiology and indications. Kidney Int. 67, 799–812.
6. Ruggenenti, P., Perna, A. & Remuzzi, G. on behalf of the GISEN Group. (1997) Ramipril in non-diabetic renal failure (REIN study). Lancet. 350, 736–7.
7. Turner, R., Holman, R., Stratton, I., Cull, C., Frighi, V., Manley, S., Matthews, D., Neil, A., McElroy, H., Kohner, E., Fox, C., Hadden, D. & Wright, D. (1998) Tight blood pressure control and risk of macrovascular and microvascular complications in type 2 diabetes: UKPDS 38. BMJ. 317, 703–13.
8. Estacio, R.O., Jeffers, B.W., Hiatt, W.R. & Biggerstaff, S.L., Gifford, N. & Schrier, R.W. (1998) The effect of Nisoldipine as compared with enalapril on cardiovascular outcomes in patients with non-insulin-dependent diabetes and hypertension. N Engl J Med. 338, 645–52.

Level C

9. Nakao, N., Yoshimura, A., Morita, H., Takada, M., Kayano, T. & Ideura, T. (2003) Combination treatment of angiotensin II receptor blocker and angiotensin-converting-enzyme inhibitor in non-diabetic renal disease (COOPERATE): a randomised controlled trial. Lancet. 361, 117–24.
10. Chrysostomou, A., Pedagogos, E., MacGregor, L. & Becker, G.J. (2006) Double-blind, placebo-controlled study on the effect of the aldosterone receptor antagonist spironolactone in patients who have persistent proteinuria and are on long-term angiotensin-converting enzyme inhibitor therapy, with or without an angiotensin II receptor blocker. J Am Soc Nephrol. 1, 256–62.
11. Mitch, W.E. (2004) Treating diabetic nephropathy—are there only economic issues? N Engl J Med. 351, 1934–6.

Case 12
Cardiovascular mortality

GRAHAME ELDER

Case history

A 67-year-old man is admitted with breathlessness. He has a long history of cigarette consumption, elevated cholesterol and hypertension treated from age 45. Chronic kidney disease (CKD) is presumed due to vascular disease but a renal biopsy has not been performed. Type 2 diabetes developed 5 years before the current admission and he commenced haemodialysis at a satellite dialysis facility 2 years before. He stopped smoking 12 months ago.

He dialyses for 5 hours three times weekly, and this is complicated by interdialytic weight gains of 3 to 4 kg, accompanied by poorly controlled hypertension and symptoms of fluid overload. His 'dry weight' has been progressively reduced and he has seen the dietician for advice on a low-salt diet and 1.2 L daily fluid restriction. However, over the last 3 months recurrent hypotension has complicated dialysis. A dobutamine cardiac echo reported positive for ischaemia and 3 weeks before this admission he developed dyspnoea, pulmonary oedema on chest X-ray and a troponin rise without electrocardiograph (ECG) changes, consistent with a non-ST-elevation myocardial infarction. At coronary angiography the right coronary artery was occluded proximally and after successful angioplasty 2 lesions were stented. The circumflex was diseased but not significantly so and the distal left anterior descending artery was significantly diseased with a long segment of approximately 60% narrowing and a 40% distal lesion.

His medications are irbesartan 75 mg daily, simvastatin 20 mg (commenced 18 months before), modified release gliclazide 30 mg day, aspirin, calcium carbonate 600 mg before each meal and darbepoetin alpha 80 μg intravenously every 2 weeks.

When examined, he is afebrile, with a weight of 89 kg (target post-dialysis 'dry weight' of 85 kg), a body mass index (BMI) of 30 kg/m^2 and waist circumference of 95 cm. His blood pressure (BP) is 165/60 mmHg and there are fine crackles in both mid and lower lung fields with clinical evidence of consolidation at the left base.

The following pre-dialysis blood results are available.

Laboratory data

	Results	Reference range
Haemoglobin	101 g/L	(120–160 g/L)
White cell count	13.0×10^9/L	($4.3–10.8 \times 10^9$/L)
Potassium	5.6 mmol/L	(3.5–5.5)
Calcium corrected for albumin	2.55 mmol/L	(2.10–2.60)
Phosphate	2.2 mmol/L	(0.8–1.4)
Ferritin	480 µg/L	(30–300)
Transferrin saturation (TSAT)	0.12	(0.11–0.45)
Intact parathyroid hormone (iPTH)	39 pmol/L	(1–7)
Glucose	7.5 mmol/L	
Cholesterol	5.7 mmol/L	
Low-density lipoprotein cholesterol (LDL-C)	3.0 mmol/L	
C-reactive protein	15 mg/L	(<10)

LEVEL A

Question 1

Which of the following statements is/are correct regarding dialysis mortality and risk factors?

(a) The annual mortality of patients on dialysis has improved dramatically over the past 15 years.

(b) Annual mortality for younger patients on dialysis is up to 10 times that of an age-matched population.

(c) Compared to patients on dialysis, patients transplanted over age 60 have neither worsened nor improved mortality.

(d) From 2000 to 2005, the reduced percentage of current and former smokers amongst new dialysis patients may reflect public anti-smoking campaigns.

Answer
None are correct

Explanation

The patient falls within the 65 to 84 age range, the most common for patients now commencing dialysis in Australia. According to the latest report from the Australian and New Zealand Dialysis and Transplant registry (ANZDATA), hypertension is considered to be the cause of end-stage kidney disease in 14% of patients commencing dialysis and diabetes the cause in 32%. Cardiovascular disease is often present: at the commencement of dialysis approximately 40% of patients have definite or suspected coronary artery disease, 24% peripheral vascular disease and 20% cerebrovascular disease. Unfortunately in 2005 the percentage who were still smoking (12%) or who were former smokers (41%) had not changed from 2000 (when figures were 11 and 31% respectively). Over that time the number of patients with type 2 diabetes increased from 28 to 38%.

For patients aged 65 to 84 years the annual mortality is 20%. This approaches the general population mortality by age 80, but for this patient at age 67 the mortality is well above the population average as seen in Figure 12.1. Not surprisingly, patients with diabetes have higher mortality rates than those without (16.6 versus 13.5 deaths per 100 patient years). Younger patients on dialysis have an extraordinarily high mortality (up to 100 times that of the background population) so that the mortality rate of a dialysis patient aged 25 is similar to that of a 70-year-old in the general population.

Cardiac events (myocardial infarcts and cardiac arrest) cause most dialysis patient deaths at around 40%, while other vascular causes comprise around 10% of deaths. Even in the age range 25 to 34 years, cardiac events cause from one-third to one-half of all deaths in Australia and New Zealand. Mortality rates for Australia and New Zealand dialysis patients in 2005 were 14.5 and 16.4 per 100 patient years respectively; almost the same as the Australian mortality rate of 15.7 per 100 patient years reported in 1992! This lack of improvement is surprising given the advances in cardiovascular therapies and dialysis technology over the past 15 years and is not fully explained by changed patient demographics. Figure 12.1 also shows that transplantation reduces mortality in *every* age

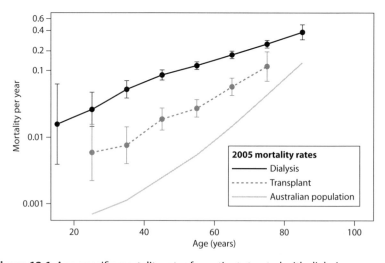

Figure 12.1 Age-specific mortality rates for patients treated with dialysis or transplantation relative to the Australian population 2005

Source: Australian Bureau of Statistics

category. Of course, healthier patients are more likely to be transplanted, but a functioning kidney transplant appears to provide significant survival advantages. These statistics suggest that the uraemic milieu is particularly harmful to cardiovascular health and that 'non-traditional' risk factors that are inadequately addressed or even exacerbated by current therapies may influence mortality.

Question 2

For patients entering dialysis programs, which of the following statements about hypertension and its management is/are true?

(a) Hypertension is present in around 45% of patients starting dialysis.
(b) Prior to dialysis, loop diuretics effectively reduce BP in most patients with CKD.
(c) Hypertension does not improve with salt restriction after patients start dialysis.
(d) Dialysis rarely improves BP control if hypertension is severe.

Answer
B

Explanation

With the development of most forms of CKD, regulation of sodium excretion fails and the total amount of sodium present in the body increases. Since sodium controls the extracellular volume, this leads to volume expansion, an increase in venous return and, while cardiac function remains normal, an increase in cardiac output. Hypertension develops when the total peripheral resistance (or vascular tone) is inappropriately high for the increased cardiac output. Factors that contribute to an inappropriate increase in the peripheral resistance include increased angiotensin II activity, increased sympathetic activity and, over time, vascular remodelling. In addition to effects that are mediated by fluid retention, sodium may *directly* influence cardiac hypertrophy and dilatation, cause vascular smooth muscle cell hypertrophy and increase reactive oxygen species.

Most patients with CKD develop salt and water overload with inappropriately elevated vascular tone, as demonstrated by the fact that around 90% of patients with end-stage renal disease have hypertension. Chronic volume overload and elevated BP are the forerunners of left ventricular hypertrophy (LVH), ventricular dilatation and cardiac failure and symptoms of fluid overload, as suffered by the patient. Prior to commencing dialysis, control of the body's sodium content can be achieved by dietary salt restriction, and by the use of loop diuretics to increase salt and water excretion. Since BP control in CKD is so dependent on salt and water balance, these measures should generally be part of the antihypertensive drug regimen.

Long-term dialysis first became possible on 9 March 1960, the date that Belding Scribner (a physician), Wayne Quinton (an engineer) and David Dillard (a paediatric heart surgeon) at the University of Washington in Seattle sutured some newly available Teflon tubing into a patient's forearm, forming an arteriovenous 'shunt', which could be opened for recurrent dialysis access. It soon became clear that removal of fluid by dialysis, together with salt restriction, could control even severe hypertension in most patients. But there is often a lag period between incremental reductions in extracellular volume and sustained BP improvements, just as there can be when prescribing antihypertensive drugs. This period may represent the time required for vascular remodelling or for the slow removal of vasoactive middle molecular weight substances.

Normal BP remains a difficult goal for many patients. Sometimes this is due to longstanding hypertension and vascular pathology, sometimes to the difficulty of adhering to salt and water restriction and, as will be seen in the next question, sometimes it is exacerbated by the dialysis prescription itself.

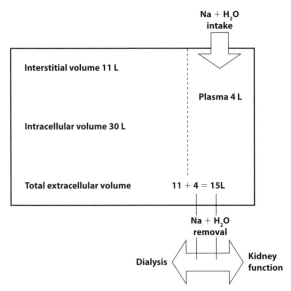

Figure 12.2 Distribution of body fluid. During dialysis the plasma compartment can be rapidly depleted causing hypotension, due to a delay in re-filling from the interstitial fluid compartment

Question 3

Why was the patient hypotensive during dialysis sessions?
- **(a)** His antihypertensive therapy may have impaired vascular compensatory mechanisms.
- **(b)** Because his interdialytic fluid gains were high.
- **(c)** Because of underlying cardiac disease.
- **(d)** Because his dialysis treatments were too short.

Answer

All may be correct

Explanation

Somewhere between 10 and 30% of patients suffer from hypotensive episodes during dialysis and its frequency has not decreased over the past 20 years despite improvements in dialysis technology. Undoubtedly an ageing dialysis population with increased comorbidity has contributed to this. However, as dialysis efficiency has increased, time on dialysis has often been reduced. This allows less time for the removal of fluid and achievement of the targeted 'dry weight': the post-dialysis weight at which a patient no longer has symptoms or signs of fluid overload or of volume depletion, and at which they are likely to have normal BP.

Assessment of the dry weight relies on clinical signs such as postural changes in BP and assessment of the jugular venous pressure when lying flat. All patients are prone to some postural hypotension or orthostatic symptoms soon after dialysis while the plasma compartment is being refilled, so assessment should be delayed some hours after a dialysis session. Plasma refilling is also influenced by neurohumoral factors (sympathetic activity, atrial natriuretic factor, nitric oxide and others) together with vascular permeability factors, and can differ markedly from individual to individual. In addition, compensatory responses to hypovolaemia rely on heart rate responses, cardiac contractility and augmentation of systemic vascular resistance, all of which may be abnormal when patients have cardiovascular disease, particularly LVH, or have been prescribed antihypertensive drugs such as beta-blockers and peripheral vasodilators that blunt compensatory mechanisms. Additional risk factors include diabetes, autonomic dysfunction, poor nutrition with a low serum albumin level and anaemia. Hypotension on dialysis can also be a clue to a significant calcific aortic stenosis, which is common in this population and which can progress rapidly (see Case 19).

Moderate dietary sodium restriction and fluid restriction assist in keeping interdialytic weight gains to a manageable level (around 2 kg), but liberal salt and water intake can result in weight gains up to or exceeding 4 kg—equivalent to the total plasma volume! Such large fluid gains usually result in pre-dialysis hypertension, and the necessity for rapid fluid removal during dialysis, which causes hypotension. Shorter haemodialysis sessions that require more rapid fluid removal will cause even worse orthostatic symptoms. Faced with this, medical staff may progressively increase a patient's dry weight to reduce symptoms during dialysis, but this is at the expense of progressive fluid overload and higher BP.

The best ways to address this situation include dietary salt and water restriction, careful use of antihypertensive agents and longer hours on dialysis, by increasing the dialysis frequency or lengthening each dialysis session. Some patients (and renal services) adjust to longer hours, but for a variety of reasons many cannot and the cycle of fluid overload, hypertension, antihypertensive drugs, inadequate dialysis hours and dialysis-related hypotension persists. When intradialytic hypotension continues to prove difficult, reducing the dialysate temperature and increasing dialysate sodium levels is sometimes useful and the use of bioimpedance to assist in adjusting the dry weight has been advocated.

Question 4

With regards to anaemia and its management and cardiovascular risk, true statements include which of the following?
(a) Patients should have haemoglobin levels in the normal range.
(b) Quality of life is improved when haemoglobin levels approach the normal range.
(c) Mortality is higher for haemoglobin levels > 130 g/L versus < 120 g/L.
(d) Left ventricular function improves when haemoglobin levels are normalised.

Answer
B and C

Explanation

Prior to the introduction of epoetin products, most patients on dialysis had poor exercise tolerance and quality of life due to chronic anaemia. Patients were often transfusion-dependent, leading to iron overload, and predisposition to transfusion-related infections and to human leucocyte antigen (HLA) sensitisation that limited opportunities for transplantation. The introduction of epoetin has allowed patients to have haemoglobin levels in the normal range. However, debate has continued regarding appropriate haemoglobin targets because correction to the normal range may increase BP, the risk of thrombosis and intravenous iron requirements.

Randomised studies in patients receiving dialysis have reported that although vitality and exercise tolerance may be improved, normalisation of haemoglobin levels does not improve left ventricular function or reduce mortality. In fact in a Cochrane review (Strippoli et al. 2004), patients with cardiovascular disease and haemoglobin levels less than 120 g/L had lower mortality than those with levels over 130 g/L. Two recent prospective studies (Drueke et al. 2006; Singh et al. 2004) assessed optimal haemoglobin targets in patients with CKD not yet on dialysis. In one, higher haemoglobin levels of 130 to 150 g/L did not reduce cardiac events, compared to levels of 105 to 115 g/L, although general wellbeing did improve. In the other, patients with haemoglobin levels of 135 g/L had a higher risk of death, myocardial infarct, hospitalisation for cardiac failure and stroke when compared with levels of 113 g/L, without improvement in quality of life.

Therefore, an appropriate haemoglobin (Hb) target for this patient would be 110 to 120 g/L; this should reduce the cardiovascular risk that might accompany higher haemoglobin levels, but should be adequate to provide reasonable vitality and quality of life. This level is also in line with current Caring for Australasians with Renal Impairment (CARI) guidelines (available at www.cari.org.au).

LEVEL B

Question 5

When should patients with CKD on dialysis (CKD-5D) be investigated for evidence of coronary artery disease and how should this be done?

(a) When coronary artery disease is suspected, coronary angiography is the preferred initial investigation.
(b) Stress echocardiography is less accurate than a nuclear myocardial perfusion study.
(c) Hypotension during dialysis may signify coronary artery disease.
(d) Framingham risk categories may not accurately identify patients with CKD who are at greatest cardiovascular risk.

Answer
C and D

Explanation

In-hospital mortality rates following acute myocardial infarction are 2%, but increase to 30% for patients with end-stage renal disease, while after a first myocardial infarct the 1-year mortality rate for patients on dialysis reaches 41 and 70% at 5 years. So there should be a low threshold for diagnostic investigations providing they lead to useful therapies. The patient displays a number of characteristics of patients likely to benefit from investigation of coronary artery disease; he has symptoms and signs of cardiac disease, hypotension during dialysis unrelated to overzealous fluid removal and had a cardiac enzyme rise. These features constitute grounds for investigation whether or not acute ECG changes are present.

For patients with suspected but unproven coronary artery disease and for patients awaiting a renal transplant, non-invasive testing is generally undertaken with a nuclear stress test or stress echocardiography. Because most patients are unable to attain an adequate exercise level, a dipyridamole or adenosine nuclear scan or a dobutamine ECG is generally performed. The cardiac echo may be preferred, because when left ventricular hypertrophy is present and coronary flow reserve is affected, nuclear myocardial perfusion studies that rely on flow distribution become less reliable, while stress echocardiography becomes more accurate. In patients with CKD, angina during dobutamine echocardiography and ischaemia with resting left ventricular dysfunction are predictive of cardiac events (death, myocardial infarction and acute coronary syndrome) over the subsequent 20 ± 14 months.

Despite the fact that patients with CKD have a high burden of coronary artery disease, the overall event rate is low and it would be useful to identify patients who are at low clinical risk. In the general population, Framingham risk categories have been shown to correlate with cardiovascular risk. Applying these to asymptomatic patients with CKD, screening has been suggested for males over 45, females over 55, patients with diabetes or with abnormal ECGs, current smokers, patients with a family history of premature cardiac disease and patients with elevated total cholesterol or low high-density lipoprotein (HDL) cholesterol. However, these traditional risk factors may not accurately identify those patients with CKD who are at greatest risk. The Brisbane scoring system was recently developed to include factors likely to influence cardiovascular risk in patients with CKD (Table 12.1). For a score of 50 or over, this model is reported to be 81% sensitive and 78% specific for prediction of cardiac events, which occurred in high-risk patients at an annualised rate of 22%. By comparison, the use of a scoring system based on Framingham risk factors was less discriminatory.

Table 12.1 The Brisbane scoring system used to identify risk of a cardiovascular event in patients with CKD

Clinical variable	High risk	Score value*
Previous CE	9.83	A = 9.83 if previous CE or 1 if no previous CE
Body mass index (kg/m²)	1.15	B = 1.15 × BMI
Duration RRT (y)	1.24	C = 1.24 × duration RRT or 1 if predialysis
Phosphate (mmol/L)	4.29	D = 4.29 × phosphate

Note: * Score = A + B + C + D, low risk <50. CE = cardiac event, RRT = renal replacement therapy
Source: Rakhit, Armstrong et al. 2006

Question 6

For patients with a positive screening test, how do revascularisation with percutaneous transluminal angioplasty (PTA) and coronary artery bypass grafting (CABG) compare?

(a) The best approach remains controversial.

(b) Short-term survival is better with PTA.

(c) Survival for patients with diabetes is better with PTA.

(d) Reinfarction and stroke rates are similar following CABG and PTA.

Answer

A and D

Explanation

Patients with proven cardiac disease or positive non-invasive investigations should undergo coronary angiography, unless there is other serious comorbidity that would preclude coronary artery bypass surgery (CABG) or percutaneous transluminal angioplasty (PTA). Nevertheless, the best approach to revascularisation of proven coronary artery disease remains controversial. A 2003 meta-analysis of trials performed using PTA (with stenting in four of the thirteen trials evaluated) or CABG showed a survival advantage for CABG at 5 years though no improvement in survival at 1, 3 or 8 years. For patients with diabetes a survival advantage was seen with CABG at 4 years and for trials that assessed multivessel disease, an advantage was seen from 5 to 8 years. Although not specifically powered for mortality outcomes, a more recent study reported that rates of reinfarction and stroke were similar following CABG and PTA with bare metal stenting, and mortality was similar to 5 years. However, there was a higher risk of requiring repeat revascularisation after PTA. With the introduction of drug-eluting stents, revascularisation rates are likely to be markedly reduced, which may tip the balance in favour of percutaneous intervention. Antiplatelet agents (aspirin plus clopidogrel) are currently recommended for 4 weeks after bare metal stents versus 3 to 6 months after insertion of drug-eluting stents, which poses a greater risk of bleeding in the event of emergency surgery (including transplantation) and increases the risk of gastrointestinal blood loss.

The 2006 United States Renal Data System (USRDS) annual report (www.usrds.org/adr.htm) assessed cardiovascular management of patients commencing dialysis in 2003. Almost a quarter of those patients were evaluated for ischaemic heart disease by stress test or coronary angiography during their first dialysis year. Despite a likely high prevalence of coronary artery disease, the cumulative percentage receiving revascularisation remained low, at <5% in the first dialysis year.

Question 7

Which of the following statements is/are true regarding risk factors that predispose patients with CKD to the development of cardiovascular disease?

(a) Cardiovascular risk rises with each stage of worsening CKD.
(b) Traditional risk factors explain most of this predisposition.
(c) Improving dialysis efficiency improves survival.
(d) Abnormal mineral metabolism is associated with increased mortality.

Answer

A and D

Explanation

The patient has a number of traditional risk factors that may have contributed to the development of CKD and cardiovascular disease: smoking, diabetes, hypertension, elevated cholesterol, borderline obesity and central adiposity. Patients with CKD have additional CKD-related risks. Using data from over a million people, Go et al. (2004) have reported a progressive increase in cardiovascular risk from an age-standardised rate of 2.1 per 100 person years in early CKD (estimated glomerular filtration rate ≥ 60 mL/min/1.73 m^2) to 11.3 per 100 person years in moderate CKD (GFR 30–44 ml/min/1.73m^2) and to 36.6 per 100 person years in CKD-5 (GFR <15 mL/min/1.73 m^2 or on dialysis). These data suggest that as renal function worsens, non-traditional factors may exert progressively more influence on cardiovascular outcomes.

For patients on dialysis, a number of studies have pointed to associations of mortality and levels of serum calcium (adjusted for albumin), serum phosphate, the calcium phosphate product and levels of PTH. Disturbances in these parameters represent the biochemical consequences of abnormal bone and mineral metabolism in CKD. Other factors associated with increased risk in this population include anaemia, fluid overload, malnutrition and chronic inflammation associated with elevated levels of C-reactive protein (as in the case of this patient) and reduced levels of Fetuin-A. Homocysteine levels, high sympathetic activity and raised plasma concentrations of the endogenous inhibitor of nitric oxide synthase, asymmetric dimethylarginine, have also been associated with cardiovascular complications, but evidence for their direct role is lacking. While inefficient dialysis has been associated with increased mortality, studies that have increased haemodialysis dose and altered the dialysis membrane characteristics (the Hemodialysis [HEMO] study) or increased peritoneal small solute clearance for patients on CAPD (the Adequacy of peritoneal dialysis in Mexico [ADEMEX] study) have not demonstrated that these changes in the dialysis prescription influence survival. However, these data *do not* prove that longer and more efficient dialysis won't improve survival; they *do* show that factors influencing survival are complex and that 'a one-size-fits-all' dialysis prescription is not enough to make a survival difference.

Table 12.2 shows the population-attributable risk for some commonly measured CKD-related parameters, based on a United States (US) nationally representative database of over 40 000 haemodialysis patients. Based on these data (and despite a lack of high-quality evidence that intervention affects cardiovascular risk or mortality), several clinical practice guidelines have suggested targets for levels of serum phosphate, adjusted serum calcium, the calcium phosphate product and for levels of iPTH. The CARI guidelines were the first of these and the most widely adopted are the US Kidney Disease Outcomes Quality Initiative (KDOQI) guidelines published in 2004. Table 12.3 indicates the CARI biochemical targets, as revised in 2006.

Table 12.2 The percentage to which commonly measured parameters contribute to the population-attributable mortality risk of CKD. For abnormalities of mineral metabolism, the risk is largely due to hyperphosphataemia

Population attributable risk	Parameter
17.5%	Mineral metabolism abnormalities
	Phosphate >1.60 mmol/L
	Calcium >2.5 mmol/L
	iPTH >64 pmol/L
11.3%	Anaemia <110 g/L
5.1%	Inefficient dialysis URR <65%

Source: Block et al. 2004

Table 12.3 Suggested target ranges from the CARI guidelines (www.cari.org.au). CARI biochemical targets are similar to those suggested by KDOQI

Parameter	Target range
Adjusted serum calcium	2.1–2.4 mmol/L
Serum phosphate	0.8–1.6 mmol/L
Calcium × phosphate product	<4 mmol^2/L^2
Intact-PTH	2–3 times the assay upper normal range*

Note: *This range may be optimal for bone turnover. However, when PTH levels are <7 times the iPTH assay upper range, therapies to achieve bone targets for PTH that compromise target levels of serum calcium, phosphate or the calcium × phosphate product should be used with caution.

Question 8

The patient is on a number of therapies to improve his lipids and to achieve proposed biochemical targets. Which of the following statements is true regarding the likelihood he will achieve the targets or that this will improve his survival?
(a) Only 45% of patients achieve all four biochemical targets (PTH, calcium, phosphate and the calcium phosphate product).
(b) Lipid lowering with atorvastatin reduces stroke.
(c) Aggressive management of traditional risk factors improves short-term survival.
(d) None of the above answers is correct.

Answer
D

Explanation

Using standard dialysis durations and therapies available from 1996 to 2001, approximately 60% achieved the target for the calcium phosphate product, less than 45% of patients achieved the targets currently suggested for serum calcium or phosphate, around 25% achieved the iPTH target and only 5 to 6% achieved all four. The reasons are complex and include difficulties in compliance with dietary restrictions and drug regimens that may demand 6 to 12 phosphate-binding tablets daily. In addition, calcium-based phosphate binders may increase serum calcium levels unacceptably, and elevation of calcium levels, phosphate levels and the calcium phosphate product are recognised side effects of using calcitriol or other vitamin D analogues to suppress secondary hyperparathyroidism.

While the patient may not achieve the biochemical targets, his treating physician undoubtedly hopes that a concerted effort to improve his biochemical parameters, improve his lipid levels and stop him smoking may improve his prospects of survival. A recent report examining cardiovascular outcomes for standard versus aggressive management of risk factors in patients with CKD 4 and 5 suggests this is not necessarily the case. The aggressively treated aspects of care were hypertension; dyslipidaemia using atorvastatin; reduction of homocystine using folic acid, vitamin B12 and pyridoxine; haemoglobin levels; phosphate levels using predominantly calcium-based phosphate binders; cessation of smoking and the use of aspirin unless contraindicated. Over the follow-up period (mean 1.8 years), levels of cholesterol (total and LDL), homocysteine, phosphate, aspirin use and smoking differed (p ≤0.05) in favour of the aggressively treated group but the groups did not differ in rates of cardiac events or in all cause mortality. Independent predictors of new ischaemia were older age, systolic BP and lower LDL-cholesterol, but not treatment group. These interesting data *do not* negate the argument to treat these factors, but suggest that more aggressive management may not influence short-term outcomes and point to the potential impact of non-targeted factors.

Another much-publicised study compared atorvastatin with placebo on cardiovascular outcomes (Wanner et al. 2005). The patients were 1255 type 2 diabetics on maintenance haemodialysis and followed for a median of 4 years. Surprisingly, and in contrast to observational analyses, atorvastatin did *not* affect cardiovascular outcomes significantly and a higher rate of fatal strokes occurred in atorvastatin-treated patients. Consequently, the authors recommended that patients with diabetes who have commenced dialysis should not be initiated on statin therapy. This remains a controversial and disputed conclusion. So the jury remains out on the degree to which standard therapies to manage this patient's risk factors will influence his survival.

LEVEL C

Case history continued ...

The patient has a chest CT on account of slowly resolving pneumonia. In addition to confirming patchy consolidation, coronary artery calcification is reported.

Question 9

Which of the following statements is/are true?

(a) Coronary artery calcification (CAC) is more common in CKD than the general population.
(b) Diabetes and smoking predict CAC in patients with CKD.
(c) CAC is associated with increased cardiovascular risk in the dialysis but not the general population.
(d) In patients on dialysis, CAC is rarely seen under age 30.

Answer

A and B

Explanation

Extensive metastatic calcification and CAC were detected at autopsy in patients with chronic renal disease long before the dialysis era. Vascular calcification and calcification of coronary arteries and valves is often visible on plain X-rays, but more recently high-speed multislice and electron beam computed tomography (MSCT and EBCT) have allowed CAC to be assessed in a quantitative fashion.

In the general population, coronary calcification is seen with ageing and calcification scores have been positively correlated with atherosclerotic plaque, plaque instability and coronary artery disease endpoints in symptomatic and asymptomatic individuals. In patients with CKD not yet on dialysis, CAC and calcification scores are reported to be up to ten times higher than in non-CKD controls. Diabetes predicts higher CAC scores both in the presence and in the absence of CKD and smoking status is an independent predictor of total CAC volume in CKD patients.

Coronary artery calcification is uncommon in normal 20- to 30-year olds, but in 2000, Goodman et al. reported CAC in 88% of dialysis patients within that age range. In those patients, calcification scores correlated positively with dialysis duration and levels of serum phosphate, the calcium phosphate product and doses of calcium-based phosphate binder. Similar risk factors have been identified in some but not all subsequent studies.

Compared to the general population, data on the natural history of dialysis patients with CAC are less robust. Patients who are transplanted and dialysis patients without calcification on baseline studies seem not to progress. Increased CAC seems to be associated with increased hospitalisation and mortality. For this patient, his age, CKD (and possibly the associated abnormalities of mineral metabolism), diabetes, smoking history, dyslipidaemia and time on dialysis may all have contributed to the CAC detected on CT. In the setting of CKD, it is not clear what independent bearing this finding has on his already high risk of further cardiovascular events.

Question 10

What factors in the uraemic milieu predispose to vascular calcification?
(a) A reduction in inhibitors of calcification
(b) An increase in promoters of calcification
(c) Cells in the blood vessel wall which start to behave like osteoblasts
(d) Systemic inflammation and reduced fetuin-A

Answer
All are correct

Explanation

Patients with CKD develop premature and accelerated atherosclerosis and vascular calcification. Calcification occurs in the intima, associated with advanced atherosclerosis, and also occurs in the arterial media, a finding otherwise associated with ageing and diabetes. In 1979, Ibels et al. demonstrated that the renal and internal iliac arteries of kidney transplant recipients had increased atheromatous/intimal disease and a thicker, more calcified media than the vessels of transplant donors. Similar findings of increased calcification and medial thickening have been reported in the coronary arteries of dialysis patients as compared to age-matched non-dialysis patients who had died of a cardiac event. These vascular changes and the accompanying reduction in vascular compliance develop progressively as renal function declines.

The extracellular fluid is normally supersaturated with calcium and phosphate ions and contains inhibitors that *prevent* soft tissue mineralisation. Recent clinical and laboratory studies have demonstrated that in CKD there is a deficiency of mineralisation inhibitors. These include, among others, matrix Gla protein (MGP), the major local inhibitor in the arterial wall, fetuin-A (a calcium-binding protein which is reduced in the presence of systemic inflammation) and bone morphogenic protein-7 (BMP-7), a protein expressed primarily in the kidney that regulates the vascular smooth muscle cell (VSMC) phenotype. BMP-7 also regulates skeletal anabolic balance and phosphate levels. Simultaneously, there is an increase in a number of mineralisation *promoters*, largely driven by elevation of the serum phosphate, but including lipids and inflammatory cytokines, calcitriol and leptin.

The process of vascular calcification is not a simple physicochemical reaction but, as shown in Figure 12.3, occurs via genomic pathways that result in transdifferentiation of vascular cells into cells that express an osteoblast (or bone-forming) phenotype. Serum phosphate levels generally increase in CKD, initiating increased transport of phosphate into VSMCs via a sodium-dependent phosphate co-transporter (*Pit-1*). Increased intracellular phosphate induces core-binding factor-1 (cbfa-1), a key transcriptional regulator of osteoblast differentiation. VSMCs (which are derived from mesenchymal progenitors

The calcification imbalance of CKD

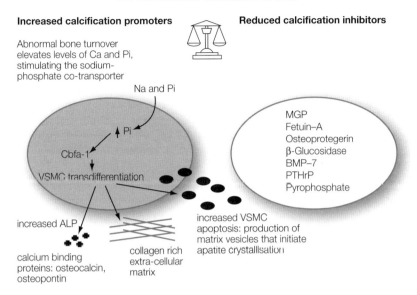

Increased calcification promoters

Abnormal bone turnover elevates levels of Ca and Pi, stimulating the sodium-phosphate co-transporter

Reduced calcification inhibitors

Na and Pi

↑ Pi

Cbfa-1

VSMC transdifferentiation

MGP
Fetuin–A
Osteoprotegerin
β-Glucosidase
BMP–7
PTHrP
Pyrophosphate

increased ALP

calcium binding proteins: osteocalcin, osteopontin

collagen rich extra-cellular matrix

increased VSMC apoptosis: production of matrix vesicles that initiate apatite crystallisation

Figure 12.3 Novel risk factors for vascular calcification. In CKD-5 there is an imbalance of calcification promoters and inhibitors

Source: Modified from Giachelli et al. 2001

capable of differentiating into adipocytes and osteoblasts) then undergo phenotypic transformation, start to express osteoblast markers and *actively* deposit bone mineral into the blood vessel walls. A recent review by Jono et al. (2006) provides further details of vascular calcification in CKD.

Question 11

What is the 'chronic kidney disease—mineral and bone disorder' (CKD–MBD)?
(a) A textbook regarded as the 'bible' of bone and mineral metabolism
(b) A classification for vascular, laboratory and bone abnormalities in CKD
(c) A means of assessing and describing cardiovascular risk
(d) Another problem for medical students

Answer

B, C and possibly D

Explanation

The term 'chronic kidney disease—mineral and bone disorder' (CKD—MBD) was adopted in 2005 to describe the interactions in patients with CKD of bone turnover, mineral homeostasis and vascular calcification that lead to cardiovascular disease, fractures and mortality. The classification system is generally to apply to adults with a GFR <60 mL/min/1.73 m^2 and is currently under development.

There are three components to CKD—MBD:

1. Laboratory biomarkers (L). This component includes abnormalities in calcium, phosphate, PTH, total and bone-specific alkaline phosphatase, 25-hydroxyvitamin D and bicarbonate. The patient has abnormalities of all the biomarkers tested, so is classified L+.
2. Bone disease (B). This includes abnormalities of bone turnover, mineralisation and volume derived from bone histomorphometry (requiring a bone biopsy), linear growth (in children) and strength. (See Case 13 for further discussion of bone histomorphometry.) Bone serum biomarkers are under consideration for inclusion but at present their use remains unsatisfactory. PTH correlates poorly with bone turnover and other bone turnover markers undergo renal excretion or have not been validated in CKD. Bone imaging techniques are also included but are problematic. X-rays of the hip, skull, hands and clavicles have been used to detect changes of hyperparathyroidism and osteomalacia but their value is limited because they do not assess the bone microstructural changes that increase fracture risk in patients with CKD. The role of dual energy X-ray absorptiometry (DXA) is also unclear. DXA provides valuable data on bone mineral density (BMD) and fracture risk in patients without CKD, but a finding of low BMD in patients with CKD may reflect complex mineralisation disorders that could be adversely affected by standard osteoporosis therapies. Other modalities that require investigation in CKD include ultrasound and radioisotope imaging and the use of micro-MRI/CT. Based on limited investigations, the patient could be categorised as B+/–. His PTH level is above the target range but this does not necessarily indicate abnormal bone turnover.
3. Extraskeletal calcification (C). Useful non-invasive imaging modalities include chest and abdominal X-rays, computed tomography scans (EBCT/MSCT) and assessment of vascular stiffness (using pulse wave velocity and pulse pressure). In the case of this patient, earlier investigation with EBCT or MSCT would have been of questionable value due to the ubiquitous nature of coronary calcification in male dialysis patients of his age. Nevertheless, for the purposes of categorisation, this patient's chest CT puts him in the C+ category and overall: CKD—MBD L+, B+/– and C+.

Currently this system is meant to be 'descriptive rather than predictive' and a prompt to evaluating the spectrum of factors influencing a patient's cardiovascular risk. Over time the CKD—MBD classification should lead to improvements in risk assessment and the facilitation of clinical decision making. A recent review of CKD—MBD edited by Drs Moe and Fadem was used as a source for some of this discussion and is suggested for further reading.

Question 12

With respect to the influence on cardiovascular outcomes of the choice of phosphate binder and the use of vitamin D or of a calcimimetic, true statements include which of the following?

(a) Sevelamer has clear advantages over calcium-based phosphate binders in normocalcaemic patients.

(b) Observational studies have reported a survival advantage for patients treated with active vitamin D.

(c) Lanthanum is a less-effective phosphate binder than calcium carbonate.

(d) Calcimimetics have been shown to reduce cardiovascular mortality.

Answer

B

Explanation

Patients having 15 hours of dialysis per week like this patient generally require calcium-based phosphate binders. These binders sometimes increase the serum calcium unacceptably. Consequently, sevelamer hydrochloride and lanthanum carbonate, two phosphate binders that contain neither aluminium nor calcium, have recently been introduced. These agents are expensive and their potential advantages remain controversial. Sevelamer has been associated with slower progression of vascular calcification compared with calcium-based binders, particularly in patients with diabetes (Galassi et al. 2006), but deficiencies in study design have resulted in criticism of these findings. A recent small study reported improved survival with sevelamer versus calcium-based binders in patients new to dialysis (Block et al. 2007) and the unpublished Dialysis Clinical Outcomes Revisited (DCOR) study is reported to show no reduction in relative risk of mortality for sevelamer versus calcium-based phosphate binders, except for the subgroup of patients over age 65 and with longer sevelamer use. Less information is available on the effects of lanthanum carbonate. It is an effective binder with a good safety record to 3 years, but given the unfortunate aluminium experience, there is some concern regarding long-term tissue accumulation of this rare earth metal.

Levels of 1,25-dihydroxyvitamin D (calcitriol) are low in CKD because activation of the 25-hydroxyvitamin D precursor occurs in the kidney. Apart from regulating PTH production and calcium–phosphate balance, calcitriol has pleiotropic effects on the breast, prostate, gastrointestinal tract, immune system and blood vessels. Few randomised trials of vitamin D or the newer (possibly less-calcaemic) vitamin D analogues have assessed patient-level outcomes. Hence, possible benefits, particularly on mortality and cardiovascular events, remain unproven. Nevertheless, in large observational studies of patients on dialysis, treatment with active vitamin D is associated with reduced mortality compared with no vitamin D treatment and the administration of doxercalciferol or paricalcitol is reported to reduce the risk of death or hospitalisation when compared with calcitriol. Although these studies have inherent limitations, the clinical advantages they suggest deserve further study.

Calcimimetics are small organic compounds that bind to the transmembrane region of the calcium-sensing receptors (CaR) on the parathyroid (and elsewhere). By increasing the CaR sensitivity to extracellular ionised calcium, they can reduce PTH responses across a wide range of calcium concentrations. Cinacalcet hydrochloride is the only calcimimetic available for patient use. It effectively reduces levels of PTH, calcium, phosphate and the calcium phosphate product and patients achieve biochemical targets more often than patients on standard therapy but, as yet, trials have not shown significant reductions in mortality or reduced rates of cardiovascular or all-cause hospitalisation. Longer studies may provide information on these important patient-level outcomes.

Bibliography

Level A

1. McDonald, S., Chang, S. & Excell, L. (eds) (2006) Australia and New Zealand Dialysis and Transplant Registry report, Adelaide, South Australia.
2. Charra, B. (2007) Fluid balance, dry weight, and blood pressure in dialysis. Hemodial Int. 11(1), 21–31.
3. Drueke, T.B., Locatelli, F., Clyne, N., Eckardt, K.U., Macdougall, I.C., Tsakiris, D., Burger, H.U. & Scherhag, A., for the CREATE Investigators. (2006) Normalization of hemoglobin level in patients with chronic kidney disease and anemia. N Engl J Med. 355(20), 2071–84.
4. Santoro, A. (2006) Cardiovascular dialysis instability and convective therapies. Hemodial Int. 10(Supp. 1), S51–5.
5. Singh, A.K., Szczech, L., Tang, K.L., Barnhart, H., Sapp, S., Wolfson, M. & Reddan, D., for the CHOIR Investigators. (2006) Correction of anemia with epoetin alfa in chronic kidney disease. N Engl J Med. 355(20), 2085–98.
6. Strippoli, G.F., Craig, J.C., Manno, C. & Schena, F.P. (2004) Hemoglobin targets for the anemia of chronic kidney disease: a meta-analysis of randomized, controlled trials. J Am Soc Nephrol. 15(12), 3154–65.

Level B

7. Go, A.S., Chertow, G.M., Fan, D. McCulloch, C.E. & Hsu, C. (2004) Chronic kidney disease and the risks of death, cardiovascular events, and hospitalization. N Engl J Med. 351(13), 1296–305.
8. Block, G.A., Klassen, P.S., Lazarus, J.M. Ofsthun, N., Lowrie, E.G. & Chertow, G.M. (2004) Mineral metabolism, mortality, and morbidity in maintenance hemodialysis. J Am Soc Nephrol. 15(8), 2208–18.

9. Eknoyan, G., Beck, G.J., Cheung, A.K., Daugirdas, J.T., Greene, T., Kusek, J.W., Allon, M., Bailey, J., Delmez, J.A., Depner, T.A., Dwyer, J.T., Levey, A.S., Levin, N.W., Milford, E., Ornt, D.B., Rocco, M.V., Schulman, G., Schwab, S.J., Teehan, B.P. & Toto, R., for the Hemodialysis (HEMO) Study Group. (2002) Effect of dialysis dose and membrane flux in maintenance hemodialysis. N Engl J Med. 19 Dec. 347(25), 2010–19.
10. Herzog, C.A., Ma, J.Z. & Collins, A.J. Poor long-term survival after acute myocardial infarction among patients on long-term dialysis. N Engl J Med. 1998, 339(12), 799–805.
11. Hoffman, S.N., TenBrook, J.A., Wolf, M.P., Pauker, S.G., Salem, D.N. & Wong, J.B. (2003) A meta-analysis of randomized controlled trials comparing coronary artery bypass graft with percutaneous transluminal coronary angioplasty: one- to eight-year outcomes. J Am Coll Cardiol. 41(8), 1293–304.
12. McCullough, P.A. (2005) Evaluation and treatment of coronary artery disease in patients with end-stage renal disease. Kidney Int Suppl. (95), S51–8.
13. Paniagua, R., Amato, D., Vonesh, E., Correa-Rotter, R., Ramos, A., Moran, J. & Mujais, S., for the Mexican Nephrology Collaborative Study Group (2002) Effects of increased peritoneal clearances on mortality rates in peritoneal dialysis: ADEMEX, a prospective, randomized, controlled trial. J Am Soc Nephrol. May, 13(5), 1307 20.
14. Rakhit, D.J., Armstrong, K.A., Beller, E., Isbel, N.M. & Marwick, T.H. (2006) Risk stratification of patients with chronic kidney disease: results of screening strategies incorporating clinical risk scoring and dobutamine stress echocardiography. Am Heart J. 152(2), 363–70.
15. Rakhit, D.J., Marwick, T.H., Armstrong, K.A., Johnson, D.W., Leano, R. & Isbel, N.M. (2006) Effect of aggressive risk factor modification on cardiac events and myocardial ischaemia in patients with chronic kidney disease. Heart. 92(10), 1402–8.
16. Serruys, P.W., Ong, A.T., van Herwerden, L.A., Sousa, J.E., Jatene, A., Bonnier, J.J., Schönberger, J.P., Buller, N., Bonser, R., Disco, C., Backx, B., Hugenholtz, P.G., Firth, B.G. & Unger, F. (2005) Five-year outcomes after coronary stenting versus bypass surgery for the treatment of multivessel disease: the final analysis of the Arterial Revascularization Therapies Study (ARTS) randomized trial. J Am Coll Cardiol. 46(4), 575–81.
17. Wanner, C., Krane, V., März, W., Olschewski, M., Mann, J.F.E., Ruf, G. & Ritz, E., for the German Diabetes and Dialysis Study Investigators (2005) Atorvastatin in patients with type 2 diabetes mellitus undergoing hemodialysis. N Engl J Med. 353(3), 238–48.
18. Wright, R.S., Reeder, G.S., Herzog, C.A., Albright, R.C., Williams, B.A., Dvorak, D.L., Miller, W.L., Murphy, J.G., Kopecky, S.L. & Jaffe, A.S. (2002) Acute myocardial infarction and renal dysfunction: a high-risk combination. Ann Intern Med. 137(7), 563–70.

Level C
19. Giachelli, C.M., Jono, S., Shioi, A., Nishizawa, Y., Mori, K. & Morii, H. (2001) Vascular calcification and inorganic phosphate. Am J Kidney Dis. 38(4 Supp. 1), S34–7.
20. Moe, S.M. & Fadem, S.Z. (eds). (2007) Chronic kidney disease-mineral and bone disorder. Adv Chronic Kidney Dis. Jan., 14(1).
21. Cunningham, J., Danese, M., Olson, K., Klassen, P. & Chertow, G.M. (2005) Effects of the calcimimetic cinacalcet HCl on cardiovascular disease, fracture, and health-related quality of life in secondary hyperparathyroidism. Kidney Int. 68(4), 1793–800.

22. Goodman, W.G., Goldin, J., Kuizon, B.D., Yoon, C., Gales, B., Sider, D., Wang, Y., Chung, J., Emerick, A., Greaser, L., Elashoff, R.M. & Salusky, I.B. (2000) Coronary-artery calcification in young adults with end-stage renal disease who are undergoing dialysis. N Engl J Med. 342(20), 1478–83.
23. Ibels, L.S., Alfrey, A.C., Huffer, W.E., Craswell, P.W., Anderson, J.T. & Weil, R. 3rd. (1979) Arterial calcification and pathology in uremic patients undergoing dialysis. Am J Med. 66(5), 790–6.
24. Jono, S., Shioi, A., Ikari, Y. & Nishizawa, Y. (2006) Vascular calcification in chronic kidney disease. J Bone Miner Metab. 24(2), 176–81.
25. Matsuoka, M., Iseki, K., Tamashiro, M. Fujimoto, N., Higa, N., Touma, T. & Takishita, S. (2004) Impact of high coronary artery calcification score (CACS) on survival in patients on chronic hemodialysis. Clin Exp Nephrol. 8(1), 54–8.
26. Qunibi, W.Y. (2007) Cardiovascular calcification in nondialyzed patients with chronic kidney disease. Semin Dial. 20(2), 134–8.
27. Strippoli, G.F., Palmer, S., Tong, A., Elder, G., Messa, P. & Craig, J.C. (2006) Meta-analysis of biochemical and patient-level effects of calcimimetic therapy. Am J Kidney Dis. 47(5), 715–26.
28. Teng, M., Wolf, M., Ofsthun, M.N., Lazarus, J.M., Hernán, M.A., Camargo, C.A. Jr & Thadhani, R. (2005) Activated injectable vitamin D and hemodialysis survival: a historical cohort study. J Am Soc Nephrol. 16(4), 1115–25.
29. Galassi, A., Spiegel, D.M., Bellasi, A., Block, G.A. & Raggi, P. (2006) Accelerated vascular calcification and relative hypoparathyroidism in incident haemodialysis diabetic patients receiving calcium binders. Nephrol Dial Transplant. 21(11), 3215–22.
30. Block, G.A., Raggi, P., Bellasi, A., Kooienga, L. & Spiegel, D.M. (2007) Mortality effect of coronary calcification and phosphate binder choice in incident hemodialysis patients. Kidney Int. 71(5), 438–41.

Case 13
Bone and mineral metabolism

GRAHAME ELDER

Case history

A 60-year-old female is admitted 1 year after a kidney transplant with sudden, sharp, left-sided chest pain after coughing. Chest X-ray shows a left rib fracture, and a thoracic vertebral compression fracture is visible on the lateral film.

She has a history of hypertension from age 50. At age 55 she developed oedema and proteinuria and a renal biopsy showed membranous glomerulonephritis plus vascular damage. After 6-months treatment with cyclophosphamide and prednisolone (1 mg/kg) her serum creatinine deteriorated from 150 to 300 μmol/L and her renal physician suggested they discuss dialysis.

She returned 6 months later with dyspnoea. An electrocardiogram showed atrial fibrillation. Laboratory investigations included the following.

Laboratory data

	Result	Reference range
Serum creatinine	750 μmol/L	53 – 105 for females
Corrected serum calcium	2.61 mmol/L	2.15 – 2.60
Serum phosphate	2.4 mmol/L	0.6 – 1.3
Alkaline phosphatase (ALP)	169 U/L	(< 120)
Intact PTH (iPTH)	55 pmol/L	(1 to 7)
25-Hydroxyvitamin D	24 nmol/L	(suggested >60)

She commenced haemodialysis and was treated with Mylanta® (aluminium hydroxide 200 mg plus magnesium hydroxide 200 mg), two tablets with breakfast and lunch plus a 600 mg calcium carbonate tablet with dinner to reduce phosphate levels. Calcitriol was started at 0.25 μg three times weekly, warfarin and digoxin were commenced and she continued antihypertensive treatment.

The serum phosphate improved to 2.0 mmol/L, calcium levels varied from 2.55 to 3.05 mmol/L and her serum aluminium level was 2.7 μmol/L (range for little risk of toxicity in CKD <2.2 μmol/L). When several painful, firm subcutaneous nodules developed on her left thigh, calcitriol, calcium carbonate and Mylanta were ceased. Her dialysis hours were increased and sevelamer (a non-calcium non-aluminium containing phosphate binder) was commenced. The pain gradually improved.

At age 59 she was transplanted with a kidney from her husband. Immunosuppressive therapy was cyclosporine A, mycophenolate mofetil and prednisolone. Two months post-transplant her creatinine was 130 μmol/L, iPTH had fallen from 49 to 27 pmol/L, serum calcium was 2.55 mmol/L and phosphate 0.45 mmol/L. She complained of bilateral upper-tibial pain, which responded poorly to paracetamol but resolved after 2 months. She then remained well until the current admission.

LEVEL A

Question 1

Which of the following diagnoses explains the predialysis laboratory results?
(a) Primary hyperparathyroidism
(b) Secondary hyperparathyroidism due to 25-hydroxyvitamin D deficiency
(c) Secondary hyperparathyroidism due to chronic kidney disease
(d) Drug-induced hypercalcaemia

Answer
C

Explanation

Despite attempted treatment of her glomerulonephritis and hypertension, the patient progressed to chronic kidney disease stage 5 (CKD-5), defined as an estimated glomerular filtration rate (eGFR) <15 mL/min/1.73 m². At this level of renal impairment, secondary hyperparathyroidism is common and explains the laboratory results. The iPTH level of 55 pmol/L is well above the maximal secretory capacity of normal parathyroid glands and would be explained by a tonic stimulus to PTH secretion plus an increased *mass* of parathyroid tissue (diffuse hyperplasia or nodular hyperplasia). Glands with nodular hyperplasia express fewer calcium and vitamin D receptors and are less responsive to normal inhibitory feedback.

The serum calcium was elevated before calcium or calcitriol was commenced and should have suppressed PTH secretion. In hyperparathyroidism this Ca–PTH interaction becomes abnormal and very high calcium levels may be necessary for any PTH suppression to occur; described as 'a shift to the right' in the calcium set-point of PTH. The set-point is the calcium level at which PTH secretion is between peak and nadir (see Fig. 13.1). In the context of hyperparathyroidism, the elevated ALP level is likely to be of bone rather than liver origin. Bone-forming cells (osteoblasts) produce ALP when stimulated into activity by PTH.

Deficiency of 25-hydroxyvitamin D, or 25(OH)D, is common in the presence of CKD and in the general community. Inadequate sunlight exposure is the usual cause, so anyone with limited mobility or a serious illness is at risk. Among patients with CKD, patients with the highest prevalence of 25(OH)D deficiency are women, patients using peritoneal dialysis and patients with diabetes. In the case of this patient, proteinuria with urinary losses of 25(OH)D bound to vitamin D binding protein may have contributed. Although 25(OH)D deficiency causes secondary hyperparathyroidism, PTH levels are lower than in this case.

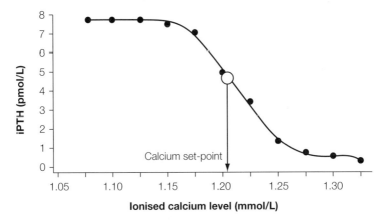

Figure 13.1 Ionised calcium levels were modulated from low to high and PTH responses were recorded. The calcium set-point is the ionised calcium level corresponding to the midpoint of the iPTH response curve. In secondary hyperparathyroidism the response curve is shifted to the right (i.e. PTH is less responsive to calcium). Calcimimetic drugs move the PTH response curve to the left (i.e. PTH levels are more responsive to calcium)

Despite a lack of renal conversion of 25(OH)D to calcitriol in severe CKD, 25(OH)D deficiency may be important. Classical actions of vitamin D affect bone, muscle and mineral metabolism, but this hormone has diverse actions, including effects on cell cycling, immunity and responses to infection. Local non-renal conversion to calcitriol may mediate these actions, as may the fact that unlike calcitriol, 25(OH)D circulates at nmol rather than pmol concentrations. Despite being less active than calcitriol, it may affect the vitamin D receptor at these concentrations.

PTH levels need cautious interpretation in patients with CKD. In the presence of renal impairment, there is an accumulation of PTH fragments that would normally be cleared by the kidneys. These fragments contribute around 50% of the PTH measured in most 'intact-PTH' assays. Unlike the full-length peptide, these fragments are not calcaemic and may even oppose the calcaemic actions of full-length PTH(1-84). This largely explains why, for patients with CKD, target values for iPTH are two- to threefold higher than levels regarded as normal in the general population.

Question 2

What is the approximate percentage of patients on dialysis with renal bone disease?
(a) 25%
(b) 50%
(c) 75%
(d) 100%

Answer
D

Explanation

In normal bone multinucleated osteoclasts are responsible for bone resorption and osteoblasts for the production and mineralisation of osteoid. The process of bone removal and replacement is called remodelling and must be tightly coupled so as to maintain bone mass. PTH and calcitriol influence the rate of bone remodelling and mineralisation while locally produced cytokines influence osteoblast–osteoclast coupling. Particularly when bone turnover is increased, the process of formation and resorption becomes uncoupled, leading to a net loss or, less frequently, a net increase in bone. By the time patients require dialysis, almost 100% have abnormalities of bone turnover, mineralisation or volume. The pathogenesis is described below.

Kidney damage leads to phosphate retention. Initially this may be caused by a reduced tubular response to the phosphaturic hormone FGF-23. This hormone is made in bone but acts in the kidney, where it requires the kidney-derived hormone Klotho for full effect. Eventually, tubular damage and reduced GFR leads to phosphate retention and, acutely at least, a reduction in levels of serum calcium is often seen. A cascade of factors then causes secondary hyperparathyroidism as shown in Figure 13.2.

These mechanisms cause a PTH-driven *increase* in bone turnover, but in some patients bone turnover is below normal. The use of calcium or aluminium-based phosphate binders and active vitamin D sterols can suppress PTH and bone turnover. However, the reduced production by the kidney of bone morphogenic protein-7 (BMP-7), a protein that is anabolic to bone, may be an important contributing factor.

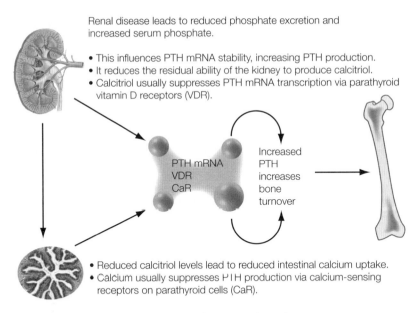

Renal disease leads to reduced phosphate excretion and increased serum phosphate.

- This influences PTH mRNA stability, increasing PTH production.
- It reduces the residual ability of the kidney to produce calcitriol.
- Calcitriol usually suppresses PTH mRNA transcription via parathyroid vitamin D receptors (VDR).

PTH mRNA
VDR
CaR

Increased PTH increases bone turnover

- Reduced calcitriol levels lead to reduced intestinal calcium uptake.
- Calcium usually suppresses PTH production via calcium-sensing receptors on parathyroid cells (CaR).

Figure 13.2 Factors causing secondary hyperparathyroidism

Question 3

Because of the fractures, a dual energy X-ray absorptiometry scan is performed. T-scores are −2.2 at the lumbar spine and −2.6 at the total proximal femur. How should these results be interpreted?

(a) She has osteoporosis.

(b) Bone mineral density is difficult to interpret in patients with CKD.

(c) She has an increased risk of fracture at both sites.

(d) The lumbar spine bone mineral density may be normal for her age.

Answer
All are correct

Explanation

Bone mineral density (BMD) increases until age 20 and then remains relatively stable in healthy individuals until around age 50, after which there is a progressive decline, which occurs more rapidly for women at the time of menopause.

Dual-energy X-ray absorptiometry (DXA) is used to measure BMD and some technical details are necessary for interpreting these results. The DXA machine uses two X-ray beams in order to derive a measurement of BMD. One beam is directed through the area of interest (e.g. a vertebra, but must also pass through surrounding soft tissues). Therefore, a second beam is directed through soft tissues adjacent to the vertebra. By subtracting the attenuation of the soft tissue beam from the attenuation of the vertebra plus soft tissue beam, the result largely represents attenuation by mineral within the vertebra. Comparing this result with the X-ray attenuation by a 'phantom' (of known density), a value can be derived for the vertebral BMD in g/cm^2.

The T-score indicates the number of standard deviations an individual's BMD differs from the mean of a young normal Caucasian population. BMD values within the age range 20 to 29 years are used for this comparison. DXA reports also include a Z-score, which indicates the number of standard deviations an individual's BMD differs from mean values for individuals of the same age, sex and (if normative data available) ethnicity. Z-scores are sometimes adjusted for weight as well, so for correct interpretation one needs to check what factors have been included when making the adjustment.

Osteoporosis is defined as a T-score of –2.5 or less at the femoral neck, total proximal femur or the lumbar spine and 'low bone density' or osteopenia is defined as a T-score less than –1 at these sites. Clinical implications of T-scores should be considered carefully. They provide an indication of fracture risk, but factors such as age are also strong determinants. Z-scores also provide useful information. If a Z-score is lower than –2, the BMD is lower than 'normal' (±2 standard deviation) for an age and sex matched population, so investigation of potential causes may be warranted.

While this patient does have osteoporosis, which increases her risk of fracture, her lumbar spine Z-score (adjusted for age, sex and ethnicity) is within the 'normal' range (i.e. within 2 standard deviations of the population mean).

Controversy abounds regarding the interpretation of BMD in patients with CKD and after transplantation, because in addition to low bone mass, the bone may have other mineralising and structural abnormalities.

Question 4

What is the effect of dialysis or transplantation on rates of fracture?
(a) Fracture is more common in both.
(b) Fracture rates return to the population mean after transplantation.
(c) Rates after kidney-pancreas transplantation are higher than after kidney transplantation.
(d) Bone mineral density falls but fracture rates do not increase.

Answer
A and C

Explanation

Properties of bone that influence the likelihood of fracture include BMD and bone quality; defined by the National Institute of Health as 'the material, architectural and mechanical characteristics of bone, which in addition to bone mass, contribute to bone strength'.

The mineral disturbances of CKD, which result in abnormal bone turnover and mineralisation, impact on bone quality and microarchitecture as well as on bone mass. Of the immunosuppressive drugs used after transplantation, glucocorticoids in particular cause bone mineral density to fall. These bone changes increase fracture risk, both before and after transplantation.

Fracture risk in patients with CKD is also related to factors that influence risk in the general population. These include: older age, Caucasian race, female sex, male or female hypogonadism (which is common in poorly nourished, under-weight or unwell patients and when high-dose glucocorticoids are used) and any history of pre-existing low trauma fracture. In addition, patients with CKD often have a metabolic acidosis or are exposed to medications such as loop diuretics and heparin, which can adversely affect bone. Fracture risk has been associated with a longer duration of dialysis and the presence of diabetes and peripheral vascular disease. These are often associated with peripheral neuropathy, reduced visual acuity and postural instability, which increase the risk of falls.

Patients with CKD are at increased risk for fracture. Prevalent vertebral fracture is found in up to 21% of patients and the relative risk of hip fracture is increased between two- and fourteenfold. Furthermore, patients on dialysis who fracture a hip have a twofold increase in mortality compared to the general population.

The fracture risk after kidney transplantation exceeds that of patients on haemodialysis and is around four times that of the general population. The annual rate of hip fracture after transplantation is 3.3 fractures/1000 patients. After kidney–pancreas transplantation, rates are higher still and several years after transplantation a fracture prevalence of 26 to 49% has been reported.

LEVEL B

Question 5

What form of renal osteodystrophy did this patient have when she was undergoing dialysis?

(a) Adynamic bone disease due to aluminium, calcium and calcitriol exposure

(b) Hyperparathyroid bone disease

(c) Osteomalacia due to 25-hydroxyvitamin D deficiency

(d) Cannot tell

Answer

D

Explanation

The term renal osteodystrophy (ROD) has been used to describe clinically and histologically diagnosed bone disease in patients with CKD. Recently it was decided to restrict the term to renal bone disease diagnosed by bone biopsy. This decision was taken because clinical diagnosis is often inaccurate, and in the hope that research results might become more standardised and therefore comparable.

As well as providing information on numbers of osteoclasts and osteoblasts in bone, the bone volume and amount of osteoid present, bone biopsies can provide information on the rate of bone formation and resorption. Prior to a bone biopsy the patient is asked to take tetracycline on two occasions, separated by a number of days. Tetracycline is deposited at the bone mineralisation front and can be viewed under ultraviolet light. Two distinct lines of tetracycline should be deposited, and the distance between these indicates the rate of bone mineralisation over the days between tetracycline doses. Absent or blurred tetracycline deposition indicates mineralisation was abnormal.

ROD is described in terms of bone turnover (T), mineralisation (M) and bone volume (V) as shown in the three-dimensional histogram shown in Figure 13.3.

The spectrum of bone turnover ranges from absent or 'adynamic bone disease' (AD), to low turnover (not illustrated), to mild hyperparathyroidism (mild HPT) through to severe hyperparathyroidism with increased fibroblasts in the bone marrow, also called osteofibrosis (OF). When mineralisation is abnormal, unmineralised osteoid is increased and there is abnormal tetracycline labelling (osteomalacia [OM]). The coexistence of abnormal mineralisation and hyperparathyroidism is termed mixed uraemic osteodystrophy (MUO). Bone volume varies with CKD-related factors as well as factors that predispose to osteoporosis in the general population.

In absence of a bone biopsy the patient cannot be classified as having a particular form of ROD, but there are clues to her possible bone pathology lurking in the history and laboratory findings:

1. Glucocorticoid exposure prior to dialysis would predispose to low bone mass.
2. 25-Hydroxyvitamin D deficiency would predispose to low bone mass and abnormal mineralisation.
3. Aluminium exposure would predispose to abnormal mineralisation.
4. Elevated levels of PTH would predispose to high bone turnover. The elevated ALP level would support this.

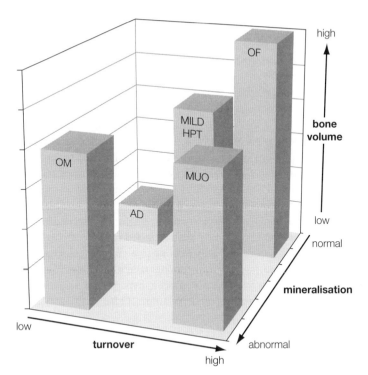

Figure 13.3 Proposed Kidney Disease Improving Global Outcomes (KDIGO) classification of bone histomorphometry

Source: Moe 2006

So a 'best guess' would be that she has mixed uraemic osteodystrophy with reduced bone volume.

Question 6

What caused the painful nodules that developed on the patient's thigh? How is this condition managed?

(a) Vasculitis

(b) Kaposi sarcoma

(c) Erythema nodosum

(d) Calciphylaxis

Answer

D

Explanation

In 1898, Bryant and White first reported features of the condition now termed calciphylaxis or calcific uraemic arteriolopathy. This condition is characterised by medial calcification of small cutaneous arteries, venules and arterioles, with intimal proliferation, fibrosis and thrombosis. These features result in ischaemia, necrosis and superinfection of the skin and subcutis. The condition is rarely seen when renal function is normal, but among patients on dialysis the incidence is estimated to be 1 to 4% annually. A possible recent increase may reflect the increased use of calcium-based phosphate binders. Dialysis patients with calciphylaxis have an overall eightfold increase in mortality (approximately 30% for non-ulcerating and 80% for ulcerating types) with most deaths within 6 months of the condition developing.

Calciphylaxis is usually a complication of uncontrolled secondary hyperparathyroidism. Nevertheless, cases have been reported in association with low bone turnover due to a loss of the capacity of bone to buffer physiological increases in levels of serum calcium and phosphate. The patient had a number of potential trigger factors including hyperparathyroidism, hyperphosphataemia, an elevated calcium phosphate product and the use of warfarin. Other factors that predispose to calciphylaxis include trauma, hypoalbuminaemia and functionally impaired protein C or S activity. These predisposing factors share a common ability to alter the balance between promotion and inhibition of calcification (as discussed in Case 12, Level C, Question 10). Obesity, diabetes, the use of iron dextran, aluminium and calcitriol have been associated with calciphylaxis, but may not be independent predictors.

Treatment of calciphylaxis requires optimal control of calcium and phosphate balance through intensified dialysis, the use of non-calcium-containing phosphate binders and possibly the use of bisphosphonates to reduce calcium and phosphate release from bone. Bisphosphonates may also act within blood vessel walls to reduce the progression of calcification. Etidronate is the oldest bisphosphonate still in clinical use and lacks the osteoclast-disrupting potency of newer amino bisphosphonates, so high doses have been used to treat osteoporosis and Paget's disease where the aim is to reduce osteoclastic resorption of bone. At high doses, etidronate also causes osteomalacia (reduced bone mineralisation), because it binds tightly to mineral crystals and by covering them up, stops their growth. This characteristic can be exploited in patients with calciphylaxis. When etidronate binds to mineral crystals within the blood vessel walls, it can reduce their growth. Recently the calcimimetic cinacalcet HCl has been used when calciphylaxis is associated with hyperparathyroidism. Sodium thiosulphate has also been advocated for calciphylaxis. Given intravenously after dialysis, sodium thiosulphate appears to dissolve precipitated calcium salts in vessels, due to a high solubility product; 250- to 100 000-fold greater than that of other calcium salts. The half-life of sodium thiosulphate is greatly increased in CKD with excretion predominantly by the biliary route.

Question 7

How do glucocorticoids influence bone turnover and bone mineral density after transplantation?

(a) By reducing the level of sex steroids
(b) By reducing osteoblastic bone formation
(c) By increasing urinary calcium excretion
(d) By reducing gastrointestinal calcium uptake

Answer

All are correct

Explanation

Glucocorticoids influence bone metabolism directly by affecting the tightly coupled balance of bone formation and resorption and indirectly by affecting calcium balance and bone active hormones. BMD often falls following glucocorticoid treatment, particularly in areas of trabecular (cancellous) bone such as the spine. Paired bone biopsies collected at transplantation and after 6 months show reductions in bone formation rates of up to 50%. Even low-dose glucocorticoids are associated with an increased risk of BMD loss and fracture.

Loss of BMD is usually most rapid in the first 6 to 12 post-transplant months when protocols often include higher glucocorticoid doses. Glucocorticoids inhibit osteoblast replication and differentiation and increase osteoblast apoptosis, and early BMD loss is caused predominantly by reduced osteoblastic activity. However, glucocorticoids also activate osteoclasts by increasing osteoblast production of RANK ligand (RANK-L, a potent osteoclast activator) and reducing the production of osteoprotegerin (OPG, a decoy receptor for RANK-L) (see Fig. 13.4).

Glucocorticoids reduce calcium absorption from the gastrointestinal tract (by opposing the action of vitamin D) and inhibit renal tubular calcium reabsorption, resulting in negative calcium balance. This may exacerbate hyperparathyroidism and bone resorption. Acting at the hypothalamus, glucocorticoids reduce secretion of gonadotrophins and hence sex steroids, which also favours bone resorption. Growth hormone secretion can be blunted, leading to a reduction of insulin-like growth factor-I transcription in osteoblasts. Reduced proximal muscle strength caused by catabolic effects of glucocorticoids on muscle may also contribute to fracture risk, because muscle weakness increases the likelihood of falls.

Of course, post-transplantation loss of BMD or fracture reflects processes in addition to glucocorticoid treatment. Most patients have pre-existing renal osteodystrophy, patients may have persisting hyperparathyroidism and 25(OH)D deficiency, and the use of calcineurin inhibitors also influences bone turnover.

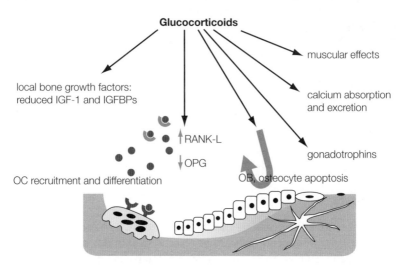

Figure 13.4 Glucocorticoid effects on bone

Question 8

What investigations would assist in establishing a cause for the rib and vertebral fracture and how might treatment be monitored?

(a) The iPTH level indicates high bone turnover is the cause.

(b) A radionuclide bone scan would indicate whether hyperparathyroidism is the cause.

(c) Bone densitometry should be repeated within 6 months to assess responses to therapy.

(d) Bone turnover markers assist in monitoring therapy.

Answer

D

Explanation

The patient's rib fracture, which has probably resulted from coughing, is a 'low trauma' fracture or 'fragility' fracture. This implies an abnormality of the underlying bone: probably a combination of low bone mass and abnormal bone quality, which would also predispose to vertebral fracture. While we cannot be sure from the history when these fractures occurred, increased uptake on an isotopic bone scan is consistent with a recent fracture (within approximately 6 months). However, bone scans are not particularly helpful in assessing ROD.

After assessing the history for risk factors, baseline investigations generally include a biochemical profile, PTH and 25(OH)D levels, lateral X-ray of the thoracic and lumbar spine and bone densitometry (DXA). If there is a family history of coeliac disease or a history suggestive of malabsorption, serum antibodies (antigliaden, endomysial or transglutaminase antibodies) should be checked. These assays assess IgA antibody levels, so a serum IgA level should be requested to exclude IgA deficiency. If non-renal pathology such as multiple myeloma is suspected, a serum and urine protein immunoelectrophoretogram should be requested. Intact-PTH levels give some indication of underlying bone histomorphology, but are not sufficiently sensitive or specific to be certain of the diagnosis.

Although in situations of very rapid bone loss, DXA examinations may be performed at intervals of 6 months, DXA examinations are generally performed every 1 to 2 years. The *average* precision of BMD measurements is around 2% at the spine and 5% at the hip, but the *range* of results is rarely reported. In fact, for an individual patient, a change between measurements of around 3% at the spine and 7% at the hip may be needed to detect truly significant changes between consecutive studies.

Bone turnover markers are products of osteoblasts or osteoclasts or result from bone matrix formation and removal. Their value is unclear in CKD, and apart from ALP and its bone-specific isoenzyme, most available markers are influenced by renal function, making interpretation difficult. For markers not affected by renal function, their correlation to bone histology is largely unproven. However, after transplantation, serum and urine bone turnover markers may be useful. It is preferable to check markers before therapy and then sequentially, in order to assess biochemical responses to therapy.

LEVEL C

Question 9

Which of the following statements is/are incorrect regarding parathyroidectomy and the patient?

(a) Parathyroidectomy was justified when she developed calciphylaxis.

(b) Parathyroidectomy was not justified due to surgical risk and recurrence rates.

(c) When she commenced dialysis, parathyroidectomy should have been considered after a trial of calcimimetic therapy.

(d) Biochemical and patient level outcomes are achieved by parathyroidectomy but only biochemical improvements are proven for calcimimetic therapy.

Answer

A, C and D

Explanation

Most patients undergoing dialysis have elevated iPTH levels, but the correlation of iPTH and bone turnover is rather poor. Bone turnover can be normal, increased or even reduced at iPTH levels up to around 50 nmol/L, although for iPTH levels >50 nmol/L bone turnover is generally increased. Hypercalcaemia and hyperphosphataemia often accompany elevated PTH levels and using standard vitamin D and calcium-based phosphate binder therapy, less than 10% of patients achieve targets for calcium, phosphate, the calcium phosphate product or iPTH that are suggested by biochemical guidelines. This has implications not just for bone, but for the development of cardiovascular disease. Numerous studies report increased relative risk for cardiovascular and all cause mortality when iPTH levels exceed 50 to 64 pmol/L and when calcium or phosphate levels exceed their target ranges.

Traditionally, parathyroidectomy has been the treatment of choice for severe hyperparathyroidism. However, the introduction of cinacalcet HCl has led to a re-evaluation of surgery. Cinacalcet is a calcimimetic, a synthetic small organic compound that binds to the transmembrane region of the parathyroid calcium-sensing receptor and increases its sensitivity to extracellular ionised calcium levels. This shifts the calcium set-point of PTH to the left and results in reduced levels of PTH for any given calcium level. By reducing PTH and bone turnover, levels of calcium and phosphate also improve towards the target range in many patients with mild to moderate secondary hyperparathyroidism and a smaller proportion of patients with severe hyperparathyroidism. There is some evidence for a reduction in fracture risk and certainly for risk of parathyroidectomy in patients treated with cinacalcet, but the effect of cinacalcet on other patient level outcomes, specifically mortality and cardiovascular risk, is currently unproven.

There is no doubt that parathyroidectomy is effective, despite relatively high recurrence rates up to 22% and postoperative hypoparathyroidism in some patients. Biochemical indices show sustained improvement up to 5 years from surgery, and despite an early increase in mortality, longer-term follow-up suggests reduced mortality compared to matched, medically (but not cinacalcet) treated controls. Patients often require high doses of calcium and calcitriol after parathyroidectomy but vascular calcification has been reported to remain stable or regress in patients who maintain a calcium phosphate product <4.2 mmol²/L². Improved levels of haemoglobin, reduced use of epoetin and improved quality of life have also been reported.

Based on these data it seems reasonable to propose a therapeutic trial of cinacalcet HCl prior to consideration of surgery if patients have iPTH levels >50 pmol/L and when standard medical management is complicated by hypercalcaemia or hyperphosphataemia. Patients who are medically unfit for surgery should also have access to cinacalcet. Prospective studies are underway that should provide data on patient-level outcomes, which are needed to assess the efficacy of cinacalcet plus standard therapy versus parathyroidectomy. When iPTH levels exceed 85 to 95 pmol/L, cinacalcet therapy is often unsuccessful in achieving adequate biochemical responses. For these patients parathyroidectomy is likely to remain an effective, long-term and relatively low-cost treatment.

Question 10

Which of the following statements is/are correct in relation to the elevated aluminium level?

(a) Aluminium-related bone disease is likely.

(b) The level reflects recent aluminium ingestion.

(c) A desferrioxamine (DFO) test or bone biopsy is mandatory.

(d) Stop aluminium-containing phosphate binders and treat with DFO.

Answer

B

Explanation

Despite serious toxicity resulting from the use of Al-containing phosphate binders over the past decades, these drugs continue to be used. Often this is because calcium-based phosphate binders have caused hypercalcaemia, and in Australia neither of the non-aluminium, non-calcium containing alternatives (sevelamer and lanthanum) was funded by the Pharmaceutical Benefits Scheme until December 2007.

Levels of plasma Al reflect recent exposure but are unreliable for diagnosing Al-related bone disease. Nevertheless, routine screening at yearly or half-yearly intervals can be justified, because elevated levels, indicating continued exposure, may identify patients at risk of toxicity. When evaluating patients receiving intravenous iron supplements, Al overload can occur despite normal plasma aluminium levels when the transferrin saturation is >60%.

The range for Al that is generally not associated with toxicity in CKD is <2.2 μmol/L. The patient's level is 2.7 μmol/L, so should she have a DFO challenge? Responses to the DFO challenge are a guide to the likely risk of Al-related bone disease and the need for a bone biopsy. When Al levels are <2.2 μmol/L, a DFO challenge is unnecessary unless Al-related low bone turnover, osteomalacia, neurological disease or anaemia due to Al is strongly suspected. For a plasma Al level from 2.2 to 3.7 μmol/L, the Al source should be identified. For this patient the source was likely to be Al-containing phosphate binders, which were withdrawn. It would be reasonable to postpone a DFO challenge but repeat the plasma Al in a further 6 months. For plasma Al levels >3.7 μmol/L the risk of Al-related disease is increased and a DFO challenge should generally be performed. For very high Al levels, the test should be withheld until the plasma Al is <4.5 μmol/L. Until then, potential sources of Al exposure (drugs and dialysate) should be withdrawn. Daily high-flux dialysis should be considered if Al levels exceed 7.4 μmol/L.

When a DFO challenge is performed, low-dose DFO is used to avoid adverse reactions. The plasma Al is measured prior to the commencement of dialysis (pre) and 5 mg/kg of DFO is given intravenously during the last hour of dialysis. The plasma Al is then measured prior to the next haemodialysis 2 days later (post). The test is positive if the increment in Al is >2 μmol/L and highly positive when the rise is >11 μmol/L. The reliability of a positive DFO test is improved when the iPTH level is below the normal target range for iPTH; approximately 85% of such patients will have Al-related adynamic bone disease.

A confirmatory bone biopsy should be performed after a positive DFO test. If Al deposition is considered positive (staining over 15 to 25% of the bone surface) and the bone formation rate/bone surface and mineral apposition rates are reduced, a course of treatment with DFO should be commenced.

Question 11

What are the possible explanations for the patient's tibial pain 6 weeks after transplantation?

(a) Stress fracture
(b) Hyperparathyroid bone disease
(c) Avascular necrosis
(d) Calcineurin-inhibitor-induced pain syndrome

Answer

D most likely

Explanation

Musculoskeletal pain is reported by 19 to 35% of patients after renal transplantation. Causes include gout, hyperparathyroidism, osteonecrosis and osteoporosis with fragility fracture. However, the symmetrical pain experienced by the patient in weight-bearing areas of the lower limbs is likely to be due to the calcineurin-inhibitor-induced pain syndrome (CIPS), also called the symmetric bone pain syndrome. Between 1 and 17% of patients describe symptoms of this condition varying from deep, aching rest pain to the sudden onset of severe, symmetrical, periarticular bone pain particularly in the feet, ankles and knees. CIPS generally occurs within the first post-transplant month and resolves within 3 months, but has occasionally been described to occur up to 14 months post-transplant with resolution over periods up to 18 months. CIPS is more common with cyclosporin than with tacrolimus and has not been reported when calcineurin-inhibitors are used to treat autoimmune disorders, possibly because higher drug doses are used for transplantation.

An important differential diagnosis of CIPS is osteonecrosis, also known as avascular necrosis or aseptic necrosis. This condition most commonly affects the femoral head followed by other weight-bearing long bones, and is particularly devastating because it often progresses to fracture and bony collapse of the articular surface. The median time from transplantation until the onset of symptoms at around 18 months is longer than CIPS and patients generally complain of unilateral hip pain with limitation of weight bearing and movement. The incidence after transplantation of 2.8 to 16% may be decreasing because lower glucocorticoid doses are used in newer immunosuppressive regimens.

The diagnosis of CIPS is generally confirmed by magnetic resonance imaging (MRI) or by radionuclide bone scan that identifies areas of hyperaemia and marrow oedema, often associated with soft tissue swelling and joint effusions. Pain may be associated with higher trough levels of cyclosporin or tacrolimus and improves as marrow oedema declines. Although the mechanism is unconfirmed, calcineurin inhibitors may cause bone pain and increase the risk of osteonecrosis by inducing vasoconstriction, leading to intraosseous venous thrombosis and marrow oedema.

Treatment should be considered against the background that CIPS generally improves over 2 to 4 months with conservative management. Simple measures include elevation of the feet and calcium channel blockers may relieve pain. Dosage reduction or withdrawal of calcineurin inhibitors can be considered and may improve symptoms. Core decompression is invasive and used infrequently, although it is reported to be effective for pain reduction.

Question 12

Which statement/s is/are correct concerning therapies to maintain bone strength and reduce fracture risk after transplantation?

(a) Prophylaxis is unnecessary with modern immunosuppressive regimens.

(b) A calcimimetic is indicated when persisting hyperparathyroidism is present.

(c) All patients should be given bisphosphonate therapy at the time of transplantation.

(d) Calcium and cholecalciferol/ergocalciferol are mandatory for all patients.

Answer

All are incorrect

Explanation

BMD falls in most patients after transplantation, but patients with lower initial BMD or severe ROD are likely to be at highest fracture risk. Therefore, prophylaxis against loss of BMD should always be considered after renal transplantation. Cinacalcet has not been proven to influence BMD in patients with secondary hyperparathyroidism after renal transplantation and cannot be recommended at present. Calcium and vitamin D supplementation is advised in all management guidelines for patients treated with glucocorticoids, but will not be suitable for some renal transplant recipients with hypercalcaemia or hypophosphataemia. Although an advantage of activated vitamin D over cholecalciferol or ergocalciferol has been reported, few studies have compared these therapies.

In a Cochrane analysis of bone therapies after renal transplantation, bisphosphonates and vitamin D analogues protected against BMD loss at the lumbar spine and the hip, with bisphosphonates appearing to be more efficacious. Bisphosphonates are reported to maintain or improve BMD at 1 year from transplantation, but at 3 to 4 years the benefits of bisphosphonate therapy are controversial and the optimal length of treatment is unclear. Studies have included oral and intravenous bisphosphonates in a variety of dosing regimens. The use of potent bisphosphonates is of some concern for patients with pre-transplant low bone turnover, or adynamic bone. On the other hand, bisphosphonates' inhibition of osteoclastic bone resorption far exceeds effects on osteoblasts and bisphosphonates may improve osteoblast survival. Although there are few reports of adynamic bone disease resulting from post-transplant bisphosphonate therapy it seems prudent to allocate patients with lower BMD, higher bone turnover and additional risk factors to bisphosphonate therapy and others to calcitriol and calcium as tolerated. All patients at risk of fracture should be encouraged to participate in weight-bearing exercise, maintain a low alcohol intake and avoid smoking. Physiotherapy to reduce the risk of falls should be considered if patients have postural instability.

Bibliography

Level A

1. Leslie, W.D., Adler, R.A., El-Hajj Fuleihan, G., Hodsman, A., Kendler, D.L., McClung, M., Miller, P.D. & Watts, N.B. (2006) Application of the 1994 WHO Classification to Populations Other Than Postmenopausal Caucasian Women: The 2005 ISCD Official Positions. J Clin Densitom. 9(1), 22–30.

Level B

2. Moe, S.M., Drueke, T.M., Cunningham, J., Goodman, W., Martin, K., Olgaard, K., Ott, S., Sprague, S., Lameire, N. & Eknoyan, G. (2006) Definition, evaluation, and classification of renal osteodystrophy: a position statement from Kidney Disease: Improving Global Outcomes (KDIGO). Kidney Int. 69, 1945–53.
3. K/DOQI: Kidney Disease Outcomes Quality Initiative. (2003) Am J Kid Dis. 42(4), supp. 3.
4. Harris, D., Elder, G., Kairaitis, L. & Rangan, G. (eds) (2005) Basic Clinical Dialysis. Sydney: McGraw-Hill.

Level C

5. Cunningham, J., Danese, M., Olson, K., Klassen, P. & Chertow, G.M. (2005) Effects of the calcimimetic cinacalcet HCl on cardiovascular disease, fracture, and health-related quality of life in secondary hyperparathyroidism. Kidney Int. 68(4), 1793–800.
6. Strippoli, G.F., Palmer, S., Tong, A., Elder, G., Messa, P., Craig, J.C. (2006) Meta-analysis of biochemical and patient-level effects of calcimimetic therapy. Am J Kidney Dis. 47(5), 715–26.
7. Elder, G.J. (2005) Parathyroidectomy in the calcimimetic era. Nephrology (Carlton). 10(5), 511–15.
8. Curtis, J.R. & Saag, K.G. (2007) Prevention and treatment of glucocorticoid-induced osteoporosis. Curr Osteoporos Rep. 5(1), 14–21.

9. D'Haese, P.C., Couttenye, M.M. & De Broe, M.E. (1996) Diagnosis and treatment of aluminium bone disease. Nephrol Dial Transplant. 11, Supp. 3, 74–9.
10. Elder, G.J. (2006) From marrow oedema to osteonecrosis: common paths in the development of post-transplant bone pain. Nephrology (Carlton). 11(6), 560–7.
11. Fan, S.L., Kumar, S. & Cunningham, J. (2003) Long-term effects on bone mineral density of pamidronate given at the time of renal transplantation. Kidney Int. 63(6), 2275–9.
12. Palmer, S.C., Strippoli, G.F. & McGregor, D.O. (2005) Interventions for preventing bone disease in kidney transplant recipients: a systematic review of randomized controlled trials. Am J Kidney Dis. 45(4), 638–49.
13. Schwarz, C., Mitterbauer, C., Heinze, G., Woloszczuk, W., Haas, M. & Oberbauer, R. (2004) Nonsustained effect of short-term bisphosphonate therapy on bone turnover three years after renal transplantation. Kidney Int. 65(1), 304–9.

Case 14
Renal vascular disease

JOHN KELLY

Case history

A 62-year-old woman is admitted to the surgical wards for peripheral angiography. She has a 6-month history of bilateral claudication pain, with a stable claudication distance of 150 metres. She has an 8-year history of hypertension, which had previously been well-controlled by a thiazide diuretic (chlorthalidone 25 mg/day) with average blood pressure (BP) readings of 132/82 mmHg in the last 12 months. She has a 40 pack-year history of cigarette smoking. Her other significant medical history is of treated hypercholesterolaemia (simvastatin 40 mg/day) and asthma. There is a family history of hypertension in both parents and one sibling. Her height is 180 cm and weight is 72 kg. Her pulse is 78/min and BP is 174/98 mmHg. There is a left carotid bruit. There are no abdominal or femoral artery bruits; however pedal pulses are absent. Urinalysis reveals protein 2+ and is negative for haematuria.

Routine investigations reveal the following.

Laboratory data

	Result	Reference range
Na^+	139 mmol/L	(136–146)
K^+	4.3 mmol/L	(3.6–5.2)
HCO_3^-	22 mmol/l	(24–31)
Urea	9.6 mmol/l	(2.5–6.5)
Creatinine	155 µmol/L	(45–90)
Glucose	5.7 mmol/L	(4.0–5.5)

Question 1

After reviewing these results, the on-call medical registrar should advise that:
(a) angiography should proceed without further delay
(b) the patient should receive intravenous hydrocortisone prior to angiography

(c) the patient should receive oral indomethacin prior to angiography

(d) the patient should be hydrated with intravenous fluids prior to angiography.

Answer

D

Explanation

The patient has significant chronic kidney disease (CKD) with an estimated glomerular filtration rate (eGFR) of 43 mL/min. Patients with a GFR <60 mL/min have an increased risk of contrast-induced nephropathy, particularly if the volume of contrast infused is >150 mL (answer A incorrect). The mechanisms of contrast toxicity may include intrarenal vasoconstriction or tubular injury due to release of vasoactive compounds or due to osmotic or oxidative stress. Evidence-based reviews of interventions which reduce the risk of contrast-induced nephropathy support the role of periprocedural hydration with isotonic saline or an isotonic sodium bicarbonate solution (answer D correct). Meta-analysis of studies examining the role of acetylcysteine variably report either no or an additional benefit of this medication compared to hydration. Prophylactic steroid therapy does not confer protection against contrast-induced nephropathy (answer B incorrect). Non-steroidal anti-inflammatory drugs (NSAIDs) and COX-2 inhibitors are nephrotoxic and should be avoided in CKD, and will potentially augment the nephrotoxic effects of contrast (answer C incorrect). Other measures which may reduce the risk of contrast-induced nephropathy include the use of non-ionic contrast, minimising the volume of contrast used or using non-iodinated contrast agents such as CO_2.

 Clinical pearls

- Patients with pre-existing renal impairment, volume depletion, congestive cardiac failure, diabetes and myeloma are at risk of contrast-induced nephropathy.
- The risk of contrast-induced nephropathy substantially increases when a patient's GFR is <60 mL/min, or when the volume of contrast infused is >150 mL.
- Periprocedural intravenous hydration is an integral component of the prevention of contrast-induced nephropathy.

Case history continued ...

The patient undergoes a right-femoropopliteal bypass. A calcium antagonist (verapamil 240 mg/day) is added to her pre-existing antihypertensive therapy.

She is reviewed in medical outpatients one month later at which time her BP is 168/92 mmHg. Grade 2 hypertensive retinopathy is evident on fundal examination. Urine microscopy shows no evidence of haematuria, hyaline or cellular casts. Her 12-lead echocardiograph shows evidence of left ventricular hypertrophy (LVH) by voltage criteria.

Biochemical tests of the patient's blood reveal the following.

Na^+	138 mmol/L	(136–146)
K^+	4.7 mmol/L	(3.6–5.2)
HCO_3^-	25 mmol/l	(24–31)
Urea	12.1 mmol/l	(2.5–6.5)
Creatinine	145 µmol/L	(45–90)
Albumin	37 g/L	(36–46)
Protein	67 g/L	(60–85)

A 24-hour urine test reveals a protein level of 0.9 g/day (reference range is 0–0.15).

Question 2

The patient's presentation with hypertension and renal impairment may be best explained by:

(a) renovascular disease

(b) white coat hypertension

(c) membranous glomerulonephritis

(d) essential hypertension.

Answer

A and D

Explanation

The age of initial onset of hypertension and positive family history is consistent with pre-existing essential hypertension (answer D correct). The recent deterioration in BP control should raise the suspicion of a superimposed secondary form of hypertension. In the context of a history of hypercholesterolaemia and smoking, physical findings of being non-obese and having peripheral vascular disease and CKD, the recent increase in BP is highly predictive of renal artery stenosis (answer A correct). White coat hypertension is more common with advancing age; however, the presence of hypertensive target organ damage (retinopathy, LVH and widespread atherosclerosis) argues against this diagnosis (answer B incorrect). Reduced GFR and proteinuria suggest the presence of renal parenchymal disease. Membranous glomerulonephritis usually causes features of nephrotic syndrome such as proteinuria >3.5 g/24 hours, hypoalbuminaemia or oedema (answer C incorrect). Atherosclerotic renal artery disease is often associated with parenchymal changes (arteriolosclerosis, glomerular sclerosis, interstitial fibrosis) which are associated with modest degrees of proteinuria.

 Clinical pearls

- Renal artery stenosis should be considered in patients with recent onset hypertension or deterioration in BP control, who have evidence of vascular disease in other territories and a GFR <60 mL/min.
- Atherosclerotic renal artery stenosis may be associated with intrarenal microvascular and parenchymal changes which result in moderate proteinuria (up to 2 g/24 hours) or reduced GFR.

LEVEL B

Case history continued ...

At the patient's initial outpatient review an ACE inhibitor (ACEi) (ramipril 2.5 mg/day) is commenced. She returns for review 1 month later at which time her BP is 154/88 mmHg. Further investigations include a renal ultrasound which reveals the right kidney is 10.3 cm in length and left kidney 9.0 cm in length.

Repeat biochemistry results of her blood are as follows.

Na^+	138 mmol/L	(136–146)
K^+	5.0 mmol/L	(3.6–5.2)
HCO_3^-	25 mmol/l	(24–31)
Urea	12.1 mmol/l	(2.5–6.5)
Creatinine	170 µmol/L	(45–90)
Albumin	37 g/L	(36–46)
Protein	67 g/L	(60–85)

A 24-hour urine test reveals a protein level of 0.8 g/day (reference range is 0-0.15).

Question 3

You decide to further investigate the patient. Which of the following investigations would you organise?

(a) Duplex Doppler of renal artery
(b) Computerised tomography renal angiogram (CTRA) with appropriate contrast prophylaxis
(c) Radionuclide renal perfusion scan with and without captopril
(d) Magnetic resonance angiogram (MRA) of the renal arteries

Answer

B or D

Explanation

The asymmetrical renal size supports the clinical suspicion of renovascular disease. A recent meta-analysis of these investigations compared to angiography suggests that both CTRA and MRA have a sensitivity and specificity of greater than 90% (answers B and D correct). The current generation of CT scanners (16-slice or greater) provide high-resolution reconstruction of the renal arteries, and allow visualisation of the abdominal aorta, renal artery walls and lumens. CTRA has the disadvantage of requiring contrast prophylaxis for CKD patients. MRA has the advantage of utilising gadolinium which is less nephrotoxic than iodinated contrast. However, access to MRA may be limited by cost or geographic location. Radionuclide scanning and duplex Doppler ultrasonography have sensitivity and specificity of about 50 to 60%, which is equivalent to the reported predictive value of a structured clinical assessment (answers A and C incorrect). Duplex Doppler ultrasonography is an operator-dependent technique and visualisation of the renal arteries can be obscured by abdominal obesity or bowel gas in up to 15% of patients.

Question 4

In order to improve the control of the patient's hypertension you should decide to:

(a) withdraw the ACEi because of the increase in serum creatinine
(b) change the ACEi to an angiotensin receptor blocker (ARB)
(c) increase the dose of ACEi and continue to monitor the patient
(d) add a beta-blocker to the patient's treatment.

Answer

C

Explanation

ACEis and ARBs are very effective agents in treating hypertension associated with renal artery stenosis. There is no evidence that one class has an advantage over the other (answer B incorrect). It is common to observe an initial 20 to 30% increase in serum creatinine following introduction of an ACEi or ARB followed by stabilisation of renal function. A progressive decline in GFR resulting in acute renal failure only occurs in about 10 to 20% of patients with bilateral renal artery stenosis. It is reasonable to continue ACEi/ARB treatment provided the patient's renal function is monitored closely and is stable (answer A incorrect, answer C correct). Hyperkalaemia is a potential complication of ACEi or ARB therapy in renal impairment. If the patient's electrolytes are monitored appropriately, measures such as dietary potassium restriction or the use of ion-exchange resins can address this problem. The selection of other antihypertensive classes is principally dictated by the patient's comorbidity and other therapy. In this case, the presence of asthma is a relative contraindication to beta-blockers and there is a potential interaction with verapamil in causing negative inotropic and chronotropic effects (answer D incorrect).

 Clinical pearls

- ACEi and ARB are effective agents in the treatment of hypertension associated with renal artery stenosis. Electrolytes and renal function need to be monitored at regular intervals to ensure the safety of these medications.
- An initial increase in serum creatinine concentration of up to 20% that then stabilises is not a contraindication to the continuation of ACEi/ARB.
- ACEi/ARB should be discontinued if the rise in serum creatinine is >20% or if the repeat value shows a progressive increase.
- If the serum potassium concentration increases to a value of >5.5 mmol/L despite precautions (low-potassium diet, ion-exchange resins) then another class of antihypertensive agent is required.

Case history continued ...

Following appropriate screening tests, renal angiography confirms the presence of an ectatic abdominal aorta and an 80% atherosclerotic stenosis near the origin of the left renal artery.

Question 5

The severity of the patient's renal artery stenosis:
(a) determines the potential risk of occlusion of the affected renal artery
(b) is the major determinant of the patient's GFR

(c)   is the major factor determining the patient's long-term risk of end-stage renal failure

(d)   is the major factor which determines the patient's risk of death.

Answer
A

Explanation

Prospective angiographic and ultrasound studies of the natural history of renal artery stenosis indicate that renal artery occlusion predominantly occurs in vessels which have >60% stenosis at the baseline examination (answer A correct). There is no relationship between the severity of renal artery stenosis and GFR (answer B incorrect). Baseline GFR, rather than the severity of the stenosis, is the major determinant of patient and renal survival (answers C and D incorrect).

Clinical pearls

- The severity of the patient's renal disease is a strong predictor of renal artery occlusion. In vessels with >60% stenosis, the 2-year risk of occlusion is 10%.
- In atherosclerotic renal artery stenosis, patient and renal survival are predicted by renal function rather than by the severity of the stenosis.

LEVEL C

Case history continued . . .

At the next clinical review, the patient has persistent hypertension with a BP of 160/80 mmHg despite treatment with maximal doses of antihypertensive therapy, with the treatment regimen including one agent which blocks the renin–angiotensin system. You discuss the option of treating the patient's renal artery stenosis by means of angioplasty and placement of a renal artery stent.

Question 6

In this discussion, you should inform the patient that renal angioplasty and stent placement is likely to:

(a)   substantially improve her BP control

(b)   result in a reduction in her requirement for antihypertensive medications

(c) significantly improve her renal function

(d) provide more than a 70% chance of the renal artery remaining patent 12 months after the procedure.

Answer

B and D

Explanation

There are many anecdotal reports suggesting the efficacy of renal revascularisation in improving BP control and renal function. However, randomised controlled studies provide a more restrained view of the benefits of this procedure. A high restenosis rate is reported in patients with atherosclerotic renal artery stenosis treated by angioplasty alone. However, 12-month patency rates of about 75% have been reported in patients treated by renal angioplasty and stenting (answer D correct). A meta-analysis of the three randomised controlled trials (RCTs) comparing angioplasty to medical therapy suggests that the average BP reduction following angioplasty is a 6 mmHg reduction in systolic and a 3 mmHg reduction in diastolic BP (answer A incorrect). While this reduction in BP may be evident at 3 months post-procedure, it may not be sustained in the long term. Short-term reductions in daily dose of medications required to control BP have been reported (answer B correct). No long-term significant differences in renal function have been reported after angioplasty (answer C incorrect). Procedural risks which include bruising, bleeding or pseudoaneurysm at the arterial puncture site, renal artery occlusion, branch dissection, stent migration, or haemorrhage have been reported in up to 6% of some case series.

At present, the total number of patients enrolled in RCTs is a little over 200. In some of these studies a significant number of 'medically treated' patients underwent angioplasty. Many patients who underwent angioplasty were not stented. These limitations may have resulted in an underestimate of the benefits of renal artery angioplasty and stenting in the RCTs completed to date.

 Clinical pearls

- Renal artery angioplasty and stenting achieves long-term arterial patency rates of 75% in patients with atherosclerotic renal artery stenosis.
- Renal artery angioplasty may achieve a short-term reduction in the number of medications required for BP control.

Question 7

Which of the following factors may be useful in predicting this patient's expected response to angioplasty?
(a) The severity of the stenosis
(b) The average renal resistive index
(c) Her systolic BP reading
(d) Her degree of proteinuria

Answer
B and D

Explanation

Although RCTs suggest that there is no or only marginal benefit obtained in comparing intervention to medical therapy, other data suggest that there is a heterogenous patient response to angioplasty. A low renal resistive index (which is a measurement of renal parenchymal perfusion obtained by duplex Doppler ultrasonography) has been reported to predict those patients who do obtain a significant reduction in BP and improvement in renal function after angioplasty (answer B correct). Among the clinical features associated with a low resistive index are a baseline creatinine clearance >50 mL/min, proteinuria <1.0 g/ 24 hours and pulse pressure <60. In multivariate analysis, only proteinuria and resistive index were independent predictors of a significant response to angioplasty (answer D correct, answer C incorrect). Stenosis severity does not correlate with resistive index or with the outcome after angioplasty (answer A incorrect).

Clinical pearl

- Low levels of proteinuria (<1.0 g/24 hours) and maintained intrarenal perfusion as measured by a low resistive index on duplex Doppler examination may identify a subset of patients with renal artery stenosis who may achieve clinical benefit from renal revascularisation.

Twelve months after the original presentation, the patient is admitted to hospital with exertional chest discomfort. The patient undergoes coronary angiography which demonstrates a 70% stenosis of the right coronary artery. One week following discharge the patient notices increasing lethargy, and muscle aches and pains and rash on both legs. Follow-up tests reveal the following:

Na+	139 mmol/L	(136–146)
K+	5.8 mmol/L	(3.6–5.2)
HCO₃⁻	22 mmol/l	(24–31)
Urea	19.6 mmol/l	(2.5–6.5)
Creatinine	320 µmol/L	(45–90)
Total creatinine kinase	150	(<140)
Haemoglobin	125 g/L	(120–150)
White blood count	10.0 × 10⁹/L	(4.0–11.0)
Platelets	263 × 10⁹/L	(150–400)
Neutrophils	5.7	(1.0–4.0)
Lymphocytes	2.0	(1.0 4.0)
Monocytes	0.7	(0.2–1.0)
Eosinophils	1.5	(<0.2)

Question 8

The patient's cardiologist rings you to discuss the merit of proceeding with coronary angioplasty next week. Your advice to the cardiologist is:

(a) proceed with the angiogram after giving appropriate prophylaxis for contrast-induced nephropathy

(b) cancel the angiogram

(c) give hydrocortisone prior to the next angiogram for a possible contrast allergy

(d) stop the patient's statin.

Answer

B

Explanation

This patient has clinical characteristics of cholesterol embolisation syndrome rather than allergy to contrast (answer C incorrect). Cholesterol embolisation is often characterised by vague constitutional symptoms, peripheral emboli or livedo reticularis rash, eosinophilia and acute renal failure. Progressive renal impairment resulting in end-stage renal disease is reported in 20 to 60% of patients. There are no RCTs of treatment; however, the recommended management of this disorder is to avoid further vascular interventions (answer A incorrect, answer B correct). The creatinine kinase does not suggest a diagnosis of rhabdomyolysis and it is important to treat the patient's vascular disease, so the statin should be continued (answer D incorrect).

Bibliography

Level A

1. Tepel, M., Aspelin, P. & Lameire, N. (2006) Contrast-induced nephropathy: a clinical and evidence-based approach. Circulation. 113, 1779–1806. This is an up-to-date review of clinical significance of and treatment options for contrast-induced nephropathy.
2. Krijnen, P., van Jaarsveld, B.C., Steyerberg, E.W., Man in 't Veld, A. J., Schalekamp, M.A.D.H. & Habbema, J.D.F. (1998) A clinical prediction rule for renal artery stenosis. Ann Intern Med. 129(9), 705–11. This describes a clinical algorithm for the detection of renal artery stenosis.

Level B

3. Vasbinder, G.B.C., Nelemans, P.J., Kessels, A.G.H., Kroon, A.A., de Leeuw, P.W. & van Engelshoven, J.M.A. (2001) Diagnostic tests for renal artery stenosis in patients suspected of having renovascular hypertension. Ann Intern Med. 135, 401–11. This provides a comprehensive meta-analysis comparing different screening modalities for the detection of renal artery stenosis.
4. Cheung, C.M., Wright, J.R., Shurrab, A.E., Mamtora, H., Foley, R.N., O'Donoghue, D.J., Waldek, S. & Kalra, P.A. (2002) Epidemiology of renal dysfunction and patient outcome in atherosclerotic renal artery occlusion. J Am Soc Nephrol. 13, 149–57. This is an elegant clinical study examining the predictive value of GFR and stenosis severity in renal artery stenosis.

Level C

5. Ives, N.J., Wheatley, K., Stowe, R.L., Krijnen, P., Plouin, P.F., van Jaarsveld, B.C. & Gray, R. (2003) Continuing uncertainty about the value of percutaneous revascularization in atherosclerotic renovascular disease: a meta-analysis of randomized trials. Nephrol Dial Transplant. 18, 298–304. This provides a meta-analysis of angioplasty versus medical treatment of renal artery stenosis.
6. Radermacher, J., Ellis, S. & Haller, H. (2001) Renal resistance index and progression of renal disease. N Engl J Med. 344, 410–17. This article describes the predictive value of resistive index in the management of renal artery stenosis.

Case 15
Renal disease in systemic lupus erythematosus

RANDALL FAULL

LEVEL A

Case history

A 22-year-old female visits her general practitioner complaining of several months of non-specific fatigue, weight loss of 5 kg over the same period, and several weeks of aching pain in her hands and fingers. She has rarely seen a doctor apart from occasional visits for immunisations, and has no past history of serious illnesses. She is not on any regular medications, and denies ingestion of alternative therapies or recreational or illicit drugs. She is a university student who works part-time as a receptionist/typist. Both her parents are Vietnamese, and the family migrated to Australia when she was 2 years of age. She thinks that her father may have mild hypertension (untreated), but otherwise her parents have no significant health problems. Both of her younger siblings are in good health. She generally copes well with study and work, although recently has struggled due to tiredness and difficulty concentrating.

On examination, she is not overtly unwell but appears tired. Her face has a flushed appearance. Other findings include that she is afebrile, her blood pressure (BP) is 130/90 mmHg in the lying position, her pulse rate is 85 beats/min and regular, and there is no respiratory distress. There is no ankle oedema and no swelling or erythema of the fingers or hands, but the small joints of the hands are tender to palpation; there is no tenderness of the feet or larger joints. Urinalysis shows blood 3+ and protein 3+.

Question 1

Which of the following is most consistent with the urinalysis?

(a) Urinary tract infection
(b) Thin glomerular basement membrane disease
(c) Proliferative glomerulonephritis
(d) Minimal change nephropathy

Answer

C

Explanation

Haematuria (microscopic or macroscopic) is usually present during a urinary tract infection, and the source of the blood is typically the inflamed, haemorrhagic wall of the bladder. Proteinuria of this degree indicates a primary glomerular/renal problem, and is not seen in urinary tract infections.

Thin glomerular basement membrane disease, which is also commonly called benign familial haematuria, is a relatively common condition where the only histopathological abnormality is thinning of the glomerular basement membrane. It is typically familial, with an autosomal dominant mode of inheritance, and is due to defects in some of the alpha 4 chains of type IV collagen in the glomerular basement membrane. Unlike Alport's syndrome, this condition generally has a benign course, although some females with thin glomerular basement membranes on electron microscopy appear to be carriers of Alport's. Thin glomerular basement membrane disease typically presents with microscopic haematuria, but little or no proteinuria.

Dipstick analysis of proteinuria is commonly reported in a range of 0 to 4+, and the 3+ in this case will be of the order of 1 to 2 g/day. This degree of proteinuria is typical of a glomerular problem, although less commonly a predominantly tubulointerstitial renal disease can cause this level of proteinuria. The additional presence of moderate haematuria (also commonly reported in the range of 0 to 4+) is further evidence of an inflammatory (i.e. proliferative) glomerular problem, known as a glomerulonephritis. Microscopy of the urine in this case would likely show features of glomerulonephritis, including irregular dysmorphic (or glomerular) red blood cells. Caution is needed, however, when interpreting a report of dysmorphic red blood cells in the urine; there is significant variability between observers. A more reliable sign of proliferative glomerulonephritis is the presence of granular or red cell casts with haematuria.

Minimal change nephropathy is the most common cause of acute nephrotic syndrome in young people. It is a striking example of a primary glomerular problem leading to heavy proteinuria (typically 4+), but it does not have the histological features of a proliferative glomerulonephritis; hence, significant haematuria is not seen in that condition.

 Clinical pearls

- Heavy proteinuria is not typical of a urinary tract infection, and other causes of proteinuria should be sought.
- Haematuria plus proteinuria equals proliferative glomerulonephritis, until proven otherwise.

Question 2

Which of the following conditions is the most likely explanation for her presentation?

(a) Rheumatoid arthritis
(b) Gout
(c) Post-viral arthropathy
(d) Systemic lupus erythematosus

Answer

D

Explanation

This young woman has symptoms and signs suggestive of a systemic disorder, although other possibilities need to be kept in mind (e.g. work-related injuries to her hands, depression causing weight loss and fatigue). Rheumatoid arthritis often presents as a symmetrical polyarthropathy in a young woman, and this inflammatory autoimmune condition could account for the weight loss and fatigue. The abnormal urinalysis is less typical, and rheumatoid arthritis is infrequently associated with glomerulonephritis. Acute polyarticular gout can present with bilateral hand pain and features of systemic inflammation, but is extremely rare in a young woman. A post-viral arthropathy could explain the pain, weight loss and fatigue, but the abnormal urinalysis would be uncommon.

Systemic lupus erythematosus (SLE) is most common in young women (nine times more common than in males), particularly of South-East Asian background, and will typically present with a non-deforming arthropathy and features of systemic inflammation. Renal involvement is very common in SLE, and the urinalysis is consistent with this. Approximately 50% of patients will have clinical evidence of renal disease (abnormal urinalysis, and/or elevated serum creatinine) at diagnosis, and renal disease will be a feature in more than 75% of patients (usually within 5 years of diagnosis). Other common symptoms of SLE include fevers, hair loss/alopecia, skin rashes (including a malar facial rash) and serositis (e.g. pleurisy, pericarditis).

Question 3

Which one of the following is likely to be of most diagnostic value?

(a) Erythrocyte sedimentation rate (ESR)
(b) Complete blood examination
(c) Rheumatoid factor
(d) Antinuclear antibodies (ANA) and double stranded DNA-antibodies

Answer

D

Explanation

Each of the investigations could give useful information, but answer D is the one that will give most specific diagnostic information. The main differential diagnoses of the patient's presentation are rheumatoid arthritis and SLE. An elevated erythrocyte sedimentation rate is expected in active forms of each of these systemic inflammatory diseases, but does not help differentiate between them. A complete blood examination might be abnormal in either condition (e.g. anaemia of chronic disease in either, or autoimmune anaemia, leucopenia or thrombocytopenia in SLE) but will not yield specific diagnostic information. Testing for rheumatoid factor will be useful to exclude or diagnose rheumatoid arthritis, but the presentation is most consistent with SLE, which is best diagnosed with a blood assay for antinuclear and double-stranded DNA antibodies.

A number of other investigations should be performed or at least considered in this scenario, including full biochemistry (including renal function), radiology of the hands, C-reactive protein, complement levels, extractable nuclear antigen (ENA), urine microscopy, quantification of urine protein and a renal biopsy.

Question 4

Which one of the following is the strongest indication for a renal biopsy in this patient?
(a) Double-stranded DNA 65 IU/mL (normal <8)
(b) Serum creatinine 130 μmol/L (normal range 50 to 120)
(c) Dysmorphic red blood cells on urine microscopy
(d) Proteinuria 1.0 g/24 hours

Answer
B

Explanation

The strongly positive double-stranded DNA antibodies is virtually diagnostic of active SLE, but does not in isolation mandate a renal biopsy or closely correlate with renal disease activity.

Answers B, C and D are each consistent with SLE glomerulonephritis. Proteinuria of 1.0 g/day and dysmorphic red blood cells on urine microscopy can occur in mild, moderate or severe glomerulonephritis, and so do not give a reliable guide to severe disease. Of most concern, though, is the abnormal renal function, which in this patient already indicates loss of a substantial proportion of her usual renal function. Typically a young woman will normally have a serum creatinine of 65 μmol/L, and the level of 130 thus would likely represent a loss of 50% of renal function. This abnormality, which is consistent with severe glomerulonephritis, is the most compelling indication for a renal biopsy.

Clinical pearls

- SLE is an important cause of inflammatory arthropathy in young women, particularly those of South-East Asian descent.
- Renal involvement is very common in SLE, and can manifest as a severe and progressive proliferative glomerulonephritis; a renal biopsy is strongly indicated when severe renal involvement is suspected.

LEVEL B

Case history continued ...

Now confident that the patient has systemic lupus erythematosus, her general practitioner starts her on Naproxen 250 mg twice daily for her arthralgias, and refers her to a renal physician. She is seen one week later. The arthralgias have improved, but she remains lethargic. Urinalysis continues to show haematuria and proteinuria. BP is 140/95 mmHg. Her serum creatinine has risen to145 µmol/L. The renal physician arranges a percutaneous renal biopsy, under ultrasound guidance, to be performed the next day.

Question 5

What is the renal biopsy most likely to show?
- **(a)** Mesangial proliferative (class II) lupus nephritis
- **(b)** Diffuse proliferative (class IV) lupus nephritis
- **(c)** Membranous (class V) lupus nephritis
- **(d)** Acute interstitial nephritis

Answer
B

Explanation

Establishing with certainty the potential diagnosis of class III or class IV glomerulonephritis is the most important reason to perform a renal biopsy in SLE. These are the most severe forms of renal involvement in SLE, and necessitate aggressive intervention with high-dose immunosuppression to prevent an inexorable decline in renal function. Each is associated with heavy (often nephrotic-range) proteinuria, an active urinary sediment with dysmorphic red blood cells and granular or red cell casts, and deteriorating renal function.

Answer A is a mild form of lupus nephritis, typically indicated by microscopic haematuria and, at the most, modest proteinuria but not by deterioration of renal function. On the other hand, a cardinal feature of answer B is abnormal renal function, as in this case. Membranous lupus nephritis (answer C) usually presents with heavy proteinuria, but does not necessarily cause renal dysfunction, and by comparison with class III or class IV has a relatively benign prognosis.

Acute interstitial nephritis, without associated glomerular lesions, is unusual in SLE. It has been reported with non-steroidal anti-inflammatory drugs (NSAIDs), including Naproxen, but does not usually evolve in this short time frame. Urine abnormalities seen in acute interstitial nephritis also are minimal, and not the active urinary sediment typical of acute glomerulonephritis in this case. Nevertheless, the Naproxen should be stopped because it is likely to worsen her renal impairment.

A widely used World Health Organization classification system for lupus nephritis was first published in 1982 and updated in 2004. Class I (minimal mesangial) and class II (mesangial proliferative) do not require specific therapy in their own right, and treatment of the SLE is dictated by extrarenal manifestations. In contrast, class III (focal) and class IV (diffuse) nephritis are strong indications for aggressive therapy, and treatment of the renal component of the SLE predominates. The management of class V (membranous) nephritis is less clear-cut. It has a more benign prognosis than class III or IV, but progressive renal impairment sometimes occurs. There is also the possibility of significant complications of the nephrotic syndrome. A common approach is to use more modest doses of immunosuppression for class V disease, and many physicians will anticoagulate the nephrotic patients because of the high incidence of thrombosis. The predominant histological feature of class VI disease (advanced sclerotic) is severe scarring and an absence of acute nephritic activity. The approach to immunosuppression is minimisation, aiming to control extrarenal disease activity, and conservative measures (e.g. BP control) to attempt to slow deterioration of renal function.

Question 6

Which of the following would you choose to treat this condition?
- **(a)** Hydroxychloroquine 200 mg twice daily plus prednisolone 25 mg/day
- **(b)** Prednisolone 1 mg/kg plus azathioprine 2 mg/kg
- **(c)** Prednisolone 1 mg/kg plus monthly IV cyclophosphamide 750 mg/m^2
- **(d)** Intravenous methylprednisolone 1 gm daily for 3 days, then option C

Answer
C

Explanation

Hydroxychloroquine is efficacious for treatment of the skin and joint manifestations of SLE, but has no role to play in treatment of the renal manifestations.

Prednisolone plus azathioprine is a widely used combination for maintenance of remission of severe (class III or IV) lupus nephritis, but is inferior to cyclophosphamide-based regimens for induction of remission. Pooled analyses of multiple trials of immunosuppressive therapy for severe lupus nephritis support the superiority of the combination of steroids plus cyclophosphamide over steroids alone. Intravenous cyclophosphamide is more commonly used than oral cyclophosphamide, although the evidence supporting its superiority is relatively sparse.

Option D is also worth careful consideration. Commencement of treatment with intravenous methylprednisolone tends to be reserved for situations where there is rapidly progressive (including crescentic) renal disease, and/or other life-threatening manifestations of severe SLE. In this case, the serum creatinine was already abnormal, and had risen further in a short time frame, but this may have been secondary to the introduction of Naproxen.

A limiting problem with use of cyclophosphamide is its numerous, worrying side effects, including bone marrow suppression (which can be quite sudden and profound), bladder toxicity (haemorrhagic cystitis and increased risk of bladder cancer) and infertility. The last side effect is often the stumbling block when discussing therapeutic options in a disease which most commonly affects young women. These limitations have driven a search for efficacious alternatives, of which the most promising currently is mycophenolate mofetil. Better known for its widespread use in solid organ transplantation, a number of studies have now shown encouraging results for both induction and maintenance treatment in severe lupus nephritis.

Clinical pearls

- A renal biopsy is invaluable for guiding therapy in SLE with renal involvement; it is one of the few conditions where a patient may have multiple renal biopsies during the course of the disease.
- Side effects increasingly limit the popularity of cyclophosphamide for treatment of SLE with renal involvement; other less-toxic treatments, such as mycophenolate mofetil, have been studied and are gaining favour.

Case history continued ...

The risks and benefits of treatment are explained to the patient. She refuses cyclophosphamide because of concerns about it inducing infertility. After further discussion she commences mycophenolate mofetil 750 mg twice daily plus prednisolone 50 mg/day. Her arthralgias and lethargy resolve quickly, and she regains her appetite and vitality. After 1 month her serum creatinine has fallen to 75 µmol/L, and BP to 110/70 mmHg. After 6 months she has only a trace of protein and 1+ blood on urinalysis. The mycophenolate mofetil is ceased and she is started on azathioprine 100 mg/day. Her prednisolone dose by then is 10 mg/day, and she is moderately cushingoid. Over the next 3 months she remains well and the prednisolone dose is gradually reduced to 5 mg/day.

Six months later she sees the renal physician for an unscheduled appointment, having failed to attend her previous scheduled appointment. She complains of several weeks of swelling of her legs, plus recurrence of arthralgias in her hands, lethargy, a malar rash and marked hair loss when she brushes her hair. On examination she is pale and has several bruises on both arms. Her BP is 165/110 mmHg. There is moderate oedema of the lower limbs to the mid-calf, but her jugular venous pressure is not elevated. Heart sounds are normal, and the apex beat is not displaced. Urinalysis shows protein 4+ and blood 3+, having been protein 2+ and blood + 3 months before. Abnormalities on biochemistry are serum creatinine 180 µmol/L, urea 12.0 mmol/L (normal range 2.7 to 8.0) and albumin 18 g/L (normal range 34 to 48). Total calcium is low, but ionised calcium is normal. Her complete blood examination shows the following new abnormalities:

- Haemoglobin 85 g/L (115–155)
- Total white cell count 3.0×10^9/L (4.0–11.0)
- Platelet count 50×10^9/L (normal range 150–400).

Question 7

Which of the following is the most appropriate action?
- **(a)** Urgent renal biopsy under platelet cover
- **(b)** Increase prednisolone dose to 50 mg/day
- **(c)** Intravenous cyclophosphamide 750 mg/m^2
- **(d)** Intravenous methylprednisolone 1 gm/day for 3 days

Answer
D

Explanation

She has had a serious relapse of her lupus nephritis and of the systemic features of SLE. It is most likely that the pancytopenia is autoimmune, but the azathioprine could also be causative (although it usually causes isolated leucopenia). Simple investigations of the pancytopenia include a Coomb's test (for autoimmune haemolysis) and reticulocyte count (high in haemolysis, low in bone marrow suppression). Poor compliance with her medications needs to be considered, but unless there is strong evidence for that, it is preferable to assume that this relapse is due to a failure of maintenance therapy. Arguments can be made in favour of each of the options in this question, but most clinicians would recommend that answer D is the most appropriate action.

A renal biopsy needs to be seriously considered, although it could reasonably be omitted or deferred for two reasons: (1) the increased risk of haemorrhage due to the thrombocytopenia; and (2) the clinical picture is once again typical of class IV lupus nephritis, and the biopsy is unlikely to change therapy. It could be reconsidered if she fails to respond adequately to therapy, and once the thrombocytopenia improves or resolves.

The key question here is how to alter her therapy and how much to increase her immunosuppression. Increasing the prednisolone back to 50 mg/day (1 mg/kg) would be a reasonable part of any alteration in her treatment, but alone may not be sufficient to rapidly bring all aspects of her SLE under control. Likewise, changing her from azathioprine back to mycophenolate mofetil, or to cyclophosphamide, needs to be seriously considered, but there will be a lag period before response. Answer D should quickly improve her systemic features, and give the best chance of doing the same to her potentially rapidly progressive renal impairment.

LEVEL C

Case history continued ...

A clinical judgement is made that the patient again has type IV lupus nephritis (relapsed), and she does not have a renal biopsy. She is given intravenous methylprednisolone 1 gm/day for 3 days, followed by prednisolone 50 mg/day. Cyclophosphamide is recommended in view of the relapse of lupus nephritis, but once again she declines this option. Mycophenolate mofetil is recommended at a dose of 750 mg twice daily. Her systemic symptoms resolve quickly, and haemoglobin, white cell and platelet count normalise within 4 weeks. Over the same time period her serum creatinine level falls to 130 µmol/L, but heavy proteinuria and low serum albumin persist.

She remains well without obvious manifestations of SLE over the next 12 months, apart from persistent proteinuria (3+ on dipstick) and low serum albumin (22 g/L). The prednisolone dose is gradually reduced to 10 mg/day, and the mycophenolate mofetil dose reduced to 500 mg twice daily due to gastrointestinal side effects. Peripheral oedema is controlled with intermittent frusemide 40 mg. She has persistent hypercholesterolaemia (total serum cholesterol 6.0 mmol/L) despite 80 mg/day of atorvastatin. Markers of lupus activity are low or negative: antinuclear factor (ANF) 1/160, double-stranded DNA 6.0 (normal <8.0), normal C3 and C4 levels, erythrocyte sedimentation rate (ESR) 10 and C-reactive protein (CRP) <4.

The patient is next brought by her family to the emergency department with a history of headache for several hours, followed by a possible seizure, then sudden onset of left-arm and left-leg weakness. She is drowsy and able to give limited details only of history, but her family says she had been well recently, apart from some mild tiredness. Vital signs are normal, including BP of 130/85 mmHg. Examination reveals weakness of the left arm and left leg, and an upward plantar response on that side. There is no neck stiffness.

Question 8

What is the most likely explanation for her presentation?
(a) Cerebral lupus
(b) Ischaemic cerebrovascular event
(c) Cerebral lymphoma
(d) Cerebral infection

Answer
B

Explanation

This patient is at risk of all of these options, but the clinical scenario most favours answer B (despite her young age). The sudden onset of clearly localising neurological deficits strongly favours an ischaemic event as aetiology, but the caring clinician needs to keep other possibilities in mind. This dramatic presentation, plus the lack of recent apparent systemic activity of her SLE, argues against cerebral lupus. The history of significant immunosuppression makes her at risk of both cerebral infection and cerebral lymphoma. While the symptoms are not typical of those of classical acute bacterial meningitis, she is at risk of a less inflammatory cerebral infection such as cryptococcal meningitis. This typically presents with more subtle neurological signs and symptoms, often without neck stiffness. Cerebral lymphoma is more common in long-term immunosuppressed patients, such as renal transplant recipients. In this case, the short-duration headache plus localising signs could be due to a haemorrhage into a previously unsuspected lymphoma.

Case history continued ...

A computerised tomography (CT) head scan, followed by a cerebral magnetic resonance imaging (MRI) scan, confirms an ischaemic cerebrovascular event. There are no peripheral stigmata of endocarditis, and the following investigations looking for an embolic source are all negative or normal: blood cultures, electrocardiogram and echocardiogram (transthoracic and transoesophageal).

Question 9

Which one of the following is the strongest risk factor for this event?

(a) Low serum albumin
(b) Normal activated partial thromboplastin time (APTT)
(c) Elevated serum total cholesterol
(d) History of hypertension

Answer

A

Explanation

The presence of low serum albumin due to the nephrotic syndrome confers an increased risk of thrombosis, both arterial and venous (particularly deep vein thrombosis in the lower limbs and the renal veins). These events occur in 10 to 40% of patients with nephrotic syndrome. Relevant abnormalities that contribute to this thrombotic tendency include decreased levels of antithrombin III (due to excess loss in the urine), increased platelet activation and excess fibrinogen (which also causes a persistently high ESR).

Other disorders of blood clotting are well described in SLE. Autoantibodies against clotting factors VIII, IX, XI, XII or XIII can interfere with coagulation assays and increase the risk of bleeding, but are very uncommon. Of more clinical importance are antibodies that are associated with a thrombotic tendency. These include the paradoxically named 'lupus anticoagulant', which is associated with thrombosis (arterial and venous), thrombocytopenia and miscarriages. A clue to its presence is prolonged activated partial thromboplastin time. Also commonly found in SLE and associated with thrombosis are antibodies to phospholipids or phospholipid-binding proteins. The best known of these are the anticardiolipin antibody (ACLA) and antibody against β2 glycoprotein I. The combination of thrombotic events and these autoantibodies is known as antiphospholipid syndrome. This can occur as an isolated syndrome (primary), or in association with SLE or other autoimmune diseases (secondary).

It is well established that hyperlipidaemia and hypertension are risk factors for cerebrovascular disease in the general community, and they are strongly associated with ischaemic cerebral events in the elderly. The young age of this patient, and relatively short duration of these events, make them less relevant to this ischaemic event.

 Clinical pearls

- Unusual conditions, and atypical presentations of common conditions, must always be considered in an unwell patient with a history of SLE and long-term immunosuppression.

- Patients with SLE can be at risk for both bleeding and thrombotic complications.

Case history continued ...

A prothrombotic screen is negative, including the absence of anticardiolipin antibodies and a negative screen for lupus anticoagulant. The clinical opinion is that her ongoing nephrotic syndrome is the underlying basis for the ischaemic event, which was probably due to an in-situ thrombosis rather than embolism. It is therefore decided that she be anticoagulated with warfarin while she remains nephrotic. Over the next few weeks she makes a good recovery, with minimal residual deficit.

Over the next 2 years she continues to have a fluctuating clinical course. While well much of the time, she has intermittent arthralgias and hair loss, and a persistent malar rash. She remains nephrotic, and her renal function slowly deteriorates to a serum creatinine of 0.20 mmol/L. A repeat renal biopsy is considered on a number of occasions, but deferred due to the ongoing anti-coagulation plus the patient's reluctance to consider alternative therapy (for example, cyclophosphamide).

She attends the next appointment with her fiancé. They are to be married soon, and are keen to start a family soon after if possible. She is aware of the risks of becoming pregnant while on warfarin, and seeks advice on alternative treatments to reduce the activity of her lupus nephritis and the associated heavy proteinuria. She is advised to consider a course of cyclophosphamide, although there is insufficient evidence to be certain that it will have additional benefit.

Question 10

Which of the following is correct with respect to the use of cyclophosphamide to treat renal disease in SLE?

(a) The risk of ovarian failure is low in women aged less than 20, but very high in women aged more than 30.

(b) Oocyte preservation is a reliable method to ensure future pregnancy in women who develop ovarian failure.

(c) The route of administration of cyclophosphamide is linked to the incidence of subsequent ovarian failure.

(d) The cumulative dose of cyclophosphamide correlates with the risk of ovarian failure, irrespective of the age of the patient.

Answer

A

Explanation

Premature ovarian failure is a feared complication of cyclophosphamide therapy for young women, the target group for SLE. In one study of lupus nephritis, the risk of ovarian failure following cyclophosphamide was 100% in women over the age of 30, approximately 50% when aged 20 to 30, and 13% in patients younger than 20. Likewise, the average cumulative dose of cyclophosphamide that induces amenorrhea decreases with age. There is no good evidence that the route of administration of the cyclophosphamide has any effect. While younger women frequently return to normal ovarian function, they remain at risk of eventually developing premature ovarian failure. The sensitivity of older women is thought to be because they have fewer residual oocytes. Strategies for preservation of fertility in women continue to evolve but are not yet reliable. Oocyte cryopreservation is not yet established due to problems of suboptimal viability and the ability to fertilise the eggs following freeze-thawing. Medical suppression of normal ovarian cycling shows promise for protecting against gonadal dysfunction, and there is experimental as well as clinical trial evidence supporting the use of gonadotrophin-releasing hormone agonist (GnRHa) (goserelin acetate) in this setting.

Case history continued ...

After explanation of the risks and benefits, her warfarin anticoagulation is reversed and she undergoes a further renal biopsy. This confirms an ongoing active proliferative glomerulonephritis (class IV), but there is also moderate glomerular sclerosis and interstitial fibrosis. While recognising that there is a degree of irreversibility of her renal damage, it is considered reasonable to attempt to suppress the active proliferative glomerulonephritis.

The mycophenolate mofetil is stopped, and she receives intravenous cyclophosphamide (750 mg/m^2) monthly for 3 months. At the same time she has a goserelin acetate implant inserted, and is commenced on trimethoprim/sulfamethoxazole prophylaxis against Pneumocystis carinii pneumonia. Her prednisolone dose is increased to 50 mg/day, tapering back to 10 mg/day over the next 3 months. Following the three cycles of cyclophosphamide, she is put back on mycophenolate mofetil. Six months after commencement of cyclophosphamide her proteinuria has diminished to 0.5 gm/day, serum albumin is back in the normal range and serum creatinine has fallen to 0.17 mmol/L. Her menstrual cycle has resumed. Her warfarin is stopped and replaced with aspirin.

The patient is also made aware of emerging and potentially less-toxic therapies for SLE, which may have a place in her treatment in the near future. Currently promising treatments include the monoclonal antibodies rituximab and abatacept.

The issue of future pregnancy is again actively discussed, and she is advised about the risks of exacerbation of her SLE, and of pregnancy with significant renal impairment. Her caring clinicians look forward to her future pregnancy with some trepidation.

Bibliography

Levels B and C

1. Weening, J.J., D'Agati, V.D., Schwartz, M.M., Seshan, S.V., Alpers, C.E., Appel, G.B., Balow, J.E., Bruijn, J.A., Cook, T., Ferrario, F., Fogo, A.B., Ginzler, E.M., Hebert, L., Hill, G., Hill, P., Jennette, J.C., Kong, N.C., Lesavre, P., Lockshin, M., Looi, L.M., Makino, H., Moura, L.A. & Nagata, M. (2004) The classification of glomerulonephritis in systemic lupus erythematosus revisited. Kidney Int. 65, 521.

2. Austin, H.A., Klippel, J.H., Balow, J.E., le Riche, N.G., Steinberg, A.D., Plotz, P.H. & Decker, J.L. (1986) Therapy of lupus nephritis. Controlled trial of prednisone and cytotoxic drugs. N Engl J Med. 314, 614.

3. Boumpas, D.T., Austin, H.A., Vaughn, E.M., Klippel, J.H., Steinberg, A.D., Yarboro, C.H. & Balow, J.E. (1992) Controlled trial of pulse methylprednisolone versus two regimens of pulse cyclophosphamide in severe lupus nephritis. Lancet. 340, 741–5.

4. Felson, D.T. & Anderson, J. (1984) Evidence for the superiority of immunosuppressive drugs and prednisone over prednisone alone in lupus nephritis. Results of a pooled analysis. N Engl J Med. 311, 1528.

5. Flanc, R.S., Roberts, M.A., Strippoli, G.F., Chadban, S.J., Kerr, P.G. & Atkins, R.C. (2004) Treatment of diffuse proliferative lupus nephritis: a meta-analysis of randomized controlled trials. Am J Kidney Dis. 43, 197–208.

6. Chan, T.M., Li, F.K., Tang, C.S., Wong, R.W., Fang, G.X., Ji, Y.L., Lau, C.S., Wong, A.K., Tong, M.K., Chan, K.W. & Lai, K.N. (2000) Efficacy of mycophenolate mofetil in patients with diffuse proliferative lupus nephritis. Hong Kong-Guangzhou Nephrology Study Group. N Engl J Med. 343, 1156.

7. Ong, L.M., Hooi, L.S., Lim, T.O., Goh, B.L., Ahmad, G., Ghazalli, R., Teo, S.M., Wong, H.S., Tan, S.Y., Shaariah, W., Tan, C.C. & Morad, Z. (2005) Randomized controlled trial of pulse intravenous cyclophosphamide versus mycophenolate mofetil in the induction therapy of proliferative lupus nephritis. Nephrology (Carlton). 10, 504–10.

8. Ginzler, E.M., Dooley, M.A., Aranow, C., et al. (2005) Mycophenolate mofetil or intravenous cyclophosphamide for lupus nephritis. N Engl J Med. 353, 2219.

9. Pendse, S., Ginsburg, E. & Singh, A.K. (2004) Strategies for preservation of ovarian and testicular function after immunosuppression. Am J Kidney Dis. 43, 772.

10. Thatayatikom, A. & White, A.J. (2006) Rituximab: a promising therapy in systemic lupus erythematosus. Autoimmun Rev. 5, 18–24.

11. Liossis, S.N. & Sfikakis, P.P. (2004) Costimulation blockade in the treatment of rheumatic diseases. Biodrugs. 18, 95–102.

12. Davidson, A., Diamond, B., Wofsky, D. & Daikh, D. (2005) Block and tackle: CTLA4Ig takes on lupus. Lupus. 14, 197–203.

Case 16
Rapidly progressive glomerulonephritis

LENA SUCCAR AND GOPI RANGAN

LEVEL A

Case history

A 53-year-old Caucasian man living in a large metropolitan city in Australia presents to his general practitioner with a 3-month history of fever, lethargy and weight loss of 5 kg. A non-specific viral or bacterial infection is initially suspected and he receives treatment with amoxycillin/clavulanate for 2 weeks. He fails to improve, and upon further review his blood pressure is found to be 170/100 mmHg, there is mild ankle oedema and urinalysis shows blood 3+, protein 2+ with leukocytes 1+. No skin rash is detected and he has been prescribed penicillin-based antibiotics without adverse effects throughout his life. Further investigations reveal that the serum creatinine is 345 μmol/L (compared to 85 μmol/L with estimated glomerular filtration rate [eGFR] of 102 mL/min/1.73 m², 6 months ago) and albumin 36 g/L. The haemoglobin is 110 g/dL, white cell count 5×10^9/L (with normal differential counts) and platelet count 233×10^9/L. The renal ultrasound shows that the kidneys are of normal appearance and size with no urinary tract obstruction.

Question 1

Which renal syndrome best describes the clinical presentation?
(a) Nephritic syndrome
(b) Nephrotic syndrome
(c) Chronic glomerulonephritis
(d) Asymptomatic urinary abnormalities

Answer
A

Explanation

Clinical presentations of glomerular diseases are classified into syndromes. These include the nephritic syndrome, the nephrotic syndrome, chronic glomerulonephritis and asymptomatic urinary abnormalities. The nephritic syndrome is the clinical correlate of acute glomerular inflammation with proliferative changes, and is typically associated with an active immunological response (cellular and antigen/antibody-mediated) within the kidney. Clinically, it is characterised by an acute onset of macroscopic ('tea/cola'-coloured urine, which suggests glomerular haematuria) or microscopic haematuria with subnephrotic-range proteinuria ('nephritic urine sediment'), hypertension (because of impaired GFR and enhanced tubular reabsorption of salt and water), progressive oliguria and acute renal impairment over days to weeks.

Rapidly progressive glomerulonephritis (RPGN) is considered under the category of the nephritic syndrome. The pathological counterpart of RPGN is crescentic glomerulonephritis (CGN), the most aggressive type of glomerular disease, characterised by severe glomerular inflammation and glomerular cell proliferation (including crescents). Patients with RPGN develop renal impairment over weeks to months in association with a nephritic urine sediment and a variable degree of hypertension, oliguria and oedema.

The nephrotic syndrome is defined as the presence of proteinuria (3.5 g/24 hrs) hypoalbuminaemia (<30 g/L and oedema) and is associated with a number of extrarenal features, including hypoalbuminaemia, oedema, hyperlipidaemia, lipiduria and hypercoagulability. This patient does not have nephrotic syndrome, as haematuria is present and the serum albumin is within the normal range. Chronic glomerulonephritis is characterised by persistent proteinuria and/or haematuria with chronic renal impairment that gradually worsens over years. In this case the patient's renal function was normal 6 months ago and the kidney size is normal. Glomerular diseases may also be diagnosed when asymptomatic haematuria or proteinuria are detected on routine examination of the urinary sediment, for example, as part of pre-employment or insurance-related medical assessment. In this case, the patient has a number of extrarenal manifestations which make this possibility incorrect.

Question 2

The differential diagnosis for the renal impairment in this patient should include which of the following?
(a) Haemolytic-uraemic syndrome
(b) Microscopic polyangiitis
(c) Minimal change disease
(d) Acute tubulointerstitial nephritis induced by amoxycillin
(e) Subacute bacterial endocarditis

Answer
B, D and E

Explanation

This patient most likely has a RPGN. The aetiology of RPGN includes small vessel vasculitis (such as microscopic polyangiitis), anti-glomerular basement membrane (GBM) disease, and immune-complex-mediated glomerulonephritides (such as systemic lupus erythematosus, which would be unusual in this case in the absence of the typical extrarenal features of lupus, and infection-related glomerulonephritis, such as with subacute bacterial endocarditis). Any cause of subacute renal failure should be considered in the differential diagnosis of RPGN. Common mimickers of RPGN include the haemolytic uraemic syndrome (HUS), renal atheroemboli, drug-induced interstitial nephritis and other connective tissue disorders, such as scleroderma. In this case, HUS would be unlikely as there is no anaemia or thrombocytopenia, and proteinuria is usually not present. However, an acute tubulointerstitial nephritis due to hypersensitivity to penicillin should be considered in the differential diagnosis. Such patients may present with acute renal impairment associated with haematuria and mild to moderate proteinuria and sterile pyuria. Although possible, the diagnosis is less likely than an acute glomerulonephritis in this patient, as there is no eosinophilia or drug rash, the patient has previously been prescribed penicillin-based antibiotics without incident and the constitutional symptoms predate the use of amoxycillin. Minimal change disease is a cause of nephrotic syndrome, most commonly in children and young adults.

Question 3

The patient is referred urgently to a nephrology clinic. Which of the following laboratory tests will most quickly help confirm the clinical diagnosis of the patient's renal condition?

(a) Examination of the urine sediment by phase-contrast microscopy
(b) Serum cryoglobulins
(c) Anti-double stranded DNA (anti-dsDNA)
(d) Anti-neutrophil cytoplasmic antibody (ANCA)
(e) Peripheral blood film

Answer
A

Explanation

Examination of the urine sediment by phase-contrast microscopy is a simple clinical tool that is used by nephrologists to diagnose the cause of a patient's kidney disease. In inflammatory glomerular diseases, damage to the glomerular capillary wall allows entry of red blood cells (RBCs) into Bowman's capsule, the tubular lumen and eventually into the urine. During their passage across the glomerular capillary wall and transit in the nephron, red blood cells undergo changes in shape (dysmorphic) and others become associated with Tamm-Horsfall protein in the distal tubule, where they form cellular casts. Some of these casts eventually dislodge from the distal tubule and are excreted in the urine, where they appear as red blood cell casts. Red blood cell casts typically occur in severe inflammatory glomerulonephritides, such as CGN. Non-inflammatory glomerular diseases, such as focal segmental glomerulosclerosis, minimal change disease, diabetic nephropathy and membranous nephropathy are not typically associated with red cell casts in the urine. The presence of red cell casts in the urine of these latter patients should raise the possibility of a superimposed inflammatory glomerulonephritis.

Examination of the urine for red cell casts and dysmorphic RBCs can be performed rapidly using phase-contrast microscopy by experienced observers. RBC morphology and casts should be examined for on a freshly passed urine sample in the clinic using phase-contrast microscopy. Alternatively, the sample may be sent to a pathology laboratory, in which case it should be collected in a fixative (such as boric acid or formalin; specific details are dependent on the laboratory) to prevent cellular elements undergoing degeneration during delay (>4 hours) in transport and processing. Testing for the presence of autoantibodies (ANCA, anti-dsDNA), complement levels (C3/C4, which are depressed in immune complex glomerulonephritides), infectious serology and cryoglobulins are all appropriate and will help determine the aetiology of RPGN and CGN, but the results usually take a few days in most laboratories. A peripheral blood film might be useful if haemolytic uraemic syndrome is suspected, where it may show evidence of red blood cell fragmentation, but this diagnosis was thought to be unlikely in this particular case.

Question 4

The patient is transferred to the emergency department of a hospital at 6.30 pm on a Friday evening. How should the patient be managed pending further definitive investigations?

(a) Intravenous methylprednisone with oral cyclophosphamide followed by a renal biopsy as soon as possible
(b) Intravenous methylprednisone followed by a renal biopsy as soon as possible
(c) Intravenous methylprednisone with oral azathioprine followed by a renal biopsy as soon as possible
(d) Intravenous methylprednisone with immediate plasmapheresis followed by a renal biopsy as soon as possible

Answer

B

Explanation

Untreated RPGN will progress to end-stage renal failure within weeks to months. Nephrologists consider this glomerulonephritis a 'renal emergency', and would favour immediate treatment with immunosuppressant medications in an attempt to prevent further progression to kidney failure. Before confirmation of the clinical diagnosis is derived from an urgent renal biopsy, the latter would initially entail corticosteroids (such as a pulse dose of intravenous methylprednisolone), which could be administered in the emergency department if the diagnosis has been suspected. Cytotoxic agents, such as cyclophosphamide, are typically used as 'induction' agents in crescentic glomerulonephritis, but a tissue diagnosis with renal biopsy is preferred before this is initiated. It is important to note that cytotoxic agents are similar to corticosteroids in inducing remission. Their main roles are the minimisation of toxicity from the use of high-dose corticosteroid (when used as a single agent) and prevention of relapses. Azathioprine is used as a 'maintenance' immunosuppressant in the management of crescentic glomerulonephritis, but it would be inappropriate to administer at this point. Plasmapheresis should be considered in patients with pulmonary-renal syndrome due to lung haemorrhage associated with anti-glomerular basement membrane (GBM) disease (Goodpasture's syndrome) or small vessel vasculitis; or disease that is refractory to conventional therapy. In addition, the European Vasculitis Study Group (EUVAS) (www.vasculitis. org) recently reported that the addition of plasmapheresis to conventional therapy with corticosteroids and cyclophosphamide should also be considered in patients who at presentation have severe renal disease (defined as a serum creatinine >500 μmol/L). In this study, plasmapheresis reduced the risk of end-stage renal failure at 12 months by 24% when compared to adjunctive treatment with pulse methylprednisolone.

 Clinical pearls

- RPGN is defined as acute or subacute renal failure (i.e. onset over weeks to months) associated with oedema, hypertension and an 'active' urine sediment (red cell casts in the urine) and proteinuria.
- RPGN is a 'renal emergency' as it is associated with rapid progression to irreversible kidney failure. The latter may be prevented by the timely treatment with immunosuppressants.
- Treatment with corticosteroids can be initiated following clinical diagnosis, with cytotoxic agents delayed until after the pathological diagnosis has been confirmed by an urgent renal biopsy.

LEVEL B

Question 5

A percutaneous renal biopsy is undertaken the following morning. What pathological features might typically be expected on light microscopy?
(a) Glomerular crescents in more than 50% of glomeruli
(b) Defects in the glomerular basement membrane
(c) Fibrinoid necrosis in arterioles
(d) Onion-skin pattern of intimal fibrosis in interlobular arteries
(e) Acute tubular necrosis

Answer
A, B, C and E

Explanation

The classical features of CGN on light microscopy include extracapillary glomerular hypercellularity (or crescents which typically affect more than 50% of glomeruli) in Bowman's space associated with fibrinoid necrosis of glomerular capillaries (defined as lytic destruction of cells and matrix with deposition of acidophilic fibrin-rich material). The composition of crescents includes parietal epithelial cells, inflammatory cells (lymphocytes and macrophages) and recent studies have identified that podocytes migrate, dedifferentiate and proliferate, contributing to crescentic lesions. Initially, proliferation and migration of the various cells are pathological mechanisms underlying cellular crescent formation. However, over time cells in crescents undergo apoptosis and are replaced by myofibroblasts, which produce matrix, leading to the development of fibrous crescent. Cellular crescents therefore transform into fibrocellular and then eventually into fibrous crescents. A renal biopsy may contain crescents in any of these stages of development. The glomerular changes are often accompanied by chronic tubulointerstitial damage, and this may include acute tubular necrosis, in addition to tubular atrophy and interstitial fibrosis and inflammation. The presence of fibrosis in both the glomerulus and the tubulointerstitium is a marker of chronicity; the severity is correlated with a poor renal prognosis and may indicate that the patient is less likely to respond to treatment with immunosuppressants. Onion-skin patterning of interlobular arteries is typical of malignant hypertension or scleroderma.

Question 6

Concerning the glomerular immunopathology of crescentic glomerulonephritis, which of the following is the most likely pattern?

(a) Linear binding of immunoglobulins
(b) Granular binding of immunoglobulins
(c) Granular binding of complement
(d) Little or no binding of immunoglobulins

Answer

D

Explanation

In addition to light microscopy and electron microscopy, renal immunopathology is a tool to further determine the specific causes of glomerular diseases. This is determined by the presence and pattern of binding of immunoglobulins (IgG, IgA, IgM), complement (C3, C1q) and fibrinogen in the glomerulus. CGN is categorised into three subtypes according to the direct immunofluorescent staining for immunoglobulins (Ig) and the type of autoantibodies that are present. Pauci-immune CGN, the most common pattern (60% of all CGN, according to data from the Chapel Hill group) (Jennette & Thomas 2007), is defined as little (less than 2+) or no staining for Ig and complement. It is usually (80% of the time) associated with anti-neutrophil cytoplasmic antibody (ANCA, against either myeloperoxidase or proteinase-3) disease with or without systemic evidence of small vessel vasculitis.

Anti-glomerular basement membrane (GBM) CGN (15% of all CGN) is defined by *in situ* binding of anti-GBM antibodies to GBM antigens (α3 chain in the C-terminal non-collagenous globular domain of type IV collagen), and is characterised by greater than 2+ linear staining for IgG. It is an acute immune disease in which local immune complexes are formed following the binding of a circulating autoantibody to a fixed natural antigen (in this case the GBM antigen). This is in contrast to an antibody binding to planted antigen (as in post-streptococcal glomerulonephritis) or a circulating antigen-antibody complex deposited in the GBM (as in subacute bacterial endocarditis). Anti-GBM disease may or may not be associated with lung haemorrhage (Goodpasture's syndrome).

Immune Complex CGN accounts for 25% of all CGN and is defined by the deposition of Ig and complement in a granular pattern, signifying immune complex deposition. Unlike pauci-immune CGN and anti-GBM disease, the disease associations of immune complex CGN are heterogeneous and common causes include systemic lupus erythematosus (SLE), IgA nephropathy/Henoch-Schönlein purpura, membranoproliferative glomerulonephritis (which may be associated with cryoglobulinaemia and hepatitis C) or post-infectious glomerulonephritis. The frequency reported for the various types of CGN is typical of patient cohorts in western countries, but may not apply to developing nations or specific communities such as indigenous Australians, where there may be a higher frequency of CGN due to nephritogenic infections such as post-streptococcal glomerulonephritis. Data on the causes and incidence of CGN in specific regions of Australia and New Zealand are currently not available.

Question 7

Glomerular crescents affecting more than 50% of glomeruli on a biopsy may be present in which of the following diseases?
(a) Henoch-Schönlein purpura
(b) Thrombotic microangiopathy
(c) Focal segmental glomerulosclerosis
(d) Light chain deposition disease

Answer
A, B and D

Explanation

Crescent formation can occur in a number of renal diseases, and is the result of acute injury to the glomerular capillary endothelium. In response to exposure to coagulant factors, such as fibrin and thrombin, this injury leads to defects in the glomerular basement membrane, extravasation and proliferation of parietal epithelial cells and podocytes, as well as inflammatory cells. The classical causes of RPGN, listed earlier, are associated with the involvement of a higher percentage (>50%) of glomeruli by crescents than other diseases. A range of conditions can less commonly (under 5%) be associated with crescent formation, including fibrillary glomerulonephritis, diabetic nephropathy, thrombotic microangiopathy and light chain deposition disease. However, it would be very rare (<0.5%) for these causes to be associated with >50% crescent formation.

Question 8

Further serological testing reveals that the patient is positive for ANCA. Concerning ANCA, which of the following statements is/are true?
(a) Antibodies against myeloperoxidase are associated with perinuclear ANCA pattern of indirect immunofluorescence of neutrophils.
(b) Antibodies against proteinase-3 are associated with perinuclear ANCA pattern of indirect immunofluorescence of neutrophils.
(c) The titre always correlates with disease activity.
(d) They have no direct role in the pathogenesis of the disease.

Answer
A

Explanation

Autoimmune serological testing provides diagnostic, prognostic and disease activity information in immune-mediated inflammatory diseases, depending on the performance characteristics of individual autoantibodies. ANCA are autoantibodies (usually of the IgG class) which react against the antigens proteinase-3 (PR3) or myeloperoxidase (MPO), in either azurophilic granules in the cytoplasm of neutrophils or lysosomes of monocytes. They are a sensitive and specific marker for ANCA-associated CGN (including Wegener's granulomatosis, microscopic polyangiitis, renal-limited vasculitis and Churg-Strauss syndrome), and overall 85% of patients with pauci-immune CGN have circulating ANCA. ANCA are characterised by the indirect immunofluorescence test (IIF) of ethanol-fixed neutrophils and by an enzyme-linked immuno-sorbent assay (ELISA) to determine the specific antigens. Using IIF, three staining patterns are identified: (1) a diffuse granular staining of the cytoplasm staining (c-ANCA) which is associated with antibodies against PR3 of the neutrophil; (2) a perinuclear staining pattern with or without nuclear involvement (p-ANCA) which is associated with antibodies against MPO; and (3) less commonly, patterns not fitting into the former two, and these include either c-ANCA (atypical) and atypical ANCA, which have less clear disease associations. The characterisation of the target molecules is undertaken by an ELISA for PR3 and MPO. The best diagnostic performance is obtained when IIF is combined with PR3 and MPO-specific ELISAs.

Disappearance of ANCA is associated with disease remission, and the presence of anti-PR3 is associated with a higher risk of relapse. However, large clinical studies have shown both a benefit as well as a lack of a clinical benefit in monitoring serial ANCA titres to predict relapse.

The lack of a consistent correlation between ANCA titres and disease relapse in all studies has also caused controversy as to whether there is a direct link between ANCA and disease pathogenesis. However, studies in the last few years have reported evidence to support this hypothesis. The Chapel Hill Group, using an animal model, showed that ANCA IgG can cause glomerulonephritis and vasculitis, possibly by direct interaction with neutrophils and monocytes, resulting in inflammatory injury to glomeruli and vessels without antibody/immune complex deposition. Furthermore, a newborn infant was reputed to have transient vasculitis post-partum, presumably through the placental transfer of ANCA from the mother who had relapsed microscopic polyangiitis. These data point to a direct pathogenic role for ANCA in CGN and vasculitis, but further interventional data in experimental studies and humans are needed to completely validate this hypothesis.

Clinical pearls

- Glomerular cellular crescents are composed of podocytes, mononuclear leukocytes and parietal epithelial cells.
- Pauci-immune CGN is the most common cause of CGN in western countries, but there are likely to be regional differences.
- Glomerular crescents occur in a wide range of kidney diseases. CGN, however, is defined when more than 50% of glomeruli are affected.
- The best diagnostic performance for ANCA is obtained when IIF is combined with PR3- and MPO-specific ELISAs.

LEVEL C

Question 9

Concerning the long-term prognosis of CGN, which of the following statements is/are true?

(a) Patients with anti-GBM antibodies *and* ANCA have more severe disease and a worse renal outcome than ANCA-positive patients.

(b) Patients with anti-GBM antibodies have more severe disease and a worse renal outcome than ANCA-positive patients.

(c) Patients with immune-complex associated CGN have fewer crescents than ANCA-positive patients.

(d) Patients with anti-PR3 have a better long-term renal prognosis than those with anti-MPO ANCA.

(e) Patients with anti-MPO ANCA have more extensive disease and chronicity on the initial biopsy than those with anti-PR3.

Answer

B, C and E

Explanation

The clinical significance of the differences among various causes of RPGN and whether immunosuppressant therapy should be tailored according to these observations remains unknown and has not been evaluated. About one-quarter to one-third of patients with anti-GBM disease are also positive for ANCA. In these cases, ANCA can be detected before or after the detection of anti-GBM antibodies, and more often by MPO-ANCA than by PR3-ANCA. Patients who are anti-GBM positive (ANCA-negative) have more severe disease at diagnosis and a worse outcome than patients with ANCA-positive (anti-GBM negative) CGN.

In contrast, patients with both anti-GBM and ANCA have less crescent formation and a better prognosis than patients with anti-GBM (ANCA negative) yet worse than those with ANCA-alone CGN. That is, the prognosis from good to bad is according to the hierarchy: ANCA alone >ANCA + anti-GBM >anti-GBM alone. The pathogenesis and aetiology for the duplex expression of these autoantibodies is unknown. This has also been noted in other autoimmune diseases. For example, patients with scleroderma can rarely develop ANCA-associated CGN. In general, anti-GBM and small-vessel vasculitis associated CGN have a higher frequency of crescent formation than immune complex CGN. Patients with MPO-ANCA may have a slightly better long-term renal survival than do patients with PR3-ANCA, even though they have more extensive disease and chronicity at presentation.

Question 10

Regarding the treatment of ANCA-associated pauci-immune CGN in this patient, which of the following statements is/are true?

(a) Induction treatment with oral cyclophosphamide is superior to intravenous cyclophosphamide in producing remission.

(b) Induction treatment with mycophenolate mofetil is equal to oral cyclophosphamide in producing remission.

(c) Induction treatment with methotrexate is equal to oral cyclophosphamide in producing remission.

(d) Maintenance treatment with azathioprine is associated with a lower rate of adverse events compared to cyclophosphamide.

(e) The risk of relapse is increased if the PR3-ANCA titre is elevated when the patient is being switched from cyclophosphamide to azathioprine.

Answer

A, D and E

Explanation

Induction treatment with cyclophosphamide and corticosteroids continue to be well-established strategies for the treatment of vasculitis-associated CGN. Recent randomised clinical trials from the EUVAS report that such a regimen is able to induce remission in nearly 90% of patients following 3 to 6 months of therapy. Although cyclophosphamide is highly effective, it is associated with significant side effects in up to 50% of patients, including myelosuppression, gonadal failure, bladder toxicity and long-term risk of carcinogenesis. This is why less-toxic agents, such as mycophenolate mofetil (MMF), are attractive but, as yet, no large randomised clinical trial has been undertaken to test this hypothesis in ANCA-associated CGN.

Regarding the route of cyclophosphamide administration, a meta-analysis of eleven non-randomised trials reported that pulse administration was associated with less toxicity but a higher relapse rate than if the drug was given by the oral route. In contrast, preliminary findings from the CYCLOPS trial (randomised trial of daily oral versus pulse cyclophosphamide as therapy for ANCA-associated systemic vasculitis) suggested that the time to remission, relapse rates and patient survival are similar with the two routes of administration (De Groot 2005). However, final reporting of these data is awaited.

The NORAM (efficacy of methotrexate versus cyclophosphamide in the treatment of non-renal Wegener's granulomatosis) trial from EUVAS demonstrated that oral methotrexate may be used as an alternative to cyclophosphamide in patients with non-life-threatening vasculitis with mild renal impairment (serum creatinine <150 μmol/L) (De Groot 2005). It is contraindicated with more severe renal impairment, and therefore would not be suitable for the patient in this case. The CYCAZREM (randomised trial of cyclophosphamide versus azathioprine during remission in ANCA-positive systemic vasculitis) study from the EUVAS group is a randomised controlled trial of 155 patients with a serum creatinine <500 μmol/L with ANCA-CGN, in which maintenance treatment with azathioprine was compared to cyclophosphamide (Jayne et al. 2003). The study showed that there was no difference in relapse rates. Although the rate of adverse events was similar in both groups, the study was not powered to provide a conclusion regarding this factor. In addition, the long-term renal outcome in patients switched to azathioprine is not known, as the study duration was only 18 months. It is also noteworthy that up to 10% of patients were intolerant of azathioprine, requiring cessation due to allergy. The role of serial ANCA testing is controversial, but at least one study demonstrated that patients with a PR3-ANCA at the time of switching from cyclophosphamide to azathioprine had a 2.6-fold increased risk of relapse compared to those who were ANCA-negative.

Question 11

Regarding the side effects of cyclophosphamide and corticosteroids in ANCA-associated CGN, which of the following is/are appropriate information to give to this patient?

(a) There is at least a 50% chance of an episode of neutropenia.

(b) There is a 10% chance of life-threatening adverse event.

(c) Alopecia is rare.

(d) The long-term risk for bladder cancer is increased by more than tenfold compared to the healthy population.

(e) The risk of cancer is increased regardless of the treatment provided.

Answer
All are correct

Explanation

The risk of side effects associated with induction therapy with oral cyclophosphamide and corticosteroids was reported most recently in the CYCAZREM study, where up to 55% of patients experienced an episode of neutropenia, despite having rigid protocols for white cell count (WCC) monitoring. Furthermore, 10% of patients experienced a severe life-threatening adverse side effect, mostly associated with leucopenia and infection. Overall, alopecia and haemorrhagic cystitis were uncommon, as was amenorrhoea (but its low frequency was due to the study population, who had a mean age of 58 years). Several studies have documented that cyclophosphamide use is associated with a nine to forty-fivefold increased risk of bladder cancer. The relative risk appears to be increased for cumulative doses of more than 25 g or an exposure of more than 12 months, and especially high if the cumulative dose or exposure exceed 100 g and 2.5 years respectively. The association of cancer in patients with Wegener's granulomatosis has been addressed in several studies. Interestingly, it seems that there is an increased risk of developing several types of cancer (bladder, renal, squamous cell skin, lymphomas, leukaemia) independent of the treatment. That is, the cancers occurred a few years prior to the diagnosis of Wegener's, before treatment with immunosuppressants. The mechanisms of this increased association are unknown and remain to be explored.

 Clinical pearls

- About one-quarter to one-third of patients with anti-GBM disease are also positive for ANCA.
- Azathioprine is suitable for use in maintenance treatment, but the long-term effects on patient and renal survival have not been evaluated.
- Patients with vasculitis may have an increased risk of cancer regardless of treatment with cyclophosphamide.

Bibliography

Level A

1. Brady, H.R., O'Meara, Y.M. & Brenner, B.M. (2005) Glomerular diseases, Chapter 264, pp. 1674–94. *Harrison's Principles of Internal Medicine*, 16th edn, Kasper, D.L., Fauci, A.S., Longo, D.L., Braunwald, E. & Jameson, J.L. (eds). New York: McGraw-Hill.
2. Isbel, N.M. (2005) Glomerulonephritis—management in general practice. Aust Fam Physician. 34, 907–13.
3. Jayne, D.R., Gaskin, G., Rasmussen, N., Abramowicz, D., Ferrario, F., Guillevin, L., Mirapeix, E., Savage, C.O., Sinico, R.A., Stegeman, C.A., Westman, K.W., van der Woude, F.J., de Lind van Wijngaarden, R.A. & Pusey, C.D; European Vasculitis

Study Group. (2007) Randomized trial of plasma exchange or high-dosage methylprednisolone as adjunctive therapy for severe renal vasculitis. J Am Soc Nephrol. 2180–8.

Level B

4. Bosch, X., Guilabert, A. & Font, J. (2006) Antineutrophil cytoplasmic antibodies. Lancet. 368, 404–18.
5. Couser, W.G. (1999) Glomerulonephritis. Lancet. 353(9163), 1509–15.
6. Jayne, D., Rasmussen, N., Andrassy, K., Bacon, P., Tervaert, J.W., Dadoniene, J., Ekstrand, A., Gaskin, G., Gregorini, G., de Groot, K., Gross, W., Hagen, E.C., Mirapeix, E., Pettersson, E., Siegert, C., Sinico, A., Tesar, V., Westman, K. & Pusey, C. (2003) A randomized trial of maintenance therapy for vasculitis associated with antineutrophil cytoplasmic autoantibodies. N Engl J Med. 349, 36–44.
7. Jennette, J.C. (2003) Rapidly progressive crescentic glomerulonephritis. Kidney Int. 63, 1164–77.

Level C

8. Atkins, R.C., Nikolic-Paterson, D.J., Song, Q. & Lan, H.Y. (1996) Modulators of crescentic glomerulonephritis. J Am Soc Nephrol. 7, 2271–8.
9. Hellmich, B., Kausch, I., Doehn, C., Jocham, D., Holl-Ulrich, K. & Gross, W.L. (2004) Urinary bladder cancer in Wegener's granulomatosis: is it more than cyclophosphamide? Ann Rheum Dis. 63, 1183–5.
10. Jennette, J.C. & Thomas, D.B. (2007) Pauci-immune antineutrophil cytoplasmic autoantibody-mediated crescentic glomerulonephritis and vasculitis. *Heptinstall's Pathology of the Kidney*, Chapter 14, Jennette, J.C., Olson, J.L., Schwartz, M.M. & Silva, F.G. (eds). Philadelphia: Lippincott. 664–72.
11. Little, M.A. & Pusey, C.D. (2005) Glomerulonephritis due to antineutrophil cytoplasm antibody-associated vasculitis: an update on approaches to management. Nephrology. 10, 368–76.
12. Morgan, M.D., Harper, L., Williams, J. & Savage, C. (2006) Anti-neutrophil cytoplasm-associated glomerulonephritis. J Am Soc Nephrol. 17, 1224–34.
13. Tipping, P.G. & Holdsworth, S.R. (2006) T cells in crescentic glomerulonephritis. J Am Soc Nephrol. 17, 1253–63.
14. Schieben, D.J., Korbert, S.M., Kimura, R.E., Schwartz, M.M. & Lewis, E.J. (2005) Pulmonary-renal syndrome in a newborn with placental transmission of ANCAs. Am J Kidney Dis. 45, 758–61.
15. Trevisin, M., Neeson, P. & Savige, J. (2004) The binding of proteinase 3 antineutrophil cytoplasmic antibodies (PR3) varies in different ELISAs. J Clin Pathol. 57, 303–8.
16. Tam, F.W. (2006) Current pharmacotherapy for the treatment of crescentic glomerulonephritis. Expert Opin Investig Drugs. 15, 1353–69.
17. De Groot, K., Rasmussen, N., Bacon, P.A., Tervaert, J.W., Feighery, C., Gregorini, G., Gross, W.L. & Lugmani, J.D.R. (2005) Randomized trial of cyclophosphamide versus methotrexate for induction of remission in early systemic anti-neutrophil cytoplasmic antibody-associated vasculitis. Arthritis Rheum. 52, 2461–9.

Case 17
Acute renal failure and rhabdomyolysis

VINCENT LEE

Case history

A 30-year-old man presents to the hospital emergency department with red-coloured urine after a training jog in preparation for a community fun-run. Apart from general myalgias, he reports no other pain. On examination his weight is 70 kg, blood pressure is 120/70 mmHg, and he is euvolaemic with no abnormalities on chest or abdominal examination. He has some mild thigh and calf tenderness but there is no swelling. Urinalysis shows large blood, no proteinuria and no other abnormality.

Question 1

What is/are likely causes of this presentation?
- **(a)** Rhabdomyolysis
- **(b)** Membranous glomerulonephritis
- **(c)** Renal calculi
- **(d)** Transitional cell carcinoma (TCC) of the bladder
- **(e)** Bladder wall tear
- **(f)** March haemoglobinuria

Answer
A, E and F

Explanation

This man presents with discoloured urine associated with myalgia starting after exercise. Haematuria in sport is common—microscopic haematuria occurs in up to 20% of marathon runners and 55% of football players, while macroscopic haematuria occurs at one stage or another in 16% of football players and marathon runners. This presentation, coined 'sports haematuria', has multiple causes but is often benign (see Table 17.1) (Patel, Torres & Greydanus 2005). Haematuria after blunt physical contact is usually due to renal trauma. Haematuria after non-contact strenuous exercise can occur due to small tears in the bladder mucosa induced by the repetitive friction on the mucosa of a partially empty bladder, and resolves after a few days (answer E correct).

Uncommonly, strenuous exercise particularly affecting the feet (e.g. running on a hard road or kendo) and hands (e.g. conga drumming) may cause mechanical trauma to the red blood cells causing haemolysis. Free haemoglobin released from lysed red blood cells is filtered into the urine, a phenomenon known as march haemoglobinuria (answer F correct). Defects in red blood cell membrane proteins have been identified in some of these patients (Banga et al. 1979).

Another consequence of intense exercise is rhabdomyolysis, which is characterised by myocyte necrosis and release of myoglobin, leading to myoglobinuria (answer A correct).

Membranous glomerulonephritis usually presents with nephrotic syndrome, characterised by peripheral oedema, proteinuria, hypoalbuminaemia and hyperlipidaemia. Haematuria, either macroscopic or microscopic, is unusual. The lack of proteinuria in this individual makes the diagnosis of membranous glomerulonephritis unlikely (answer B incorrect).

Renal calculi usually presents with painful (rather than painless) macroscopic haematuria (answer C incorrect). TCC of the bladder usually affects older men and women, especially those with a past history of smoking or analgesic abuse (answer D incorrect).

Table 17.1 Causes of haematuria associated with exercise

- Myocyte damage: rhabdomyolysis
- Haemolysis: march haemoglobinuria
- Kidney damage: blunt trauma
- Bladder wall damage: due to repetitive friction from exercise
- Urethral injury: more common in cyclists
- Benign: relatively common and self-limiting, mechanism unknown, not associated with long-term renal damage

 Clinical pearls

- Self-limiting haematuria after exercise is common and usually benign.
- Persistent haematuria after exercise mandates further investigation of the renal tract looking for structural abnormalities, signs of glomerulonephritis (such as accompanying proteinuria) or pigmenturia (myoglobinuria or haemoglobinuria).

Question 2

What laboratory blood abnormalities are likely to be present in this man?

(a) Elevated creatine kinase

(b) Hyperkalaemia

(c) Hypouricaemia
(d) Elevated bicarbonate
(e) Elevated creatinine

Answer

A, B and E

Explanation

In a young man with haematuria after exercise, it is important to consider the diagnosis of rhabdomyolysis. In rhabdomyolysis, disruption of myocytes leads to release of creatine kinase and creatinine, leading to a rise in their serum levels (answers A and E correct). Hyperkalaemia and hyperuricaemia may be present due to cellular release of potassium and uric acid respectively (answer B correct, answer C incorrect). Patients with rhabdomyolysis usually develop a metabolic acidosis associated with reduction in serum bicarbonate (answer D incorrect).

Clinical pearl

- Rhabdomyolysis is accompanied by elevated creatine kinase (sometimes over 100 000 U/L), often with hyperkalaemia, hyperuricaemia, metabolic acidosis and disproportionately elevated serum creatinine (compared to serum urea) due to the breakdown of myocytes.

Case history continued ...

The patient's blood results show the following:

Serum creatinine	150 µmol/L	(60–120 in males)
Haemoglobin	135 g/L	(130–180)
Creatine kinase	150 000 U/L	(30–135)
Blood film normal		

Question 3

Based on these results, which of the following is/are likely to be present?
(a) Urinary red blood cells
(b) Plasma discolouration
(c) Myoglobin in urine
(d) Haemoglobin in urine

Answer

C

Explanation

The clinical picture of myalgia, haematuria and elevated serum creatine kinase level suggests the diagnosis of rhabdomyolysis. Haematuria is usually associated with detectable haem in the urine on a dipstick. Causes of a negative haem test in combination with discoloured urine include drugs such as rifampicin, ingestion of beet and acute intermittent porphyria.

In rhabdomyolysis, myocyte necrosis occurs leading to release of myoglobin which is freely filtered by the glomerulus. This man has myoglobinuria (answer C correct). In everyday practice, testing for myoglobin is cumbersome. The currently available assays (immunochemistry, haemagglutination inhibition, radioimmunoassay, complement fixation) are expensive and time-consuming. In addition, myoglobin is rapidly metabolised into bilirubin and cleared from plasma through the glomerulus, so it is more difficult to 'capture' the peak concentration of serum myoglobin and thus estimate total myocyte damage. Myoglobin is rapidly cleared from plasma; it is a monomer of 17 000 daltons and is thus smaller than haemoglobin, which is protein-bound and a combination of a tetramer of 69 000 and dimer of 34 000 daltons. Because it is smaller and not protein bound, myoglobin is more easily filtered through the glomerulus, so provided renal failure does not limit filtration, plasma retains its normal colour. Urinary myoglobin appears when the serum myoglobin level exceeds 1.5 to 3 mg/L (normal <0.01 mg/L). In contrast, haemoglobin is bound to haptoglobin in the plasma and is a larger molecule. Only the unbound dimer is filtered and haemoglobinuria does not occur until the filtered load exceeds the ability of the proximal tubule to reabsorb haemoglobin. Retention of free haemoglobin (both unbound and bound) leads to a red-brown discolouration of the plasma, generally at levels exceeding 1 to 1.5 mg/L (Rose 2006). Myoglobinuria is not associated with plasma discolouration. In this man, the haemoglobin level and blood film are normal, making the possibility of haemoglobinuria associated with haemolytic anaemia highly unlikely (answers B and D incorrect).

The standard urinary benzidine dipstick detects the presence of haem (in red blood cells, myoglobin and haemoglobin) and is as sensitive as urine microscopy in detecting abnormal amounts of red blood cells in urine (the equivalent of 1 to 2 red blood cells per high power field). Conventional urinary dipstick is unable to detect myoglobin concentrations below 60 mg/L. Both myoglobinuria and haemoglobinuria are associated with the dual finding of positive blood detection on standard urine dipstick coupled with negative urine microscopy for red blood cells (answer A incorrect).

 Clinical pearls

- Urinary dipstick is as sensitive as urine microscopy for the detection of haematuria.

- Pigmenturia is detectable by a positive urinary haem dipstick test, accompanied by lack of red blood cells on urine microscopy.

Question 4

Which of the following is/are indicated in this man?
(a) Watch and wait
(b) Aggressive intravenous fluid hydration
(c) Sodium bicarbonate to correct acidosis
(d) Steroids

Answer

B and C

Explanation

This patient has impaired renal function due to rhabdomyolysis. The main goals in this case are to prevent death and further worsening of renal function. This is achieved by correcting volume depletion and preventing intratubular cast formation. Volume replacement by intravenous hydration addresses the two main causes of early death in rhabdomyolysis: hypovolaemic shock and hyperkalaemia causing fatal cardiac arrhythmias. Studies of the use of intravenous hydration in rhabdomyolysis in earthquake victims suggest that early treatment of rhabdomyolysis prevents the establishment of renal failure. He has a severely elevated serum creatine kinase, suggesting that a lot of his muscle is affected by rhabdomyolysis. This patient requires immediate intravenous fluid hydration (answer A incorrect, answer B correct). It is desirable to achieve a high urine flow rate (200 to 300 mL/hour) to wash out excess tubular casts and myoglobin. Intravenous fluid administration rates of 1 L or higher per hour are initially required, especially as sequestration of fluid into 'third space' compartments occurs early after injury. Fluid resuscitation should continue until the patient is volume replete; in this man there is a risk of fluid overload due to his existing renal impairment. Coexisting metabolic acidosis and the use of loop diuretics such as frusemide acidify the urine, which enhances the tubular toxicity of myoglobin. Correction of both the systemic acidosis and urine pH can be achieved with careful administration of sodium bicarbonate (answer C correct). Acetazolamide prevents proximal tubular reabsorption of bicarbonate and thus alkalinises the urine; however, it should only be used when the blood pH is not acidic as it can exacerbate systemic acidosis. Care must be taken to prevent overalkalinisation, which favours precipitation of intrarenal calcium and phosphate. The infusion of mannitol with sodium bicarbonate is beneficial in maintaining adequate urinary flow but only works if acute tubular necrosis (ATN) is not yet established. Additionally, overzealous infusion of mannitol may cause overdiuresis, hypernatraemia, hyperosmolality and fluid overload, especially in individuals with renal impairment. Steroids have not been shown to improve outcomes in this condition and may cause or exacerbate rhabdomyolysis (answer D incorrect).

Clinical pearl

- The treatment of rhabdomyolysis involves early administration of fluids, urinary alkalinisation (by bicarbonate and acetazolamide) and increasing urinary flow (using mannitol and loop diuretics) to prevent the development of acute renal failure and to avoid mortality due to hypovolaemia and hyperkalaemic cardiac arrest.

LEVEL B

Case history continued ...

The patient has developed rhabdomyolysis associated with prolonged running, complicated by acute renal impairment. He is currently being treated with intravenous fluids and sodium bicarbonate. On further history-taking, he reveals that he is taking medication.

Question 5

Which of the following can cause rhabdomyolysis?
- **(a)** Simvastatin
- **(b)** Colchicine
- **(c)** Alcohol
- **(d)** Phenytoin

Answer
All are correct

Explanation

Physical injury and drugs are the two most common causes of rhabdomyolysis (see Table 17.2) (Walsh & Amato 2005). There are many drugs that cause rhabdomyolysis through a variety of different mechanisms. 3-hydroxy-3-methylglutaryl coenzyme A (3-HMG-CoA) reductase inhibitors (e.g. simvastatin) cause a generalised necrotising myopathy which can range in severity from an asymptomatic rise in serum creatine kinase to acute renal failure with myoglobinuria (answer A correct). Colchicine inhibits the polymerisation of intracellular tubulin into microtubular structures; this is the basis for its therapeutic effect (against gout) as well as its toxic effect (on muscle) (answer B correct). Phenytoin is associated with hypersensitivity reactions such as fever, rash, lymphadenopathy and inflammatory myositis (answer D correct). Alcohol and other illicit drugs together cause approximately one-third of cases of drug-induced rhabdomyolysis (answer C correct). Alcohol is directly toxic to the muscle; it can cause a range of effects including acute necrotising myopathy, acute hypokalaemic myopathy, chronic alcoholic myopathy and asymptomatic elevation in creatine kinase. Rhabdomyolysis may also result from physical injury due to alcohol's effects on a person's behaviour or conscious state. Other mechanisms by which drugs can cause rhabdomyolysis are mitochondrial toxicity (e.g. zidovudine), hypokalaemia (e.g. diuretics), and amphiphilia (ability of certain drugs that contain a positively charged amine group on its hydrophobic region to interact with the anionic phospholipids of cell membranes and organelles, such as amiodarone).

Table 17.2 Drug causes of rhabdomyolysis

Pathologic process	Examples
• Necrotising myopathy	• Cholesterol-lowering drugs — 3-hydroxy-3-methylglutaryl coenzyme A reductase inhibitors — Fibric acid derivatives — Niacin • Alcohol • Cyclosporine
• Amphiphilic	• Amiodarone • Chloroquine
• Antimicrotubular	• Colchicine • Vincristine
• Mitochondrial myopathy	• Zidovudine
• Inflammatory myopathy	• L-tryptophan • Phenytoin
• Hypokalaemic myopathy	• Diuretics • Laxatives
• Unknown	• Corticosteroids • Omeprazole

Source: Walsh & Amato 2005

 Clinical pearl

• As there are numerous drugs (many in common use) that can cause rhabdomyolysis, be suspicious of a drug- or toxin-related cause in a person presenting with rhabdomyolysis.

Case history continued ...

The patient is immediately treated with intravenous normal saline and sodium bicarbonate. Over the next 24 hours he passes only 50 mL of urine.

Question 6

Which of the following are true statements regarding this man's prognosis?
- **(a)** His renal function will more likely than not return to normal.
- **(b)** He is likely to require long term dialysis.
- **(c)** His risk of death is approximately 10%.
- **(d)** The cause of rhabdomyolysis has no bearing on the risk of acute renal failure (ARF).

Answer

A and C

Explanation

Rhabdomyolysis associated ARF causes acute tubular necrosis (ATN) and has a good prognosis with appropriate therapy. In hospitalised patients, approximately three-quarters survive and renal function recovers to normal in the majority of survivors (answer A correct). Even if dialysis is required, patients will normally only require dialysis for at most 1 to 2 months while the kidney 'recovers' from ATN (answer B incorrect). Regardless of cause, the prognosis of ARF is worse in patients who are older, have renal impairment at presentation, oliguria and higher creatine kinase levels. In large series, death rates have ranged from 3 to 21% depending on the population studied. In this man with his young age and lack of comorbid conditions, the risk of death is low (answer C correct). Prognosis varies with the cause of ARF: individuals with rhabdomyolysis due to muscle disorders such as polymyositis have a low risk of ARF whereas patients with drug- or trauma-related rhabdomyolysis do less well (answer D incorrect) (Melli, Chaudhry & Cornblath 2005).

 Clinical pearls

- The prognosis of rhabdomyolysis is similar to that of acute tubular necrosis of any cause: potentially reversible if treated early enough.
- Prognostic factors for the development of acute renal failure in rhabdomyolysis include older age, oliguria, renal impairment at presentation, higher creatine kinase and aetiology.

Question 7

Which of the following may explain the mechanism of renal injury in rhabdomyolysis?

(a) Tubule blockade by myoglobin casts
(b) Tubular toxicity by free iron
(c) Complement deposition
(d) Renal vasoconstriction and ischaemia

Answer

A, B and D

Explanation

About half of individuals who develop ARF in association with rhabdomyolysis develop acute tubular necrosis, which is a direct consequence of ischaemia (induced by hypovolaemia and hypotension), direct tubular toxicity of myoglobin and myoglobin tubular cast formation (answers A, B and D correct) (see Fig. 17.1) (Malinoski, Slater & Mullins 2004). Complement deposition does not occur in rhabdomyolysis (answer C incorrect).

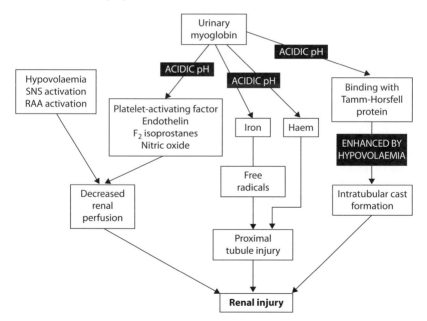

Figure 17.1 Pathogenesis of renal injury in rhabdomyolysis. Urinary myoglobin is a key player in the pathogenesis of renal injury

Note: SNS = sympathetic nervous system, RAA = renin–angiotensin–aldosterone system, acidic pH = reactions enhanced by an acidic environment, which may also be inhibited by urinary alkalinisation thereby reducing renal injury

Clinical pearl

- Renal injury in rhabdomyolysis is due to renal hypoperfusion, myoglobin-induced renal injury and intratubular cast formation. By ameliorating these pathways of injury through fluid resuscitation and urinary alkalinisation, renal injury may be prevented.

LEVEL C

Question 8

This patient has developed acute renal impairment due to rhabdomyolysis induced by exercise. Which of the following metabolic derangements are likely to be present in myocytes undergoing rhabdomyolysis?
(a) Raised intracellular calcium
(b) Raised intracellular adenosine triphosphate (ATP) levels
(c) Early mononuclear cell infiltration
(d) Free radicals

Answer
A and D

Explanation

Muscle cells depend on fine control of sodium and calcium concentration within the sarcoplasmic reticulum by ATP-dependent calcium pumps within the sarcoplasmic membrane. Disruption of the membrane or ATP depletion leads to a rise in intrasarcoplasmic calcium levels (answer A correct). This leads to cell contraction by the myosin-actin filaments. If uncontrolled, ATP is consumed leading to further Ca influx, forming a vicious cycle leading to muscle cell necrosis (answer B incorrect). Damaged muscle is invaded by neutrophils which release proteases and free radicals further perpetuating injury (answer D correct). Muscle cell ischaemia is usually present; however, only when blood flow is restored do the majority of leucocytes migrate and cause damage in this region by further release of free radicals and proteases (answer C incorrect). The above description applies to both traumatic and non-traumatic rhabdomyolysis (Vanholder et al. 2000).

Question 9

Which of the following can cause rhabdomyolysis?
(a) Hypokalaemia
(b) Hypophosphataemia

(c) Hypermagnesaemia
(d) Hyperchloraemia

Answer

A and B

Explanation

About 10% of cases of rhabdomyolysis are due to metabolic abnormalities (Amanzadeh & Reilly 2006). Phosphorus is an essential element with roles in cell structure (e.g. nucleic acids), cellular metabolism (ATP and ADP metabolism), regulation of subcellular processes (phosphorylation of key enzymes) and maintenance of acid–base homeostasis (urinary buffering). Severe hypophosphataemia (particularly at serum levels <0.3 mmol/L, normal 0.8 to 1.6 mmol/L) is associated with rhabdomyolysis (answer B correct) (see Table 17.3). The treatment of hypophosphataemia is replacement therapy with inorganic phosphate. Concern has been raised that the intravenous route of administration may cause a precipitous fall in serum calcium, hypotension, defects in tissue oxygenation (due to increased erythrocyte 2,3-diphosphoglycerate) and ARF. However, the majority of case reports suggest that intravenous phosphorus therapy is safe. Intravenous phosphorus should be administered in cases of severe hypophosphataemia (serum level <0.3 mmol/L) at approximately 0.08 to 0.16 mmol/kg body weight every 2 to 6 hours.

Hypokalaemia is associated with rhabdomyolysis, particularly at serum levels <2.0 mmol/L (normal 3.5 to 5.0 mmol/L) (answer A correct). Patients who take long-acting diuretics (e.g. chlorthalidone) or diuretics in combination with other influences that lower potassium (e.g. liquorice, underlying primary aldosteronism) are susceptible to rhabdomyolysis (see Table 17.3). Potassium may be administered orally in mild deficiency or intravenously if serum levels are low enough to cause symptoms of cardiotoxicity (especially at levels <3.0 mmol/L).

Clinical rhabdomyolysis has not been reported in humans with selective magnesium deficiency. However, low magnesium levels are commonly accompanied by other risk factors for rhabdomyolysis such as alcoholism, hypophosphataemia, hypokalaemia or malabsorption. Hypermagnesaemia is not associated with rhabdomyolysis (answer C incorrect). There are no clinical reports of rhabdomyolysis that are clearly attributable to abnormalities in sodium, chloride or calcium levels (answer D incorrect).

 Clinical pearl

- Electrolyte abnormalities that cause rhabdomyolysis include hypophosphataemia and hypokalaemia, through perturbations in muscle cell electrical activity, metabolism and blood flow.

- Alcoholism is the most common cause of rhabdomyolysis induced by phosphate depletion. Diuretics and malabsorptive states are the main causes of hypokalaemia-induced rhabdomyolysis.

Table 17.3 Electrolyte abnormalities and rhabdomyolysis

Electrolyte abnormality	Common causes leading to rhabdomyolysis	Mechanism of muscle damage
Hypophosphataemia	• Decreased absorption (alcoholism, malabsorption) • Redistribution of phosphorus (alcoholism, respiratory alkalosis, rapid correction of respiratory acidosis [e.g. commencing mechanical ventilation], sepsis, diabetic ketoacidosis, refeeding syndrome during hyperalimentation) • Increased urinary excretion of phosphorus (alcoholism)	• Alterations in muscle cell transmembrane potential • Alterations in intracellular sodium, chloride and water • Impaired mitochondrial function
Hypokalaemia	• Enhanced potassium loss (diuretics particularly thiazides, mineralocorticoid excess, heat stress, malabsorption syndrome, villous adenoma of rectum, chronic laxative use, chronic vomiting, thyrotoxicosis, renal tubular acidosis, amphotericin B)	• Alterations in muscle cell transmembrane potential • Decreased muscle blood flow • Defective muscle glycogen metabolism

Question 10

The patient now tells you that he has had multiple similar attacks in the past, especially after prolonged exercise. His sister has a similar history. What possible underlying causes may explain this?

(a) Carnitine palmityltransferase deficiency
(b) Neuroleptic malignant syndrome
(c) Serotoninergic syndrome
(d) McArdle's disease

Answer
A and D

Explanation

The history suggests that this man has an inherited predisposition to rhabdomyolysis. The most common conditions are disorders of glycolysis and glycogenolysis (e.g. McArdle's disease [answer D correct], phosphoglycerate kinase deficiency and phosphofructokinase deficiency), fatty acid oxidation (e.g. carnitine palmityltransferase deficiency [answer A correct]) and purine nucleotide cycle (myoadenylate deaminase deficiency) (see Table 17.4 for details about the most common of these disorders). Disorders affecting the Krebs cycle, pentose phosphate pathway (glucose-6-phosphate dehydrogenase deficiency) and mitochondrial respiratory chain are also associated with an inherited predisposition to rhabdomyolysis. The final common pathway of these disorders is inadequate muscle supply of ATP leading to muscle cell breakdown. These disorders usually present with myalgias, rhabdomyolysis and occasionally acute renal failure after prolonged exercise, fasting or infection. Family history is usually positive in one-third of cases with an identifiable enzyme defect. Diagnosis is based on a standardised forearm ischaemic exercise test, electromyography and muscle biopsy (with histopathology and biochemistry with measurement of muscle enzyme activities) (Bonnefont et al. 2004; Darras 2006). About 40% of patients with unexplained recurrent rhabdomyolysis will have an enzyme defect.

Neuroleptic malignant syndrome (NMS) is a distinctive clinical syndrome of mental status change, rigidity, rhabdomyolysis, fever and dysautonomia. It is associated with the administration of dopamine-blocking agents such as phenothiazines, inhibitors of striatal dopamine production (e.g. lithium) and abrupt withdrawal of dopaminergic agents, and is not associated with excessive exertion (answer B incorrect). Severe rigidity and tremor cause excess heat production which leads to muscle breakdown, probably exacerbated by dysfunctional hypothalamic-driven thermoregulation. Another related condition is malignant hyperthermia which is associated with the use of inhalational anaesthetic agents. Familial clusters of both NMS and malignant hyperthermia have been reported.

The serotoninergic syndrome occurs when excess serotonin activity leads to altered mental state, neuromuscular irritability, autonomic instability and rhabdomyolysis with renal failure. The use of selective serotonin reuptake inhibitors in combination with monoamine oxidase inhibitors (MAOIs) is most commonly the cause, although other combinations (MAOIs with pethidine, tricyclic antidepressants and lithium) and individual drugs (e.g. 'Ecstasy' 3,4-methylene-dioxymetamphetamine) are also causes (answer C incorrect). There are no known genetic predispositions to the serotoninergic syndrome.

Table 17.4 Metabolic myopathies commonly associated with rhabdomyolysis

Type	Persons affected	Inheritance	Clinical features	Pathophysiology	Diagnosis	Treatment
Carnitine palmityltransferase II (CPT II) deficiency, adult onset type	Males, starting at 6–20 years of age	Autosomal recessive	Recurrent attacks of muscle pain and weakness, recurrent myoglobinuria. Precipitated by exercise, fasting, high fat intake, cold, infection, fever, emotion, anaesthesia, drugs (diazepam, ibuprofen, valproate)	Defective transport of long-chain fatty acids (e.g. acylcarnitine) through the outer and inner membranes of mitochondria causing defective conversion of long chain fatty acids into ketones. Multiple (>40) mutations described	Elevation of long chain fatty acids in blood and urine, particularly during an acute attack, CPT II levels in muscle, normal glucose levels in blood, provocation test (e.g. effect of fasting on production of ketone bodies)	Dietary restriction of long-chain fatty acids, medium–chain triglycerides, carbohydrate loading before and during exercise, avoidance of triggers
McArdle's disease (glycogen storage disease V)	Childhood	Autosomal recessive	Exercise intolerance, pain/cramps/fatigue in exercised muscle, exacerbation by brief intense activity, rhabdomyolysis with exercise	Defect in myophosphorylase, an enzyme essential for glycogenolysis	Ischaemic forearm exercise test: increase in ammonia but not lactate after exercise, muscle biopsy. Increased glycogen stores on muscle biopsy, absent myophosphorylase staining and enzyme activity	Graded exercise, oral sucrose, exercise conditioning programs

Clinical pearls

- Recurrent rhabdomyolysis or isolated rhabdomyolysis (i.e. no obvious precipitating cause) should prompt a search for inherited metabolic myopathies. These are characterised by a positive family history and a history of poor exercise tolerance.
- The most common causes are mitochondrial enzyme defects in glucose, glycogen or fatty acid metabolism.
- Diagnosis is difficult using non-invasive testing. Therefore, muscle biopsy is usually required to make the diagnosis, using histology, immunostaining of muscle enzymes and measurement of enzyme activity.

Bibliography

Level A

1. Patel, D.R., Torres, A.D. & Greydanus, D.E. (2005) Kidneys and sports. Adolesc Med Clin. 16, 111–19, xi.
2. Banga, J.P., Pinder, J.C., Gratzer, W.B., Linch, D.C. & Huehns, E.R. (1979) An erythrocyte membrane-protein anomaly in march haemoglobinuria. Lancet. 2, 1048–9.
3. Rose, B.D. (2006) Red urine: hematuria; hemoglobinuria; myoglobinuria, *UpToDate*, Rose, B.D. (ed.) UpToDate: Waltham, MA.

Level B

4. Walsh, R.J. & Amato, A.A. (2005) Toxic myopathies. Neurol Clin. 23, 397–428.
5. Melli, G., Chaudhry, V. & Cornblath, D.R. (2005) Rhabdomyolysis: an evaluation of 475 hospitalized patients. Medicine (Baltimore). 84, 377–85.
6. Malinoski, D.J., Slater, M.S. & Mullins, R.J. (2004) Crush injury and rhabdomyolysis. Crit Care Clin. 20, 171–92.

Level C

7. Vanholder, R., Sever, M.S., Erek, E. & Lameire, N. (2000) Rhabdomyolysis. J Am Soc Nephrol. 11, 1553–61.
8. Amanzadeh, J. & Reilly, R.F. (2006) Hypophosphatemia: an evidence-based approach to its clinical consequences and management. Nat Clin Pract Nephrol. 2, 136–48.
9. Bonnefont, J.P., Djouadi, F., Prip-Buus, C., Gobin, S., Munnich, A. & Bastin, J. (2004) Carnitine palmitoyltransferases 1 and 2: biochemical, molecular and medical aspects. Mol Aspects Med. 25, 495–520.
10. Darras, B.T. (2006) Approach to the metabolic myopathies, *UpToDate*, Rose, B.D. (ed.) UpToDate: Waltham, MA.

Case 18
Acute renal failure and drug-induced nephrotoxicity

ROB WALKER

LEVEL A

Case history

A 74-year-old man presents with a three-day history of nausea, vomiting and diarrhoea. On examination he is afebrile; he has a tachycardia at 110 beats/min; his blood pressure (BP) is 110/80 mmHg lying and falls to 88/60 mmHg upon standing; his jugular venous pressure (JVP) is only visible when his bed is tilted head down and measures 1 cm below the right atrium (a negative value); his mouth is quite dry; his weight on admission is 72 kg and he normally weighs 75 kg. He states he has only passed urine twice in the last 24 hours and estimates the amount to be about 200 mL. His bladder is not palpable. His admission blood tests show a plasma creatinine of 540 μmol/L and urea of 34 mmol/L, his potassium is 6.5 mmol/L and arterial blood gases demonstrate a metabolic acidosis with a pH of 7.10, HCO_3^- 12 mmol/L, PCO_2 25 mmHg, PO_2 110 mmHg, and base excess of –12. His haemoglobin is 110 g/L, white blood count 9.6×10^9/L. Past medical history includes osteoarthritis, hypertension and occasional angina on exertion. Medications are bendrofluazide 5 mg daily, ramipril 5 mg daily, atenolol 50 mg daily, diclofenac SR 75 mg twice a day and omeprazole 20 mg daily.

Question 1

This man is in acute renal failure. Which of the following is/are correct?
- **(a)** On the information given you can exclude a rapidly progressive glomerulonephritis as the cause for his acute renal failure.
- **(b)** Urinary tract obstruction is the most likely cause of the low urine output.
- **(c)** It is possible that he has developed acute tubular necrosis.
- **(d)** He must be catheterised to measure his urine output.
- **(e)** The major cause for his acute renal failure is reduced renal perfusion.

Answer
C and E

Explanation

This is a typical presentation of acute renal failure. This man has evidence of significant intravascular volume depletion which in turn has reduced his renal perfusion. His antihypertensive therapy will further compromise his ability to maintain adequate renal perfusion. The background of long-standing hypertension and antihypertensive therapy will have significantly reduced the kidneys' normal autoregulatory response to maintain adequate perfusion in the face of a reduced systemic perfusion pressure. If renal hypoperfusion persists, it is highly likely that acute tubular necrosis secondary to ischaemia will develop.

A rapidly progressive glomerulonephritis cannot be excluded. Urinalysis would be helpful. The absence of an active urinary sediment (haematuria, red cell casts, proteinuria) would make this diagnosis much less likely.

The absence of a palpable bladder would make obstruction less likely but it cannot be completely ruled out. It is most likely that he is oliguric because of the hypotension, and acute reduction in renal perfusion and the compensatory retention of sodium and water by the kidney attempting to correct the reduced intravascular volume. Increased activation of the renin–angiotensin–aldosterone axis, arginine vasopressin (antidiuretic hormone) and sympathetic nerve activity all contribute to increased salt and water retention and hence the oliguria. He is alert and conscious and therefore able to pass urine when necessary. The insertion of a urinary catheter will not change management and will only increase the risk of complications such as urethral stricture and urinary tract infection.

 Clinical pearls

- The rule of three is used to assess aetiology of acute renal failure (ARF):

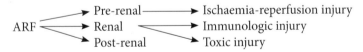

ARF
- Pre-renal ⟶ Ischaemia-reperfusion injury
- Renal ⟶ Immunologic injury
- Post-renal ⟶ Toxic injury

- Pre-renal causes are related to a reduction in renal perfusion for whatever cause: low intravascular volume due to fluid loss, poor cardiac output, or drugs lowering systemic BP. Over 75% of cases of ARF have a major pre-renal element.
- Post-renal causes are obstruction to the urinary tract from tubular obstruction as can occur with the tumour lysis syndrome and high concentrations of uric acid precipitating out in the tubular lumen, intrinsic ureteric obstruction (tumour or calculi), extrinsic compression of ureters (retroperitoneal tumours or fibrosis) and bladder outflow obstruction (prostatic hypertrophy, invasive pelvic malignancies).

- Renal causes: second rule of three:
  — Ischaemic injury secondary to prolonged reduced perfusion plus free-radical injury associated with reperfusion.
  — Immunologic: acute glomerulonephritis, acute interstitial nephritis.
  — Toxic: drug-induced injury (direct toxic effect on the tubular epithelial cells).
- 'A reasonable definition of acute renal failure is an acute and sustained increase in serum creatinine concentration of 44.2 µmol/L if baseline is less than 221 µmol/L or an increase of more than 20% if the baseline serum creatinine is more than 221 µmol/L' (Lameire, Van Biesen & Vanholder 2006).
- Acute kidney injury is now the preferred terminology for ARF.

Question 2

Urinalysis from this case demonstrates a benign urine with no haematuria, white cells or proteinuria. Renal ultrasound demonstrates no dilated pelvicalyceal systems. Which of the following is/are correct?

(a) Diclofenac does not contribute to the acute renal failure.
(b) Atenolol is safe to use in renal failure as it is excreted by the liver.
(c) Omeprazole does not cause any renal injury.
(d) An urgent renal biopsy is indicated.
(e) Immediate management is resuscitation with intravenous normal saline.

Answer

E

Explanation

The urinalysis makes an immunological cause for the acute renal failure less likely but it does not rule it out completely. The absence of any pathology on renal ultrasound effectively excludes lower urinary tract obstruction. Non-steroidal anti-inflammatory drugs (NSAIDs) (diclofenac in this case) can have a critical impact on renal function. Under normal conditions with normal renal function, renal prostaglandins play little or no role in the maintenance of renal perfusion. Under stress conditions, with activation of vasoconstrictors (angiotensin II, arginine vasopressin, sympathetic nerve activity and catecholamines), the vasodilatory prostaglandins are required to modulate the effects of the vasoconstrictors. If these are blocked by NSAIDs inhibiting cyclo-oxygenase, then there is unopposed vasoconstriction intensifying the reduction in renal perfusion. Normally with fluid losses such as vomiting or diarrhoea, the kidneys retain sodium and water to help replete the intravascular volume. The angiotensin-converting enzyme inhibitor (ACEi), ramipril, and diuretic will block sodium and hence water reabsorption, further adding to the reduction in intravascular volume.

Atenolol is the only beta-blocker that is excreted by the kidneys. The dosage needs to be modified in renal failure or preferably an alternative beta-blocker should be used. The dose needs to be withheld or substantially reduced over this acute period.

Omeprazole can produce acute renal failure in the form of an acute interstitial nephritis (AIN). The proton pump inhibitors are now the most common agents implicated in drug-induced nephritis (Roger 2006). It is unlikely in this case as most forms of AIN present with a progressive decline in renal function with a maintained urine output or even polyuria. Urinalysis (microscopy and Wright's stain) usually demonstrates the presence of white cells and eosinophils.

At this stage, the most likely diagnosis is acute renal failure on a pre-renal basis made worse by this man's medications. In the absence of an active urinary sediment, a renal biopsy is not necessary and would not modify initial management.

Initial management is urgent correction of this man's depleted intravascular volume and the restoration of his systemic BP which in turn will restore renal perfusion. In most cases, correction of the intravascular volume with intravenous normal saline will also correct the metabolic acidosis and hyperkalaemia. Unless there are obvious electrocardiogram abnormalities of hyperkalaemia, no additional therapy is required to correct the hyperkalaemia. However, frequent monitoring should be used to confirm correction of these parameters.

Clinical pearls

- Pre-renal (hypotension/hypoperfusion) factors leading to ischaemia are the predominant cause of the acute renal impairment seen in usual clinical settings. In a community setting acute tubular necrosis was responsible for 45% of cases and pre-renal failure for 21% of cases admitted to hospital (Liano & Pascual, Madrid Acute Renal Failure Study Group 1996). In a hospital setting, drug-induced acute kidney injury is a substantially greater contributor.
- Always assess BP (lying and standing), the JVP (the most accurate clinical manometer of intravascular volume) and the individual's body weight as the most important markers of the body's intravascular volume status. The reduction in weight will give an estimate of the extent of fluid loss. In this case 3 kg of weight loss equals 3 L of fluid.
- Always consider the role of drugs in precipitating or contributing to the acute renal failure.

Case history continued ...

On admission, the admitting registrar requests urinary biochemistry tests on the first urine obtained. The urinary sodium is 50 mmol/L and urinary osmolality is 420 mosm/kg.

Question 3

Which of the following statements is/are correct?
(a) These results exclude a pre-renal aetiology for his acute renal failure.
(b) The presence of a diuretic interferes with the validity of this test.
(c) These values could be consistent with acute tubular necrosis.
(d) It is important to know what the baseline renal function was prior to the onset of the illness.
(e) Urinary creatinine would allow the calculation of the fractional excretion of sodium (FENa).

Answer
B, C, D and E

Explanation

If the acute renal failure is due to pre-renal causes alone, the kidneys will be avidly retaining sodium and water to try and correct the low intravascular volume. Under conditions of marked intravascular volume depletion and previously normal renal function, a urinary osmolality of greater than 600 mosm/kg and a urinary sodium concentration of less than 20 mmol/L would be consistent with a pre-renal aetiology for the acute renal failure which would be more accurately confirmed with FENa <0.01 (1%).

$$FENa\% = \frac{UNa \times PCr}{PNa \times UCr} \times 100$$

A urinary osmolality approximating the plasma osmolality (300 mosm/kg) and a urinary sodium concentration greater than 40 mmol/L are consistent with acute tubular injury and the loss of the medullary concentration gradient. However, there are limitations to the interpretation of the results. Diuretics will make the values uninterpretable because they block sodium reabsorption.

 Clinical pearl

- Although urinary biochemistry may be helpful, the results need to be interpreted with respect to the clinical context. Diuretics and ACEi will negate the validity of urinary biochemistry results.

LEVEL B

Case history continued ...

After making a full recovery, the patient presents 2 years later with acute chole-cystitis associated with vomiting and abdominal pain. He is febrile, hypotensive and mildly jaundiced. His medications on admission are an ACEi, a thiazide diuretic, an NSAID and omeprazole. Admission biochemistry demonstrates a plasma creatinine of 130 µmol/L along with deranged liver function tests. He is commenced on gentamicin (standard dosing of 5 mg/kg/24-hourly), metro-nidazole (500 mg 8-hourly) and amoxicillin (2 gm 8-hourly). He undergoes an urgent CT scan with contrast which confirms the diagnosis of acute cholecystitis. He is subsequently taken to theatre for a laparoscopic cholecystectomy. Post-operatively he continues to lose about 200 mL/hour via nasogastric drainage. His BP post-operatively remains low at 106/60 mmHg.

Question 4

Which of the following statements is/are correct?

(a) This man has near normal renal function on admission with a glomerular filtration rate (GFR) greater than 70 mL/min.

(b) His GFR is moderately impaired.

(c) A 24-hour dosage interval for gentamicin is appropriate to prevent toxicity.

(d) Contrast toxicity is unlikely to be a problem in this setting.

(e) Metronidazole does not require dose modification in renal failure.

Answer
B and E

Explanation

Assuming a normal weight of 70 kg this man's calculated creatinine clearance is 44 mL/min. With his underlying comorbidities he is at a high risk of developing a significant deterioration in his renal function.

Gentamicin is excreted only by the kidneys. The use of once-a-day dosing regimens for gentamicin, along with drug monitoring, has reduced the incidence of gentamicin-induced nephrotoxicity. However, the computer programs for drug monitoring assume a steady-state condition for the calculation of the area under the curve for gentamicin pharmacokinetics. Drug sampling is usually 1 hour post-dose and 6 hours post-dose and values are used to calculate the area under the curve for pharmacokinetics of the drug and when it would be expected that the drug has been cleared from the blood stream. The program calculates when the trough level is less than 0.5 mg/L (the lower limit of detection for the assay) and recommends the timing of the next dose. If renal function is unstable, it is essential to confirm that the trough level is in fact <0.5 prior to administration of the next dose. If the level is elevated, then accumulation is occurring consistent with deteriorating renal function. In addition, gentamicin drug monitoring has only been extensively validated in individuals with normal to mildly impaired renal function (GFR ≥60 mL/min). Clearly this man is clinically unstable and his renal function is likely to deteriorate due to a number of contributing factors. These include sepsis, hypotension, the residual effects of his medications and exposure to contrast material.

Metronidazole is eliminated by hepatic routes.

 Clinical pearls

- It is essential to determine an individual's estimated creatinine clearance or GFR when prescribing potentially nephrotoxic drugs.
- Appropriate changes to the amount of drug administered and/or dosage intervals need to be made according to kidney function.
- Confirm gentamicin trough levels have been reached before administering the next dose. Gentamicin has a prolonged post-dose effect and does not that require that a minimum plasma concentration be maintained for bactericidal activity.
- Changes in plasma creatinine are late manifestations of renal injury.
- Remember that the unstable sick patient will have additional factors related to the illness which will compromise renal function.

Case history continued …

Over the weekend, gentamicin levels are obtained only after the first 24 hours and no change in the dosage interval was made. He remains hypotensive. His plasma creatinine is measured on day three and is now 285 μmol/L. Gentamicin monitoring recommends a new dosage interval of greater than 48 hours.

Question 5

Which of the following statements is/are correct?
- **(a)** An elevated plasma creatinine due to contrast nephrotoxicity is usually evident within 24 hours.
- **(b)** Gentamicin toxicity produces acute tubular necrosis.

(c) Gentamicin toxicity will only occur when trough level concentrations are elevated.

(d) Peak levels of gentamicin are more relevant to the risk of ototoxicity.

Answer
B and D

Explanation

The rise in plasma creatinine due to either contrast- or gentamicin-induced toxicity is a late manifestation of injury. Gentamicin has a small molecular weight of 500 daltons and is freely filtered at the glomerulus with little tubular handling. Gentamicin clearance is comparable to the GFR. The urinary concentration of gentamicin can be two- to fivefold higher than plasma concentrations. There is some uptake of gentamicin predominantly in the S1 and S2 segments of the proximal tubule. Gentamicin binds to the phospholipids (megalin) of the apical membrane and is taken up into cells via receptor-mediated endocytosis. There is subsequent sequestration in the lysosomes leading to lysosomal rupture with disruption of intracellular metabolism resulting in acute tubular necrosis. Accumulation of gentamicin is consistent with development of nephrotoxicity.

 Clinical pearl

- Risk factors for gentamicin nephrotoxicity are:
  - renal impairment (all causes): reduced clearances and greater accumulation
  - volume depletion and diuretics: reduced urine flow rate leads to a higher urinary concentration at the level of the proximal tubule as well as a prolonged contact time leading to a greater uptake of gentamicin by proximal tubular cells
  - other nephrotoxic agents: synergistic injury
  - recent aminoglycoside therapy
  - hypokalaemia: predisposes tubular epithelial cells to injury.

Question 6

With respect to the use of contrast in this patient's acute renal failure, which of the following is/are correct?

(a) In the absence of an elevated plasma creatinine, contrast nephrotoxicity is unlikely.

(b) Contrast-induced toxicity is not associated with long-term sequelae.

(c) The use of iso-osmolar contrast media is associated with a lower risk of nephrotoxicity.

(d) NSAIDs are unlikely to enhance the risk of contrast nephrotoxicity.

(e) Adequate hydration with intravenous (IV) saline pre- and post-contrast exposure is the most reliable renal protective intervention.

Answer

C and E

Explanation

Contrast-induced nephrotoxicity (CIN) has an incidence of 1.6 to 2.3% with all diagnostic interventions and is more common with intra-arterial contrast. Major risk factors include chronic kidney disease (CKD), diabetes, increasing age, intravascular volume depletion, underlying atherosclerotic vascular disease, smoking, cirrhosis and the nephrotic syndrome. A plasma creatinine in the normal range does not exclude CKD (see above). There is a higher incidence of toxicity associated with hyperosmolar contrast media. Of those individuals who develop acute renal impairment (usually defined as a 25% increase in plasma creatinine or greater than 44 μmol/L increase in plasma creatinine within 2 to 7 days following contrast exposure), up to 7% will require dialysis (the overall incidence of developing dialysis-dependent acute renal failure is 0.5 to 1.0%). Individuals with diabetes and CKD are at highest risk of contrast nephrotoxicity (3 to 20% incidence). Although dialysis is infrequently required, contrast nephropathy is by no means a benign complication as up to 30% of individuals will have a degree of residual impairment following the development of contrast nephropathy. The development of contrast-induced nephrotoxicity is associated with an increased length of hospital stay and a 5.5-fold increased risk of short- and long-term mortality.

Contrast media induces renal injury via the development of intense arteriolar vasoconstriction associated with increased endothelin and decreased nitric oxide production as well as a direct cellular-mediated injury via oxidative stress and increased intracellular calcium. Cellular toxicity is enhanced under hypoxic conditions. NSAIDs can potentiate vasoconstriction and increase ischaemia reperfusion-mediated injury (see above).

There have been a large number of randomised controlled trials examining strategies for reducing the incidence of contrast-induced nephrotoxicity. Most recent trials have used N-acetylcysteine as a protective agent with variable results. Several meta-analyses have produced inconclusive results due to significant unexplained heterogeneity resulting from differences in contrast media, definition of acute renal impairment, co intervention with other agents, the dose of N-acetylcysteine used, route of administration (oral or IV), as well as the timing of procedure. Recent reviews (Barrett 2006) recommend the use of pre-hydration with N-saline to establish high urine flow rate. In an in-patient setting, use IV saline 1 to 2 hours pre- and 6 to 24 hours post-procedure. For an outpatient-based procedure, oral hydration pre- and IV saline for 6 hours post-procedure is recommended. There is no evidence for the use of mannitol or frusemide to increase urine flow rate. A small number of studies have demonstrated increased morbidity when frusemide was added to N-saline (Solomon et al. 1994). Frusemide should not be used to prevent contrast-induced nephrotoxicity.

Clinical pearls

- Contrast-induced nephrotoxicity is common in clinical practice. All at-risk individuals need adequate hydration prior to, as well as after, contrast exposure to maintain a high urine output.
- Current evidence-base favours the use of IV N-saline to reduce the risk of contrast induced nephrotoxicity.
- The role of N-acetylcysteine as a renoprotective agent remains uncertain.

LEVEL C

Question 7

With respect to the pathophysiology of this man's acute renal failure, which of the following is/are correct?

(a) A renal biopsy will demonstrate a patchy non-continuous acute tubular necrosis.

(b) The anatomical location of the acute tubular necrosis is predominantly in the cortex in the region of the distal collecting tubules.

(c) A proposed mechanism by which intravenous hydration prevents contrast-induced toxicity is via a reduction in renal tissue oxygen consumption.

(d) A cyclo-oxygenase 2 (COX2) inhibitor is less likely to enhance renal injury in this setting.

Answer
A and C

Explanation

There is a marked oxygen gradient from the renal cortex to the medulla related to the counter-current mechanism necessary for the development of the medullary concentration gradient. Portions of the renal medulla function normally under marginal hypoxic conditions. Under conditions of intense renal vasoconstriction, perfusion via the vasa recta is reduced with a consequent reduction in the oxygen gradient. If this is sustained hypoxic-ischaemic injury can occur. Ischaemic injury has a characteristic distribution along the medullary rays which explains the patchy areas of acute tubular necrosis seen on renal biopsy. Injury is predominantly confined to proximal tubular epithelial cells (especially in the S3 segment) (Lieberthal & Nigam 1998).

COX2 is constitutively expressed in the kidney and therefore the use of a COX2-specific inhibitor is not renal sparing.

 Clinical pearls

- Maintenance of systemic BP and hence renal perfusion combined with a high urine flow rate will reduce renal oxygen requirements, minimising the potential for hypoxic injury.
- A COX2 inhibitor can induce changes in renal haemodynamics and renal tubular function under conditions of duress similar to that seen with non-specific COX inhibition.

Case history continued ...

The patient's kidney function continues to decline. His urea is now 44 mmol/L, creatinine is 556 µmol/L and his potassium is 6.4 mmol/L. He has a metabolic acidosis with a pH of 7.12. With aggressive re-hydration his BP is now 142/86 mmHg and his JVP is 5 cm.

Question 8

Which of the following is/are correct?

(a) Continuous veno-venous haemofiltration (CVVH) is the preferred management for his ARF.

(b) Standard intermittent haemodialysis (IHD) has been shown to be ineffective in this clinical setting.

(c) Acute peritoneal dialysis is no longer a preferred therapy.

(d) The early use of frusemide and/or dopamine or theophylline would have prevented the need for dialysis.

Answer

C

Explanation

There have been a number of randomised controlled trials (RCTs) comparing different modalities to treat ARF in the ICU setting which have failed to demonstrate that one modality is better than another. On the basis of current evidence, CVVH and IHD should be considered equivalent (Ricci, Bellomo & Ronco 2006). Acute peritoneal dialysis is now very rarely used.

Clinical studies have failed to demonstrate any benefit of frusemide in the prevention and treatment of acute renal failure. A recent meta-analysis of nine RCTs (involving 849 patients) did not demonstrate any difference in any outcome measure, including mortality and the need for dialysis (Ho & Sheridan 2006). Additionally, administration of frusemide may cause further depletion of the intravascular volume and compromise renal perfusion. The role of low-dose dopamine to produce renal vasodilatation and maintain renal perfusion has not been supported in clinical trials. Likewise, the role of theophylline to enhance renal perfusion and improve outcomes in acute renal failure has not been supported in clinical trials.

Bibliography

Level A
1. Lameire, N., Van Beisen, W. & Vanholder, R. (2006) The changing epidemiology of acute renal failure. Nat Clin Pract Nephrol. 2, 364–77.
2. Roger, S. (2006) Proton pump inhibitors: indigestion for nephrologists. Nephrology. 11, 379–80.
3. Liano, F. & Pascual, J. (1996) Epidemiology of acute renal failure: a prospective, multicenter, community-based study. Madrid Acute Renal Failure Study Group. Kidney Int. 50, 811–18.

Level B
4. Barrett, B.J. & Parfrey, P.S. (2006) Preventing nephropathy induced by contrast medium. N Eng J Med. 354, 379–86.
5. Solomon, R., Werner, C., Mann, D., D'Elisa, J. & Silva, P. (1994) Effects of mannitol and frusemide on acute decreases in renal function induced by radiocontrast agents. N Engl J Med. 331, 1416–20.

Level C
6. Lieberthal, W. & Nigam, S.K. (1998) Acute renal failure. I. Relative importance of proximal vs. distal tubular injury. Am J Physiol Renal Physiol. 275, F623–31.
7. Ricci, Z., Bellomo, R. & Ronco, C. (2006) Dose of dialysis in acute renal failure. Clin J Am Soc Nephrol. 1, 380–8.
8. Ho, K.M. & Sheridan, D.J. (2006) Meta-analysis of frusemide to prevent or treat acute renal failure. BMJ 333, 420–3.

9. Walker, R.J. (2000) The cellular mechanisms of drug nephrotoxicity. *The Kidney: Physiology and Pathophysiology*, 3rd edn. Seldin, D.W. & Giebeish, G. (eds). New York: Raven Press Inc.. Chapter 101, 2835–60.

10. Walker, R.J. & Kay, I.P. (2004) Who should not go to the cathlab? *Cardiac catheterisation and percutaneous intervention*. Kay, I.P., Sabate, M. & Costa, M. (eds). London: Martin Dunitz. Chapter 1, 1–7.

Part C
Haemodialysis

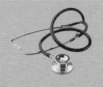

Case 19
Dialysis hypotension

CARMEL HAWLEY

Case history

A 75-year-old woman has end-stage kidney failure secondary to autosomal dominant polycystic kidney disease. She also has a history of type 2 diabetes mellitus managed by diet. She has been on dialysis for 3 years, dialysing in a hospital-based centre for 4 hours three times per week. Three hours into one of her 4-hour dialysis sessions, her blood pressure (BP) drops to 80/60 mmHg. She is sweaty and has central chest pain. There is no definite history of ischaemic heart disease or other vascular diseases. Her routine medications include metoprolol 50 mg twice daily, vitamin B once daily, folic acid 5 mg/day, erythropoietin 4000 U twice weekly intravenously (IV), iron polymaltose 50 mg weekly IV, caltrate one with each meal and calcitriol 0.25 µg daily.

Question 1

In relation to the low BP during dialysis described above, which of the following statements is/are true?

(a) Repeated episodes of hypotension on dialysis occur in <10% of patients on haemodialysis for 4 to 5 hours three times a week.
(b) Hypotension when it occurs is accompanied by muscle cramps, nausea and vomiting.
(c) The patient is very likely to have persistently low BP even when not on dialysis.
(d) It is related to the removal of salt and water rather than to solute clearance during dialysis.

Answer
B and D

Explanation

Intradialytic hypotension (IDH) occurs commonly, complicating 20 to 30% of dialysis treatments in standard in-centre dialysis (usually 4 hours of treatment per session) (answer A incorrect). *IDH is the commonest complication of haemodialysis and one of the most serious.* Symptoms and signs of cardiac and/or cerebral ischaemia are not uncommon in patients with recurrent IDH. Muscle cramps, nausea and vomiting frequently accompany the hypotensive events (answer B correct). It is important to distinguish this syndrome from the entity of persistently low BP seen in patients with comorbid conditions such as cardiac failure or severe autonomic dysfunction (answer C incorrect). Hypotension occurs because patients cannot cope with the hypovolaemic challenge that occurs during dialysis: an inability to compensate for the amount of fluid being removed during dialysis. The clearance of other solutes and resultant changes in electrolytes that occur during dialysis is not responsible for the syndrome of IDH (answer D correct).

Although hypotension during dialysis is most commonly related to the patient's inability to compensate in a timely manner to cope with the effect of volume removal on BP, other diagnoses need to be considered. A careful history, physical examination and ancillary tests are necessary to exclude other serious causes such as an acute coronary syndrome and uncommon but important causes such as pericardial tamponade and air embolism. The possibility of sepsis or bleeding, particularly from the gastrointestinal tract, also needs to be considered.

Clinical pearls

- Hypotension during dialysis is primarily related to a reduction in circulating plasma volume during the procedure.
- It is important to distinguish between persistent hypotension and hypotension that occurs only during the dialysis procedure.
- Hypotension is often accompanied by cramps, nausea and vomiting.
- Less common causes, particularly acute coronary syndromes, pericardial disease, sepsis and gastrointestinal or other causes of bleeding, need to be considered in the differential dialysis of hypotension during dialysis.

Question 2

In relation to the occurrence of IDH which of the following statements is/are true?
(a) Patients with diabetes mellitus are at higher risk of IDH.
(b) Left ventricular hypertrophy increases the risk of IDH.
(c) Younger patients complain of IDH more often.
(d) Patients who do not experience IDH very often usually vasoconstrict and increase cardiac output effectively during dialysis.

Answer
A, B and D

Explanation

In all patients on standard short dialysis, the ultrafiltration rate from the plasma space exceeds the ability to 're-fill' the plasma space from interstitial space. However, most patients do not have repeated episodes of IDH. This is because compensatory mechanisms occur to prevent IDH in most patients: these include autonomic responses which result in peripheral vasoconstriction and increased cardiac output (answer D correct). The most important causes of any inadequate compensatory response to reduced plasma volume include autonomic or baro-receptor failure (leading to excessive venous pooling or aberrant vasodilatation) or impaired cardiac function (primarily related to preload dependence of both systolic and diastolic dysfunction). Autonomic and baroreceptor failure is more common in diabetes mellitus and in the elderly (answer A correct and answer C incorrect). Left ventricular hypertrophy increases the risk of IDH by interfering with the cardiac response to hypotension (answer B correct). These principles are outlined in Figure 19.1.

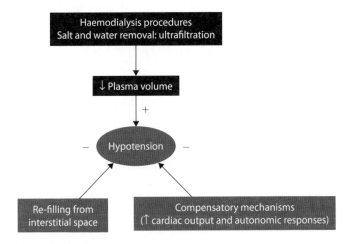

Figure 19.1 The principles of intradialytic hypotension

 Clinical pearls

- In most patients during dialysis the rate of ultrafiltration exceeds the rate at which re-filling of the plasma space can occur from the interstitial space.
- Cardiac and vascular mechanisms prevent IDH from occurring in most patients.
- Patients who develop IDH do not compensate appropriate to ultrafiltration and are reduced in plasma volume during dialysis.

Question 3

Appropriate treatment strategies for this patient when IDH develops would be to:

(a) undertake saline infusion to correct plasma volume
(b) withhold metoprolol before the next dialysis
(c) terminate the dialysis session early
(d) shorten this and all future dialysis sessions to avoid this occurring.

Answer

A, B and C

Explanation

Saline infusion is generally given to correct the intravascular volume depletion that leads to this adverse event (answer A correct). Saline has been shown to be just as effective as 5% albumin. Patients are also generally placed in a head-down tilt position to avoid cerebral symptoms and supplemental oxygen should be administered. Although antihypertensive medication is generally withheld before dialysis in an attempt to avoid IDH, not all experts agree that this should be done and the evidence-base for doing this is not strong (answer B correct). However, in general most antihypertensives are withheld pre-dialysis by most units. Care must be taken with the withholding of beta-blockers in patients with coronary artery disease.

For a particular dialysis session during which IDH has occurred, shortening the dialysis may be useful, particularly if the event is refractory to usual measures (answer C correct). However, in general this *leads to underdialysis* if it is recurrent and is therefore not recommended (answer D incorrect). Encouraging the patient to reduce fluid consumption and hence the amount of fluid that has to be removed in each dialysis session is a more effective strategy.

 Clinical pearls

- Saline is generally given for severe IDH.
- Generally, antihypertensive agents are withheld pre-dialysis but anti-anginal medication may need to be continued.
- Avoiding large weight gains between dialysis sessions is important.

LEVEL B

Case history continued ...

The patient continues to develop hypotension during dialysis, with these episodes occurring generally on the day after the weekend break from dialysis and on one of the other two dialysis days. Management includes withholding antihypertensive medication pre-dialysis. During this time the patient's weight gains are generally in the order of 2 kg, except over the weekend when the average weight gain is 3.5 kg. At this stage the patient's BP is 150/95 mmHg on average pre-dialysis. Post-dialysis BP is generally 110/70 mmHg (if the patient has not had dialysis terminated early).

Question 4

Which of the following would be the best approach/es in this patient?

(a) Counsel/educate the patient in relation to salt and water intake in an attempt to reduce the weight gains, particularly over the weekend.

(b) Try to reduce the patient's post-dialysis target weight ('dry weight').

(c) Ensure the patient abstains from eating during the dialysis procedure.

(d) Use isolated ultrafiltration to correct fluid overload before performing standard dialysis.

Answer

A, C and D

Explanation

Reducing the weight gain, particularly during the 'long break' from dialysis in patients on only three sessions per week, is important but difficult. If the weight gain is less, the ultrafiltration rate required to correct the volume overload in the patient is therefore slower and generally better tolerated. Education of the patient about ways to reduce salt and water intake is important as early as possible in the patient's treatment course (answer A correct).

Although finding the correct 'dry weight' is important in patients with recurrent episodes of IDH, this may be difficult to achieve. In this instance reducing the dry weight to correct the hypertension is likely to make the episodes of IDH worse. The greater the dialytic reduction in weight, the greater the refilling from the interstitial space. Thus, although it is important to achieve the 'dry weight' if possible, this is not the correct time to do so for this patient (answer B incorrect). The theoretical concept of 'dry weight' is important. This is the weight at which a patient has an ideal volume status (BP is close to normal and no peripheral oedema or pulmonary oedema can be detected) and below which patients will develop symptoms and signs of volume depletion. This weight needs to be reassessed regularly by nursing and medical staff. An inappropriately low 'dry weight' can lead to IDH.

Withholding food during dialysis of patients who develop IDH may reduce the risk of these adverse events by reducing splanchnic vasodilatation and decreased peripheral resistance. One small study demonstrated this to be a successful strategy in symptomatic patients (answer C correct).

Performing ultrafiltration as an isolated procedure before and after standard dialysis is generally better tolerated. This is best done as an extra dialysis session in a 'one-off' attempt to correct the patient's volume overload status in a patient such as the one described (answer D correct).

 Clinical pearl

- Strategies to reduce the frequency of IDH include:
  — reduce weight gains between dialysis
  — abstain from eating during dialysis
  — allow the patient to be at or a bit above their 'ideal weight'
  — consider 'isolated' ultrafiltration.

Question 5

The patient's haemoglobin is noted to be to 90 g/L during the period in which these episodes of IDH were occurring. Which of the following would be potentially helpful to avoid the recurrent intradialytic hypotensive episodes?

(a) Change the dialysis membrane
(b) Correct the haemoglobin to >100 g/L
(c) Change the blood flow and dialysate flow rates
(d) Lengthen each dialysis session from 4 hours to 5 hours
(e) Switch the patient to peritoneal dialysis

Answer

B, D and E

Explanation

Severe anaemia can confound the problem by resulting in poor oxygen delivery with consequent poor cardiac function. Correction of anaemia is likely to improve the patient's symptoms (answer B correct).

Blood flow rate, dialysate flow rate and choice of dialyser appear to have no appreciable effect on the incidence of IDH (answers A and C incorrect).

A good strategy is to lengthen dialysis time, for example from 4 to 4.5, or even better to 5, hours, allowing a *slower ultrafiltration rate* to remove the necessary volume of fluid. The longer the dialysis and slower the ultra-filtration rate, the more time there is for plasma refilling and hence the less the drop in plasma volume. However, this may not be feasible logistically and the patient may not be willing to have longer dialysis sessions (answer D correct).

Peritoneal dialysis is a good option to be considered in a patient where IDH is very troublesome (answer E correct).

Clinical pearls

- Lengthening the time for each dialysis session, to allow a slower rate of fluid removal, can reduce the incidence of IDH.
- Anaemia may confound the situation and should be corrected to the accepted target levels of haemoglobin.
- Peritoneal dialysis should be considered for patients who are intolerant of haemodialysis because of IDH.

LEVEL C

Case history continued ...

The patient increases her dialysis times to 5 hours and successfully reduces her weight gains between dialysis. She has very infrequent episodes of IDH over the next 12 months. However, she suffers an anterior myocardial infarction. During her convalescence from this, recurrent IDH again becomes problematic.

Question 6

Which of the following statements is/are true?

(a) High-flux dialysis is superior at reducing the frequency of IDH episodes to low-flux dialysis.
(b) The recurrence of IDH relates to poor cardiac reserve.
(c) Raising the dialysate temperature may improve the problem.
(d) Changing the patient to haemodiafiltration may improve the situation.

Answer

B and D

Explanation

Dialysis flux does not alter the frequency of IDH (answer A incorrect). Prior to the near-universal use of bicarbonate dialysate, the use of acetate-based dialysate was associated with a higher incidence of IDH.

In this patient, it is highly likely that the recent myocardial infarction has resulted in a reduction in the ability of the left ventricle to increase cardiac output in response to the reduction in circulating plasma volume that occurs during dialysis. This is likely to be the reason why the problem has recurred. In such patients, other strategies to reduce the risk of IDH need to be employed (answer B correct).

During dialysis, blood vessels vasoconstrict in order to maintain their peripheral resistance and hence their BP. One of the downsides to this vasoconstriction is that it results in an elevated core body temperature. A point is reached where the temperature rises so high that it results in reflex vasodilatation, thus resulting in hypotension. The main strategy for preventing this is to use *cool dialysate* to reduce the body temperature and thus avoid the vasodilatation (see Fig. 19.2). Cool dialysate has clearly been shown to be beneficial (answer C incorrect). A systematic review by Selby and McIntyre (2006) concluded that cooled dialysate reduced IDH by 7.1 (95%CI 5.3 to 8.8) times. By this approach, blood is returned to the patient in thermal equilibrium with the dialysate. Even one degree difference in body temperature has a measurable effect on the incidence of IDH. Manipulations include setting a fixed temperature reduction or utilising a device which allows a biofeedback temperature control to deliver 'isothermic' dialysis. A recent systematic review of the manipulation of dialysate temperature concluded its efficacy. However, further documentation of the tolerance of cold symptoms during dialysis is required. Changing to haemodiafiltration does help in many patients and this is considered to be because of the lower body temperature achieved with this therapy (answer D correct). Thus, avoiding the rise in core body temperature and consequent IDH risk can be achieved currently by using conventional dialysis with cool dialysate, using a biofeedback temperature device or using the technique of haemodiafiltration.

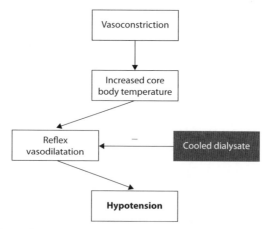

Figure 19.2 Controlling body temperature during dialysis

 Clinical pearl

- Dialysate cooling prevents the rise that usually occurs in a patient's core body temperature during dialysis and is an effective strategy to reduce the frequency of IDH.

Question 7

Which of the following statements is/are true?
(a) A higher dialysate sodium is an effective strategy for IDH.
(b) Sodium profiling is a very effective strategy for IDH.
(c) Blood volume monitoring is helpful to reduce IDH.
(d) A higher dialysate calcium results in a higher BP during dialysis.
(e) A higher dialysate calcium reduces frequency of IDH episodes.

Answer
A and D

Explanation

The strategy of using a higher dialysate sodium has been used successfully for many years to help maintain BP stability during dialysis (answer A correct). Dialysate sodium levels affect the change in blood volume that accompanies any given amount of fluid removal. Sodium profiling is variably successful. It often requires much trial and error in order to find a profile of dialysate sodium that works for an individual patient. In general there remains some controversy about whether sodium profiling alone is useful in this setting (answer B incorrect). Similarly there is debate about how valuable blood volume monitoring is in this setting because of difficulties in interpretation and prediction of hypotensive events (answer C incorrect). However, biofeedback systems using combined ultrafiltration and sodium profiling have shown more promising results. In addition, dialysate calcium modification has also been trialled: higher dialysate calcium has been shown to result in a higher BP throughout dialysis (answer D correct) but in clinical studies this does not seem to change the frequency of symptomatic IDH events (answer E incorrect).

 Clinical pearls

- Increasing dialysate sodium improves cardiovascular stability during dialysis.
- The roles of sodium profiling and blood volume monitoring remain controversial.

Question 8

Which of the following pharmacological agents has been shown to be effective for treating IDH in clinical trials?
(a) Vasopressin
(b) Midodrine (alpha-1 adrenergic agonist)
(c) Sertraline hydrochloride (selective serotonin reuptake inhibitor)

(d) Adenosine A1 receptor antagonists

(e) Carnitine

Answer

All are correct

Explanation

All of the above agents have been shown to reduce the occurrence of IDH (all answers correct). However, the data demonstrating efficacy are not robust as most studies have small numbers of patients and other study-design deficiencies. Of these agents, midodrine is the most used and has been subjected to systematic review (Prakash, Garg & Heidheim 2004). Although this review concluded that midodrine given 15 to 30 minutes before dialysis appears to have a role in the treatment of haemodialysis patients experiencing IDH, it was also concluded that the data needed to be interpreted with caution because of the quality and sample size of the studies it examined. Drug therapies should only be tried once all other manipulations of the dialysis prescription and other conservative approaches have been exhausted. There has been a recent study with the use of an adenosine A1 receptor antagonist which demonstrated efficacy. *However, caution must be exercised with the use of any of these agents in this context and non-pharmacological measures should always be used first.* These agents are contraindicated in the setting of coronary ischaemia.

 Clinical pearls

- Pharmacological therapies should only be used for IDH when all other more conservative measures have failed.
- Internationally, midodrine is the most widely used agent for this purpose.

Bibliography

Level A

1. Cameron, J.C., Grunfeld, J.P., Ponticelli, C., Ritz, E., Winearls, C. & van Ypersele, C. (2005) Oxford Textbook of Clinical Nephrology, 3rd edn, Davidson, A.M. (ed.). Oxford: Oxford University Press. (3) pp. 1943–4.

Level B

2. Daugirdas, J.T. (2001) Pathophysiology of dialysis hypotension: an update. Am J Kidney Dis. 38(Supp. 4), S11–17.

Level C

3. Sherman, R.A. (2002) Intradialytic hypotension: an overview of recent, unresolved and overlooked issues. Semin Dial. 15, 141–3.

4. Donauer, J. (2004) Hemodialysis-induced hypotension: impact of technologic advances. Semin Dial. 17, 333–5.
5. Selby, N.M. & McIntyre, C.W. (2006) A systematic review of the clinical effects of reducing dialysate fluid temperature. Nephrol Dial Transplant. 21, 1883–98.
6. Prakash, S., Garg, A.X., Heidenheim, A.P. & House, A.A. (2004) Midodrine appears to be safe and effective for dialysis-induced hypotension: a systematic review. Nephrol Dial Transplant. 19, 2553–8.

Case 20
Haemodialysis adequacy

PETER KERR

LEVEL A

Case history

A 56-year-old man has been receiving haemodialysis for 2 years, having developed renal failure due to IgA nephropathy. However, he now complains of poor energy and diminished appetite. There have been no other systemic symptoms, nor fever. However, he has lost some weight, with the dialysis team making two downward adjustments to his target weight in the last 3 months, each of 0.5 kg. Blood tests reveal elevated predialysis urea (28 mmol/L), creatinine (750 µmol/L), potassium (6.4 mmol/L) and phosphate (2.45 mmol/L) but a low serum albumin (31 g/L).

Question 1

You are concerned about the level of predialysis urea. You understand that dialysis patients do not have normal values for urea but feel this level is too high. Which of the following could explain this?

(a) Excessive protein intake
(b) Intravascular volume depletion
(c) Under-dialysis
(d) Catabolic state
(e) All of the above

Answer

A and C

Explanation

Urea is derived from protein degradation. This includes exogenous (ingested) and endogenous (body tissue) protein. In the steady state, input/production and output are balanced and the blood urea level is relatively stable. Urea removal is through the kidney, predominantly by glomerular filtration; however, up to 10 to 15% of filtered urea may be reabsorbed in the proximal tubule depending on tubular flow rates. In volume depletion, with low tubular flow and sodium delivery to the distal tubule, reabsorption of urea is at its highest. In renal failure, with no effective kidney function, removal of urea is essentially totally dependent on dialysis efficiency. For this scenario, answer A is possible, as is answer C. Answer B is not likely given the lack of renal function and answer D is unlikely given the clinical scenario.

Question 2

If you consider the possibility of excessive intake of protein in this man as an explanation for his results, which of his blood test results would support this?

(a) Elevated urea
(b) Elevated creatinine
(c) Elevated potassium
(d) Elevated phosphate
(e) Low albumin

Answer

A, B, C and D

Explanation

Protein is a major nutrient group in our diet. However, we do not eat (as a rule) pure protein but rather protein-rich foods including meats, dairy products and many vegetables. Thus eating a lot of meat would provide urea (from the protein degradation), creatinine as this is derived from muscle, and potentially potassium and phosphate as these are intracellular ions. Vegetable protein is often particularly associated with potassium. Thus in this scenario, any of answers A to D could be found in a dialysis patient who is not complying with the usual dietary restrictions, including eating excess protein. E is more likely to represent undernutrition.

Question 3

Given the results, and after some discussion with the patient, you become more concerned that rather than having excess protein intake, he may be under-dialysed. What should you measure to assess how much dialysis this patient is receiving?

(a) Pre- and postdialysis creatinine
(b) Pre- and postdialysis urea
(c) Pre and postdialysis beta-2 microglobulin
(d) Serum albumin
(e) Serum potassium

Answer

B

Explanation

Dialysis adequacy is usually considered in terms of the removal of a solute in the course of dialysis. Most of the dialysis membranes in common usage do not remove large molecules, and indeed do not readily remove molecules above a molecular weight of about 5000 (such as vitamin B12); although, so-called high-flux membranes have reasonably good removal of beta-2 microglobulin (molecular weight 11 800). Thus, dialysis adequacy usually concentrates on small molecule removal with the archetypical small molecule being urea, as it readily crosses biological and dialysis membranes. Typically, dialysis urea removal is assessed using pre- and postdialysis measurements (answer B). This is most commonly expressed as the urea reduction ratio (URR), with the calculation being (pre – post)/pre, typically expressed as a percentage. Creatinine is not usually measured in this way because it does not dialyse as readily as urea, despite its small molecular weight (approximately twice that of urea). Even though beta-2 microglobulin is removed with high-flux membranes, this is still not at the efficiency of urea removal. Albumin levels may have some relationship to dialysis adequacy but are influenced by nutrition and inflammation (as a negative acute-phase reactant). Potassium is also related to dialysis efficiency but will be influenced by diet, cell turnover and breakdown, as well as acid–base status.

 Clinical pearls

- Serum levels of urea and creatinine are not expected to be 'normal' in dialysis patients.
- Serum urea (and creatinine levels) in dialysis patients are influenced not only by dialysis but also by nutritional status and catabolism.

LEVEL B

Case history continued ...

The man in question has the following biochemistry measured: predialysis urea 28 mmol/L and postdialysis urea 12 mmol/L. Hence, the calculated URR is 57% with an estimated Kt/V of 0.9.

Question 4

On the basis of these results, it is reasonable to assume the following:

(a) The postdialysis urea suggests he is well dialysed.

(b) The predialysis urea suggests he is underdialysed.

(c) The URR value suggests he is adequately dialysed.
(d) The Kt/V value suggests he is poorly dialysed.
(e) No assumptions regarding the adequacy of dialysis can be made.

Answer
D

Explanation

The adequacy of dialysis in terms of urea removal is most correctly assessed using Kt/V, which is the normalised (to total body water) clearance of urea during a dialysis session. K is the dialyser clearance, t stands for time and V is total body water (approximately equalling the volume of distribution of urea)—this is a unit-less number. An analysis of the National Cooperative Dialysis Study (NCDS) in the late 1980s suggested that Kt/V values below 0.8 were associated with increased mortality. Subsequently, a value of 1.0 was set as a minimum to ensure a safety margin. However, further studies have suggested values below 1.2 may be associated with increased mortality. The recent Hemodialysis (HEMO) study did not show any additional benefit in terms of mortality if the target Kt/V was set at 1.6 compared to 1.2. Kt/V is cumbersome to calculate accurately, so simpler bedside techniques were developed to assess urea clearance, URR being the most popular as it simply reflects (as a percentage) the reduction in urea level from pre- to postdialysis. A value of 65% correlates with a Kt/V of 1.2. The predialysis urea may be high because of chronic underdialysis but may also reflect good dialysis with a high protein intake. Similarly, a low postdialysis urea may reflect good dialysis or poor dialysis in the setting of poor protein intake. The correct answer is D.

Question 5

If you then assume this patient is underdialysed, what may be the cause of this?
(a) An arterial stenosis in the fistula
(b) Inadequate anticoagulation during dialysis
(c) Use of a low-flux dialyser
(d) Early sign-off from dialysis
(e) Prescription of too short a dialysis time

Answer
A, B, D and E

Explanation

There are many possible causes for underdialysis, the most obvious being under-prescription; that is, prescribing a dialysis combination inadequate for the patient's circumstance. This may be too short a time, too small a dialyser, too low a blood flow or even too low a dialysate flow. Other factors may be missed time due to the patient completing their dialysis session early (e.g. due to cramps), fistula problems which limit the blood flow (such as an arterial stenosis) and clotting of fibres in the dialyser due to coagulation problems. A low-flux dialyser per se should not greatly influence the clearance of small molecules such as urea. Therefore answers A, B, D and E are possible.

> ### Case history continued ...
>
> The nursing staff report that our patient frequently signs off early from dialysis, sometimes even one hour early. After some discussion, the patient admits to this and vows to correct it. However, over the next month, despite completing 4 hours of dialysis every session, he does not feel better. His URR is 61%. Since it was last measured, his serum albumin has dropped further to 29 g/L. His protein catabolic rate (PCR) is measured at 0.85 g/kg/day.

Question 6

In this setting, the low serum albumin is likely to be due to:
- **(a)** loss of albumin across the dialyser
- **(b)** on-going nephrotic syndrome
- **(c)** overdialysis
- **(d)** poor protein intake
- **(e)** covert inflammation.

Answer
D and E

Explanation

The majority of dialysers in clinical use are impermeable to albumin, making loss of albumin across the dialyser unlikely. Similarly, after 2 years of dialysis, ongoing urinary losses of protein are unlikely. Overdialysis is probably a non-entity, given that conventional dialysis only provides 10 to 15% of normal renal function equivalent. Albumin is reflective of protein intake, as such a low serum albumin may indicate poor protein intake. However, albumin is also a negative acute phase reactant, meaning that levels drop rapidly in the setting of inflammation.

 Clinical pearls

- Dialysis adequacy is commonly assessed in terms of urea clearances, representing small molecule clearance.
- Urea clearances are assessed using the unitless number Kt/V, or the urea reduction ratio (URR).

- Nutrition influences the assessment of dialysis adequacy. In particular, undernutrition with poor protein intake makes assessment of Kt/V unreliable.
- There are many technical reasons for underdialysis, including reduction in session duration, fistula problems and clotted dialyser fibres.

LEVEL C

Case history continued …

On the basis of the previous results, a decision is made that the patient is deficient in protein intake.

Question 7

Which of the following manoeuvres is/are likely to improve his serum albumin?

(a) Use of a high-flux dialyser

(b) Adoption of a high-protein diet

(c) Intradialytic parenteral nutrition

(d) Increasing the dialysis session duration by 1 hour

(e) Increasing the blood flow rate during dialysis

Answer

B, D and E

Explanation

Although serum albumin is linked to nutrition, very few manoeuvres have been shown to influence positively the serum albumin. A high-flux dialyser is unlikely to influence the albumin level, although theoretically some small proteins and amino acids may be lost across a high-flux dialyser. The use of a high-protein diet, especially one containing mostly high biological value protein (containing all the essential amino acids), would be expected to produce a rise in the serum albumin in this setting (answer B). Intradialytic parenteral nutrition, administering the nutrient solutions only during the dialysis sessions, is controversial. Some small studies have demonstrated benefit of this manoeuvre; however, the weight of opinion suggests that this is an expensive exercise with little benefit. Both D and E represent options that will provide for increased dialysis clearance; the expectation of manoeuvres such as these is that wellbeing and appetite will improve, resulting in an improvement in serum albumin over time.

Case history continued ...

In attempting to determine the reason for his underdialysis, you examine his dialysis records. You discover that he is now regularly receiving 4½ hours dialysis per session. His measured blood flow rate during dialysis is 225 to 275 mL/min over recent weeks, with venous pressures of 100 to 150 mmHg. The 'arterial' pressure during dialysis is normal. You note he has a native fistula in his left forearm, constructed prior to the time when he first started dialysis, 2 years ago.

Question 8

What is your interpretation of the blood flow and pressure parameters?
(a) They are normal and appropriate.
(b) It is likely there is a proximal venous stenosis.
(c) There is likely to be an arterial/anastomotic stenosis.
(d) Recirculation may explain the poor URR.
(e) Stenosis of the fistula may explain the poor URR.

Answer
B and E

Explanation

The parameters given above suggest that the blood flow rate is lower than one might typically prescribe and hence may be adversely impacting on the URR. The venous pressure is high for a native arteriovenous (AV) fistula (AV grafts, usually made of PTFE GORE-TEX®, tend to have higher venous pressures, often of this order). In this setting, it is often difficult to determine if there is an arterial (or inflow) problem as the more proximal venous stenosis protects the inflow problem via a dam effect. Certainly, the venous stenosis may cause the restricted blood flow rate and the low URR but the issue of recirculation is more vexed. The traditional thinking was that a venous stenosis produced a dam-wall effect with likely recirculation of blood into the capacious fistula; however, since the introduction of fistula blood flow measurements this concept has been challenged with true intrafistula recirculation being rare.

Case history continued ...

The patient went on to have his fistula repaired—a venous stenosis was patched with a piece of saphenous vein. No arterial stenosis was found. He is still struggling a little (URR is 65%) but he frequently has potassium levels over 6.0 mmol/L and despite large doses of phosphate binders, his serum phosphate is in the order of 2.0 to 2.5 mmol/L. He complains of itch and his appetite is only fair. The predialysis blood pressure (BP) is 155/90 mmHg. Interdialytic weight gains are in the order of 3.0 kg.

Question 9

Apart from the URR (or Kt/V), what other indicators may be used to assess dialysis adequacy?

(a) Elevated predialysis phosphate
(b) Elevated predialysis potassium
(c) Interdialytic weight gain
(d) Predialysis BP
(e) Predialysis beta-2 microglobulin

Answer
D

Explanation

Many alternative approaches to dialysis adequacy have been proposed, rather than adopting the concept of small molecule clearance exemplified by urea clearances. Both potassium and phosphate serum levels may reflect dialysis dose but must be considered in conjunction with assessments of diet and compliance with the entire dialysis and drug regimens. Similarly, a large interdialytic weight gain may indicate a good diet, although more frequently represents poor compliance with fluid and salt restrictions. The beta-2 microglobulin levels are more influenced by the flux of the dialyser (high versus low flux), although for a given high-flux dialyser the levels will reflect dialysis dose as well. The BP is often quoted as another indicator of dialysis adequacy reflecting a combination of fluid management and unmeasured haemodynamic factors.

Question 10

What techniques could now be used to deliver more clearance for the patient?

(a) Use of short daily dialysis
(b) Use of second daily nocturnal dialysis
(c) Use of nocturnal dialysis six times a week
(d) Change to peritoneal dialysis
(e) Transplantation

Answer
A, B, C and E

Explanation

The major thrust in this man should be to increase his dialysis hours; this will particularly increase his clearance of molecules such as phosphate and the so-called middle molecules. These techniques have been associated with a considerable increase in wellbeing in dialysis patients, although a translation to improved mortality has not been definitively demonstrated yet. Answers A, B and C all offer longer dialysis hours and should offer improved clearances. Peritoneal dialysis is unlikely to offer any improvement; 2 years of haemodialysis will have most likely eliminated any residual renal function and peritoneal dialysis in this circumstance rarely offers improved clearances over haemodialysis. Transplantation, of course should be the aim for all suitable dialysis patients.

 Clinical pearls

- Nutritional status requires constant attention in dialysis patients and remains a trap in interpreting tests for dialysis adequacy.
- Fistula stenosis is a common cause of poor dialysis clearances.
- Dialysis adequacy assessment should also involve consideration of other biochemical parameters, as well as wellbeing, volume control and BP control.
- Longer-hours dialysis offers significant advantages in solute and volume control.

Bibliography

For a broad discussion of both dialysis adequacy and nutrition, see:
Levy, J., Morgan, J. & Brown, E. (2004) *Oxford Handbook of Dialysis*, 2nd edn. Oxford: Oxford University Press.

Case 21
Access insufficiency

KEVAN POLKINGHORNE

LEVEL A

Case history

A 65-year-old woman has progressive chronic kidney disease due to diabetic nephropathy. She is referred to a nephrologist for assessment and planning for dialysis. She is feeling well and has a good appetite. Her serum urea and creatinine are 35.5 mmol/L and 290 µmol/L respectively. Her weight is 75 kg and height 145 cm giving a body mass index (BMI) of 36 kg/m². She has no past history of ischaemic heart disease or peripheral vascular disease but is a smoker with a 40-pack-year history. She prefers to have haemodialysis. On examination of her upper limbs, her radial pulses are present although slightly reduced in volume. Her forearm veins are not easily visible.

Question 1

In relation to planning for dialysis in this patient, which of the following is true?
(a) She should be referred as soon as possible to a vascular surgeon for assessment and placement of vascular access.
(b) The serum creatinine of 290 µmol/L indicates moderate kidney failure.
(c) She should be advised to conserve her arm veins and if possible prevent any intravenous cannulation of the forearms veins.
(d) Early referral to a nephrologist well before dialysis is important to enable timely access placement.

Answer
A, C and D

Explanation

The assessment of the severity of her kidney failure requires the calculation of her estimated glomerular filtration rate (eGFR). Currently the best and most validated formula for eGFR is the abbreviated Modification of Diet in Renal Disease (MDRD) formula, which requires serum creatinine, gender, race (if African-American) and age. The eGFR in this case is 15 mL/min/1.73 m² indicating severe kidney failure (answer B incorrect). The patient should be referred to a vascular surgeon for assessment and placement of vascular access for haemodialysis (answer A correct).

Patients who have chronic kidney disease and who are dialysis candidates should be advised to conserve their arm veins for future dialysis access. The insertion of intravenous cannulae in the forearms should be avoided if possible, especially in the non-dominant arm (answer C correct). Ideally patients with established chronic kidney disease who are dialysis candidates should be referred to a nephrologist once the eGFR is <30 mL/min (or earlier depending on the diagnosis and/or rate of progression) to enable adequate time for dialysis planning, education and vascular access placement (answer D correct).

Clinical pearls

- Early referral to a nephrologist well before dialysis is important to enable timely vascular access placement.
- Calculation of the eGFR is important to assess the level of renal failure.
- Patients who are considered dialysis candidates should be advised to conserve their forearm veins for future vascular access.

Question 2

The most appropriate vascular access for this patient is:
(a) native arteriovenous fistula (AVF)
(b) saphenous vein forearm loop graft
(c) PTFE forearm loop graft (AVG)
(d) tunnelled jugular central venous catheter.

Answer

A

Explanation

Long-term haemodialysis requires the creation of permanent access to the circulation (Fig. 21.1). This is best achieved by the construction of the native AVF using either the radial artery and the cephalic vein at the wrist (the radiocephalic fistula) or the brachial artery and the cephalic vein at the elbow (the brachiocephalic fistula). Alternative permanent access can be by the AVG, which is usually placed as a loop between the brachial artery and the cephalic vein at the elbow. The central venous catheter, either tunnelled or not, is considered only a temporary vascular access until permanent access can be constructed. The AVG is utilised as permanent access in patients in whom an AVF cannot be constructed.

The AVF is the vascular access of first choice for a number of reasons (answer A correct). Firstly, the intervention-free patency of the AVF is significantly longer than that of AVG or central venous catheters (NKF-K/DOQI 2001; ANZSN & KHA 2003). This means that patients with AVF are less likely to be admitted to hospital to maintain function of the vascular access, thus reducing morbidity associated with the haemodialysis treatment. Secondly, given the synthetic nature of the catheter (and graft) material, both patients with catheters and AVG have a higher risk of infection compared to patients with an AVF. Finally, new patients commencing haemodialysis with a catheter have a two to three times increased risk of death (all cause and infectious mortality) compared to those with an AVF (Polkinghorne et al. 2004). The saphenous vein forearm loop is an alternative to the AVG; however, it is still associated with a higher risk of complications compared to the AVF.

 Clinical pearls

- The AVF is the first-choice vascular access for haemodialysis patients due to the lower morbidity and mortality risk.
- Every attempt should be made to establish a well-functioning AVF in patients intending to have haemodialysis treatment.

Question 3

In relation to the construction of the native AVF in this patient, which of the following is/are true?
(a) AVF usually can be used within 2 weeks of construction.
(b) Type II diabetes is associated with a lower prevalence of AVF use.
(c) There is a substantial risk that the AVF will fail to mature adequately for dialysis.
(d) Early (in the first 24 hours postcreation) hand ischaemia or steal occurs more frequently in AVF than in AVG.

Answer
C

Explanation

In order for the AVF to be mature and ready to use prior to commencing haemodialysis, it must be constructed well in advance of the anticipated need for haemodialysis (NKF-K/DOQI 2001). In general, a maturation time of at least 4 weeks and ideally 2 to 3 months is needed prior to first use of the AVF (answer A incorrect).

While numerous studies from the United States demonstrate a lower prevalence of AVF in subjects with diabetes mellitus, studies from Australia and

Figure 21.1 Vascular access for haemodialysis:
(a) native AVF, (b) AVG and
(c) central venous catheter

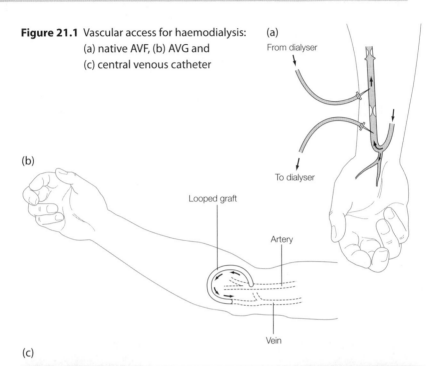

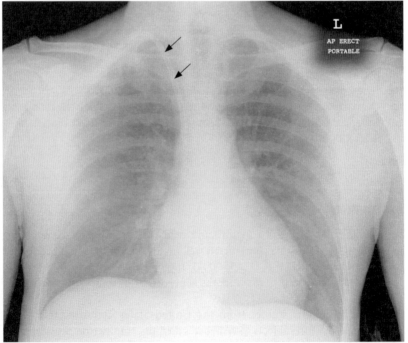

Europe where the overall prevalence of AVF use is much higher, demonstrate that subjects with diabetes do not have a lower prevalence of AVF compared to non-diabetic patients (answer B incorrect). Thus an AVF should be attempted in patients with or without diabetes.

The primary failure rate, defined as failure or need of further intervention to the vascular access before ever being used for dialysis, ranges from 28 to 58% for AVF (answer C correct). However a significant proportion can be salvaged and this reinforces the need for early AVF creation especially in patients with significant vascular disease or diabetes mellitus (Asif, Roy-Chaudhury & Beathard 2006).

Vascular steal occurs when the arteriovenous shunt diverts sufficient blood flow away from the distal limb to cause ischaemia. The early onset 'immediate type' occurs in the first 24 hours after creation of the access and is invariably associated with AVG creation in which blood flow in the graft reaches its peak almost immediately. A second type, 'delayed onset steal', tends to occur in patients with AVF months to years following construction (answer D incorrect). Whether this late onset reflects a gradual increase in blood flow as the AVF matures or a progression of underlying distal vascular disease is not clear, although it probably is a combination of both.

 Clinical pearls

- AVFs typically require a maturation time of at least 4 weeks and ideally 2 to 3 months before they can be used.
- AVFs have a high primary failure rate and therefore often need further intervention before an adequate AVF is ready for dialysis.

LEVEL B

Case history continued ...

The patient initially had a radiocephalic AVF created which thrombosed 4 days after creation. A Doppler ultrasound of the arms was ordered and after assessment, a brachial cephalic AVF was created and matured without incident. She was maintained on haemodialysis without major incident for 14 months. On the morning of her usual afternoon dialysis session, she presents to her general practitioner complaining of a tender AVF. There is a recent history of low blood pressure (BP) at the end of dialysis (110/60 mmHg) as well 2 days of diarrhoea. Examination of the AVF reveals loss of the bruit suggesting thrombosis of the fistula. Her last haemoglobin 2 weeks ago was 135 g/L.

Question 4

Which of the following should be done in this patient?
(a) Urgent ultrasound of the AVF to assess the blood flow.
(b) Urgent referral to her nephrology unit for assessment.
(c) Urgent assessment of the serum potassium.
(d) Arrange appointment with her vascular surgeon at the next available clinic.

Answer

B and C

Explanation

Acute thrombosis of AVF is a medical emergency and is recognised clinically by the loss of the characteristic AVF bruit. A diagnostic ultrasound is rarely needed (answer A incorrect). Occasionally thrombosis can occur in a venous side branch of an AVF, and in this situation an ultrasound scan can be useful. The patient needs to be referred urgently to her nephrologist who would arrange admission for assessment by the vascular surgical team (answer B correct). Urgent declotting of the AVF is required to enable minimal interruptions to the dialysis treatment (answer D incorrect). Urgent assessment of the patient fluid state and serum potassium are also required to assess the need for dialysis before any operative procedure (answer C correct). Thrombosis is the major cause for failure of haemodialysis vascular access accounting for up to 80% of failures (Schwab et al. 1999).

 Clinical pearls

- The acute thrombosis of the AVF is a medical emergency and is recognised clinically by the loss of the characteristic AVF bruit.
- Thrombosis is the major cause of failure of haemodialysis vascular access.

Question 5

The possible underlying cause/s or contributing factors for AVF thrombosis are:
(a) the haemoglobin of 135 g/L
(b) the low BP at the end of dialysis
(c) the history of diarrhoea
(d) a stenosis within AVF.

Answer

B, C and D

Explanation

The Achilles heel of both AVF and AVG is the development of vascular stenosis leading to thrombosis of the access (answer D correct). In AVF, stenotic lesions tend to occur at branch points in the venous system, particularly in areas of turbulent flow but also at the anastomosis. It is clearly apparent that the development of vascular stenosis occurs at a faster rate in AVG and the most common site for this development is at or just distal to the venous anastomosis.

A haemoglobin of 135 g/L is unlikely to be a cause of vascular access thrombosis (answer A incorrect). Erythropoietin therapy has been associated with an increased risk of AVG thrombosis in some studies but not AVF thrombosis (Besarab 2004). The reported mechanism is thought to be due to the resultant increased haematocrit and blood viscosity. However, the use of erythropoietin to maintain the haemoglobin at current accepted targets is not associated with any increased risk.

Other potential contributing factors to vascular access thrombosis include hypotension; for example, due to poor cardiac function (often manifest by low BP during dialysis) and/or hypovolaemia (e.g. due to diarrhoea). While by themselves they cause access thrombosis, they can often help unmask an underlying access stenosis (answers C and D correct).

Clinical pearls

- The majority of vascular access thrombosis is due to an underlying stenosis.
- Potential contributing factors for AVF thrombosis include hypotension and hypovolaemia.

LEVEL C

Case history continued ...

The patient was admitted to hospital and at thrombectomy a significant AVF stenosis just distal to the anastomosis was found. The AVF stenosis was corrected and dialysis was continued using the AVF. After 7 months she was referred for fistulography due to the clinical suspicion of a further AVF stenosis on access surveillance. A significant stenosis was seen on the cephalic vein 3 cm distal to the arteriovenous anastomosis.

Question 6

Which of the following pharmacological agents has been shown to reduce the incidence of AVF or AVG thrombosis in clinical trials?

(a) Aspirin
(b) Dipyridamole
(c) Fish oil
(d) Warfarin
(e) Aspirin/clopidogrel

Answer

B and C

Explanation

There are surprisingly few data assessing the efficacy of anti-platelet or other agents in reducing access thrombosis (Kaufman 2000). The majority of randomised controlled trials (RCTs) are small, short term and were performed in the 1970s to mid-1980s, with only three published since 2002. Studies in AVF have primarily been focused on the prevention of primary failure following AVF creation using anti-platelet agents. The data for aspirin in preventing AVF or AVG thrombosis is conflicting with one study of ninety-two AVF patients demonstrating a reduced thrombosis rate at 1 month post-AVF creation while in another study aspirin was associated with a non-significant doubling of AVG thrombosis (answer A incorrect). In that same study, dipyridamole (either alone or in combination with aspirin) reduced the risk of thrombosis (answer B correct). Fish oil has been assessed in a small RCT of twenty-four patients demonstrating an impressive reduction in AVG thrombosis rate over 12 months (24 versus 85%, p <0.05) (answer C correct) (Schmitz 2002). Low dose warfarin aiming for International Normalised Ratio (INR) 1.4 to 1.9 did not reduce thrombosis rates despite a higher incidence of bleeding problems in the warfarin group (answer D incorrect) (Crowther et al. 2002). A trial of aspirin and clopidogrel was stopped prematurely due to bleeding problems in the treatment group with no reduction in AVG thrombosis (answer E incorrect) (Crowther et al. 2002).

 Clinical pearls

- There are surprisingly few data assessing the efficacy of anti-platelet or other agents in reducing access thrombosis.
- Aspirin has not been associated with a clinically proven benefit in reducing vascular access thrombosis, while both warfarin and the combination of aspirin and clopidogrel have been associated with increased bleeding events without any benefit on vascular access thrombosis.

Question 7

Regarding the measurement of vascular access blood flow for vascular access surveillance, which of the following is/are true?

(a) Vascular access blood flow can be measured by three different techniques: Doppler ultrasound, magnetic resonance angiography (MRA) or using dilution principles.

(b) Dilution principles can measure access blood flow by assessing a change in blood properties using indicators such as blood temperature, haematocrit or conductivity.

(c) The most investigated and validated dilution technique is based on blood temperature changes.

(d) The dilution techniques are performed between dialysis sessions so as to avoid any possible haemodynamic effect of the dialysis treatment on access blood flow.

(e) The gold standard technique for assessing vascular access blood flow is Doppler ultrasound.

Answer

A and B

Explanation

Vascular access blood flow can be measured by three different techniques: dilution, Doppler ultrasound or MRA (answer A correct). MRA is expensive and not freely available. Doppler ultrasound is available, although is relatively expensive when used to screen asymptomic subjects and is operator dependent. The most investigated and validated techniques are those utilising dilution principles.

Krivitski elegantly described and validated the application of dilution principles to measure vascular access blood flow (Krivitski 1995). According to the dilution method, blood flow (Q) is given by:

$$Q = V/S$$

where V is the amount of injected indicator that completely mixes in the blood flow stream Q; S is the area under the dilution curve which is equal to the average concentration of indicator in the blood multiplied by the duration of the curve. He was able to demonstrate that by reversing the dialysis blood lines (inducing access recirculation) and measuring both the blood flow in the tubing and the changes in ultrasound velocity induced by a saline bolus (using ultrasound probes attached to the blood line), access blood flow (Qa) is equal to:

$$Qa = Qb \times (Sv/Sa - 1)$$

where Qb is the venous line blood flow and Sv/Sa is the ratio of areas under the dilution curves recorded by matched arterial (Sa) and venous dilution sensors generated by the saline bolus injection. The above equation can be then rewritten into the now widely recognised form:

$$Qa = Qb * (1/R - 1)$$

where R is the fractional access recirculation caused by the reversal of the dialysis lines. Following the initial description of the technique by Krivitski using saline as the indicator, others demonstrated the measurement of access blood flow based on different blood properties such as electrical impedance (conductivity), optical properties (haematocrit) and temperature (answer B correct).

The ultrasound saline dilution velocity method is the best validated method for measuring access blood flow and is considered the gold standard method (answer C incorrect) (NKF-K/DOQI 2001). The dilution techniques are performed during the dialysis session and therefore are dependent on the haemodynamic status of the patient at the time of the test. It is recommended that the measurements be performed during the first hour of the dialysis session when the BP of the patients is stable (answer D incorrect) (NKF-K/DOQI 2001). While Doppler ultrasound can be used to measure access blood flow, it is operator dependent and there is poor agreement between Doppler ultrasound measurements and ultrasound dilution (answer E incorrect).

 Clinical pearls

- Access blood flow can be measured by a variety of techniques of which saline ultrasound dilution is the gold standard.
- Dilution techniques are performed during the dialysis session and results are dependent on stable haemodynamics at the time of the test.

Question 8

Which of the following is/are true regarding vascular access surveillance for AVF and/or AVG?

(a) Randomised controlled trials have demonstrated an increase in AVG survival with AVG blood flow surveillance.

(b) Randomised controlled trials have demonstrated an increase in AVF survival with AVF blood flow surveillance.

(c) Doppler ultrasound screening for AVG stenosis does not increase AVG survival.

(d) Static venous pressure is superior to dynamic venous pressures for vascular access monitoring.

(e) Access recirculation is useful for the surveillance of AVF and AVG.

Answer

B and C

Explanation

Three well-designed RCTs have been published since 2001 assessing the effect of blood flow surveillance using ultrasound dilution on AVG survival (Smits et al. 2004; Ram et al. 2003; Moist et al. 2003). While in all three studies there were more interventions performed in the Qa surveillance group compared to the control group, demonstrating that more stenoses were detected, there was no overall benefit seen with blood flow surveillance (answer A incorrect). In all three studies the intervention performed was angioplasty and therefore the results question the efficacy of angioplasty in the treatment of AVG stenosis. In contrast to AVG, the only RCT to assess AVF demonstrated a superior survival rate with Qa surveillance using angioplasty as the intervention in the majority of subjects (answer B correct).

The results of anatomical screening using Doppler ultrasound have been mixed (all studied AVG). Six randomised controlled trials (Ram et al. 2003; Mayer, Zingale & Tsapogas 1993; Sands et al. 1997; Malik et al. 2005; Robbin 2006; Lumsden et al. 1997) have been published since 1993, three of which reported a prolongation of AVG survival while three did not (answer C correct). Interventions were by angioplasty in all but one of the studies.

Static venous pressures are measured using the venous drip chamber transducer with the blood pump flow off, normalising the reading for the height between the access and the drip chamber. Despite suggestive observational data, they were not shown to be superior to dynamic venous pressures in the surveillance in the only published randomised controlled trial (answer D incorrect).

Access recirculation occurs when the dialysed blood, returning to the systemic recirculation via the venous needle of the extracorporeal circuit, is taken up again through the arterial needle, bypassing the systemic circulation. The presence of access recirculation will therefore reduce the efficiency of any haemodialysis treatment and can only occur once blood flow within the AVG or AVF is less than the dialyser blood flow (Qb). Therefore, the presence of access recirculation signifies reduced access blood flow resulting from the presence of a haemodynamically significant stenosis. The clinical usefulness of recirculation measurements in AVG surveillance is limited, as the risk of thrombosis in AVG is high once access blood flow is reduced to 500 to 800 mL/min, a range of blood flow which is too high to cause access recirculation (NKF-K/DOQI 2001). Unlike AVG, AVF blood flow can decrease to a dialyser blood flow lower than prescribed while still maintaining patency. Thus the measurement of access recirculation can be a useful tool to detect AVF stenosis (answer E incorrect) (NKF-K/DOQI 2001).

Clinical pearls

- Access blood flow surveillance has been shown to be beneficial in AVF but not AVG.
- Screening for AVG stenosis using Doppler ultrasound does not prolong AVG survival.
- Static venous pressures are not superior to dynamic venous pressure in AVG surveillance.
- Vascular access recirculation is useful for the surveillance for AVF but not AVG, although it is a relatively late sign of access dysfunction.

Bibliography

Level A

1. National Kidney Foundation's Kidney Disease Outcomes Quality Initiative. (2001) NKF-K/DOQI clinical practice guidelines for vascular access: update 2000. Am J Kidney Dis. 37, S137–81.
2. Council of the Australian and New Zealand Society of Nephrology (ANZSN) & the Board of Kidney Health Australia (KHA). (2003) The Caring for Australasians with Renal Impairment (CARI) guidelines: vascular access. www.cari.org. au/guidelines.php
3. Polkinghorne, K.R., McDonald, S.P., Atkins, R.C. & Kerr, P.G. (2004) Vascular access and all-cause mortality: a propensity score analysis. J Am Soc Nephrol. 15, 477–86.
4. Asif, A., Roy-Chaudhury, P. & Beathard, G.A. (2006) Early arteriovenous fistula failure: a logical proposal for when and how to intervene. Clinical Journal of the American Society of Nephrology. 1, 332–9.

Level B

5. Schwab, S.J., Harrington, J.T., Singh, A., Roher, R., Shohaib, S.A., Perrone, R.D., Meyer, K. & Beasley, D. (1999) Vascular access for hemodialysis. Kidney Int. 55, 2078–90.
6. Besarab A. (2004) Treatment of anaemia in dialysis patients. *Principles and Practice of Dialysis*, W.L. Henrich (ed.). Philadelphia: Lippincott Williams & Wilkins, 464–501.

Level C

7. Kaufman, J.S. (2000) Antithrombotic agents and the prevention of access thrombosis. Semin Dial. 13, 40–6.
8. Schmitz, P.G., McCloud, L.K., Reikes, S.T., Leonard, C.L.& Gellens, M.E. (2002) Prophylaxis of hemodialysis graft thrombosis with fish oil: double-blind, randomized, prospective trial. J Am Soc Nephrol. 13, 184–90.
9. Crowther, M.A., Clase, C.M., Margetts, P.J., Julian, J., Lambert, K., Sneath, D., Nagai, R., Wilson, S. & Ingram, A.J. (2002) Low-intensity warfarin is ineffective for the prevention of PTFE graft failure in patients on hemodialysis: a randomized controlled trial. J Am Soc Nephrol. 13, 2331–7.
10. Krivitski, N.M. (1995) Novel method to measure access flow during hemodialysis by ultrasound velocity dilution technique. ASAIO J. 41, M741–5.

11. Smits, J.H., van der Linden, J., Hagen, E.C., Modderkolk-Cammeraat, E.C., Feith, G.W., Koomans, H.A., Van Den Dorpel, M.A. & Blankestijn, P.J. (2001) Graft surveillance: venous pressure, access flow, or the combination? Kidney Int. 59, 1551–8.
12. Ram, S.J., Work, J., Caldito, G.C., Eason, J.M., Pervez, A. & Paulson, W.D. (2003) A randomized controlled trial of blood flow and stenosis surveillance of hemodialysis grafts. Kidney Int. 64, 272–80.
13. Moist, L.M., Churchill, D.N., House, A.A., Millward, S.F., Elliott, J.E., Kribs, S.W., DeYoung, W.J., Blythe, L., Stitt, L.W. & Lindsay, R.M. (2003) Regular monitoring of access flow compared with monitoring of venous pressure fails to improve graft survival. J Am Soc Nephrol. 14, 2645–53.
14. Mayer, D.A., Zingale, R.G. & Tsapogas, M.J. (1993) Duplex scanning of expanded polytetrafluoroethylene dialysis shunts: impact on patient management and graft survival. Vascular Surgery. 27, 647–58.
15. Sands, J., Gandy, D., Finn, M., Johnson, A., Burrows, S. & Miranda, C. (1997) Ultrasound-angioplasty program decreases thrombosis rate and cost of PTFE graft maintenance. J Am Soc Nephrol 8, 171A (abstr).
16. Malik, J., Slavikova, M., Svobodova, J. & Tuka, V. (2005) Regular ultrasonographic screening significantly prolongs patency of PTFE grafts. Kidney Int 67, 1554–8.
17. Robbin, M.L., Oser, R.F., Lee, J Y., Heudebert, G.R., Mennemeyer, S.T. & Allon, M. (2006) Randomized comparison of ultrasound surveillance and clinical monitoring on arteriovenous graft outcomes. Kidney Int. 69, 730–5.
18. Lumsden, A.B., MacDonald, M.J., Kikeri, D., Cotsonis, G.A., Harker, L.A. & Martin, L.G. (1997) Prophylactic balloon angioplasty fails to prolong the patency of expanded polytetrafluoroethylene arteriovenous grafts: results of a prospective randomized study. J Vasc Surg. 26, 382–90; discussion 390–2.

Case 22
Access infection

KEVAN POLKINGHORNE

Case history

A 65-year-old woman has end-stage kidney disease due to diabetic nephropathy. She is currently treated with haemodialysis using a right tunnelled central venous jugular line for the last 4 months. She presents with an acute onset of fevers and rigors. There is no history of abdominal or loin pain but she has a dry cough. Her blood pressure on admission is 110/60 mmHg with a pulse of 115 beats/min. Her temperature is 38.5°C. The catheter exit site is clean and without inflammation.

Question 1

With regards to the diagnosis of catheter-related bacteraemia, which of the following statements is/are true?

(a) A diagnosis of definite catheter-related bacteraemia is made by culturing blood taken solely from the catheter.

(b) A diagnosis of definite catheter-related bacteraemia is made by culturing blood taken solely from a peripheral vein.

(c) A clean catheter exit site makes the diagnosis of catheter-related bacteraemia unlikely.

(d) The risk of catheter-related bacteraemia in dialysis patients is higher compared to other tunnelled catheters.

Answer

D

Explanation

Catheter-related bacteraemia is suspected when a haemodialysis patient who has a dialysis catheter in situ presents with fevers without any other possible source of infection. To make the diagnosis, blood cultures must be taken separately from both the catheter lumen/s and a peripheral vein at the same time prior to the administration of any antibiotics. The diagnosis is confirmed if the cultures taken from the catheter and the peripheral vein grow the same organism. Growth of an organism from the blood but not the catheter suggests an alternative source of the bacteraemia. Growth of an organism from the catheter blood cultures but not from the peripheral blood cultures suggests bacterial colonisation of the catheter and not necessarily catheter-related bacteraemia. Probable catheter-related bacteraemia is diagnosed if the peripheral blood culture results are positive with negative catheter blood cultures, there is defervescence of symptoms after antibiotic therapy (with or without catheter removal) and there is no evidence for a source of infection other than the catheter. A diagnosis of catheter-related bacteraemia is made when the patient's fever resolves after antibiotic therapy or catheter removal when blood culture results are negative and there is no evidence for a source of infection other than the catheter.

While the occurrence of an exit site infection can suggest that the catheter is a likely source for the presentation, a clean exit site does not rule out the diagnosis. The risk of bacteraemia in dialysis patients is significant and compared to other catheter types may be higher as the number of catheter connections and disconnections is greater, leading to potential catheter contamination.

 Clinical pearls

- The diagnosis of catheter-related bacteraemia is made in a febrile patient if blood cultures taken from both the catheter and the peripheral blood grow the same organism without any other apparent source of infection.
- Probable catheter-related bacteraemia is diagnosed if the peripheral blood culture results are positive with negative catheter blood cultures, there is defervescence of symptoms after antibiotic therapy (with or without catheter removal) and there is no evidence for a source of infection other than the catheter.

Question 2

Common organisms causing catheter-related bacteraemia include:

(a) *Staphylococcus aureus*

(b) *Staphylococcus epidermidis*

(c) *Enterococcus*

(d) gram-negative organisms.

Answer

All are correct

Explanation

Multiple studies demonstrate a wide range of organisms causing catheter-related bacteraemia. Gram-positive bacteria are most commonly cultured ranging between 61 and 95% of infections in published series. The most common gram-positive organisms include *Staphylococcus aureus*, *S. epidermidis* and *Enterococci*. Infections by gram-positive organisms such as *S. aureus* and *S. epidermidis* are typically thought to result from propagation of skin flora around the exit site, along the external surface of the catheter and into the bloodstream. Gram-negative organisms such as *E. coli* are responsible for a significant minority of infections ranging from 5 to 45% of infections. As such, empiric antibiotic therapy should be broad-spectrum covering both gram-positive and gram-negative organisms pending culture results.

Clinical pearls

- Gram-positive organisms are the most common cause of catheter-related bacteraemia.
- Gram-negative organisms are responsible for a significant minority of infections.
- Empiric antibiotic therapy should be broad-spectrum covering both gram-positive and gram-negative organisms.

Question 3

Which of the following statements regarding catheter-related bacteraemia and its possible complications is/are true?

(a) Use of tunnelled dialysis catheters is not independently associated with mortality.

(b) Metastatic infection does not occur from central venous catheters used for dialysis.

(c) Severe sepsis or septic shock is extremely rare (less than 1%).

(d) Infection rates in tunnelled catheters are significantly lower than with non-tunnelled catheters.

Answer
D

Explanation

The use of tunnelled catheters in haemodialysis has been consistently demonstrated to be an independent risk factor for morbidity and mortality compared to the native arteriovenous fistula in dialysis patients. This increased risk in mortality is thought to be due in part to the increased rates of sepsis as a result of the catheter and complications such as metastatic infection. Metastatic infection (infection at another site arising as a result of the catheter infection) is not rare with reported rates between 3.2 and 9.7%. Septic shock, where there is hypotension that cannot be corrected by infusing fluids, is a particularly feared complication as patients often succumb despite aggressive therapy. Reported rates of severe sepsis range between 2.9 and 10.1%. The use of a tunnelled catheter compared to that of non-tunnelled catheters is associated with a reduced incidence of infection. However, despite this the risk of bacteraemia is significant with tunnelled catheters and their use can only be considered as temporary before permanent dialysis access can be established.

 Clinical pearls

- Catheter-related bacteraemia is a major cause of morbidity and mortality in haemodialysis patients.
- Metastatic infection is a major complication of catheter-related bacteraemia and complicates between 3 and 9% of episodes.
- Infection rates with tunnelled catheters are significantly lower than with non-tunnelled catheters.

LEVEL B

Case history continued ...

Both peripheral and catheter blood cultures taken at the time of presentation grow methicillin-sensitive *Staphylococcus aureus* and antibiotic therapy with flucloxacillin is commenced. After 48 hours the patient's temperature is 37.6°C and she has mild lumbar back pain.

Question 4

Which one of the following describes the best course of action for this patient?
(a) The catheter should be removed and replaced with a new catheter exchanged over a guidewire.
(b) The catheter should be removed and a tunnelled line placed in the left internal jugular vein.
(c) Further blood cultures should be performed and the catheter should be removed only if they are positive.
(d) The catheter should be removed without the immediate replacement of a dialysis line.

Answer

D

Explanation

Antibiotics alone will fail to definitively treat the infection in a majority of subjects with catheter-related bacteraemia as the infection cannot be cleared until the synthetic material is removed. A new tunnelled line should not be placed into the patient, either at the same exit site using guidewire exchange or at a new site, as the ongoing bacteraemia will likely lead to infection of the new catheter. To enable the continuation of dialysis therapy, a new temporary uncuffed catheter can be placed after a 'plastic free' period of 48 hours depending on the need for dialysis. Once the patient has negative peripheral blood cultures with resolution of fevers for at least 48 hours, a new tunnelled line can be re-inserted.

 Clinical pearls

- Catheter removal is needed in the vast majority of episodes of catheter-related bacteraemia in order to cure the infection.
- A new permanent catheter should not be placed until the infection has cleared.

Question 5

In relation to further management of this patient, which of the following statements is/are true?

(a) The presence of positive blood cultures 48 hours after commencing appropriate antibiotic therapy with or without catheter removal suggests the presence of metastatic infection.

(b) A radionuclide bone scan, computerised tomography (CT) scan or magnetic resonance imaging (MRI) scan of the spine is indicated.

(c) If the fever immediately settles with catheter removal, parenteral antibiotic can be switched to oral after 24 hours.

(d) Uncomplicated *Staphylococcus aureus* bacteraemia should be treated for 10 days.

Answer

A and B

Explanation

Blood cultures should be performed at 48 to 72 hours after the commencement of antibiotic therapy to ensure that they have become negative, even if the patient is afebrile. Ongoing positive blood cultures in the face of appropriate antibiotic therapy raise the possibility of metastatic infection such as endocarditis. Other sites of metastatic infection documented in catheter-related bacteraemia include osteomyelitis, septic arthritis and epidural abscess. The back pain is suggestive of osteomyelitis and a radionuclide bone scan, CT scan or MRI scan should be performed. Antibiotic therapy for *Staphylococcus aureus* bacteraemia should be parenteral and for at least 2 weeks if uncomplicated. Parenteral therapy for uncomplicated coagulase-negative staphylococcus is usually 1 week and gram-negative organisms at least 2 weeks or longer depending on the organism. Oral antibiotic therapy is not appropriate for the treatment of catheter-related bacteraemia.

Clinical pearls

- Blood cultures should be performed at 48 to 72 hours after the commencement of antibiotic therapy to ensure that they have become negative.
- Ongoing positive blood cultures in the face of appropriate antibiotic therapy raise the possibility of metastatic infection such as endocarditis.
- Antibiotic therapy for *Staphylococcus aureus* bacteraemia should be parenteral and for at least 2 weeks if uncomplicated.

LEVEL C

Case history continued …

The patient is now well and dialysing with a new tunnelled central venous catheter. She has a new arteriovenous fistula (AVF) constructed in the right upper arm (maturing well). She presents with an erythematous catheter exit site of which a swab demonstrates profuse growth of *Staphylococcus aureus*.

Question 6

In regard to the use of exit-site ointment for the prevention of catheter-related bacteraemia, which of the following statements is/are true?

(a) Rates of catheter-related bacteraemia are lower with the use of exit-site ointments compared to antibiotic lock solutions.

(b) Mupirocin is the most commonly used ointment.

(c) Polysporin ointment is superior to mupirocin as it is effective against a broad range of gram-positive and gram-negative bacteria.

(d) Honey is superior to mupirocin in the prevention of catheter-related bacteraemia.

Answer

B

Explanation

Three randomised controlled trials (RCTs) have addressed the effect of exit-site antibacterial ointments on catheter-related bacteraemia (see Table 22.1). One study compared mupirocin to no treatment; another compared polysporin ointment to a placebo and one compared mupirocin to medicated honey. Mupirocin is a topical antibiotic with solely gram-positive cover while polysporin is composed of three different antibiotics (bacitracin, gramicidin and polymyxin B) and therefore is effective against a broad range of gram-positive and gram-negative bacteria. In an open-labelled randomised trial that included fifty subjects, mupirocin was effective in reducing rates of catheter-related bacteraemia compared to no treatment, although rates of bacteraemia in the 'no treatment group' of this study were unusually high. As might have been expected, the treatment effect was entirely due to a reduction in staphylococcal infections.

Likewise, polysporin ointment compared to a placebo was also effective in reducing bacteraemia rates. In a study of 169 patients, the use of polysporin was associated with a 60% relative risk reduction in bacteraemia with only seven catheters needed to be treated to prevent one episode of catheter-related bacteraemia. While polysporin ointment has a wider antibacterial spectrum, no direct comparison of mupirocin to polysporin has been performed. A third study by Johnson et al. (2005) investigated the use of medicated honey in the prevention of catheter-related bacteraemia. Honey has broad-spectrum antibacterial properties and unlike mupirocin has not been associated with the development of bacterial resistance. In this RCT, there was no significant difference between the bacteraemia rates in the two groups over a median follow-up of 95 days. While a larger study would be required to confidently demonstrate therapeutic equivalence, the lack of antibiotic resistance when using honey makes it an attractive agent for prophylaxis of catheter-related bacteraemia.

Table 22.1 RCTs of exit site ointments as prophylaxis against cuffed catheter-related bacteraemia in haemodialysis patients

Study	Number	Intervention	Control	Result (treatment versus control)[a]
Johnson et al. 2002	50	Mupirocin	No mupirocin	1.6 versus 10.5*
Lok et al. 2003	169	Polysporin	Placebo	0.63 versus 2.48[†]
Johnson et al. 2005	101	Honey	Mupirocin	0.97 versus 0.85

Note: [a] Rates of catheter-related bacteraemia per 1000 catheter days, * $p < 0.01$, [†] $p < 0.001$

Clinical pearls

- The application of antibacterial ointments to the cuffed catheter exit site appears to be effective in reducing catheter-related bacteraemia.
- Medicated honey appears to be as effective as mupirocin and has not been associated with the occurrence of antibacterial resistance.

Question 7

With regard to antibiotic lock solutions for the prevention of catheter-related bacteraemia, which of the following statements is/are true?

(a) Gentamicin/citrate is the most efficacious solution.

(b) Both citrate and cefotaxime antibiotic locks have been demonstrated to reduce patient mortality.

(c) Citrate-containing solutions are currently the optimal antibiotic lock solution in terms of efficacy and side effects.

(d) The risk of ototoxicity from gentamicin is negligible.

Answer

B

Explanation

A number of recent RCTs have compared the effect of various catheter lock solutions and standard heparin on the incidence of catheter-related bacteraemia (see Table 22.2). Compared to heparin, rates of catheter-related bacteraemia were reduced using these solutions but whether any particular lock solution is superior remains unknown. In addition, whether the use of exit site ointments or antibiotic lock solutions is the superior approach has not been tested.

Two studies also reported lower mortality due to catheter-related bacteraemia in the antibiotic lock group, despite not being powered for this outcome. Gentamicin ototoxicity and fatal arrhythmias due to high-dose citrate have been reported and these potential serious side effects should be balanced against the possible benefits of using this treatment.

Clinical pearls

- The use of antibiotic lock solutions has consistently demonstrated a reduction in bacteraemia compared to standard heparin locks.
- The optimal antibiotic lock solution has yet to be determined.

Table 22.2 RCTs of prophylaxis against cuffed catheter-related bacteraemia in haemodialysis patients

Study	Number	Intervention	Control	Result (treatment versus control)[b]
Dogra et al. 2002	108	Gentamicin/citrate	Heparin	0.3 versus 4.2[†]
McIntyre et al. 2004	50	Gentamicin/heparin	Heparin	0.3 versus 4.0*
Betjes & van Agteren 2004[a]	76	Citrate/taurolidine	Heparin	0 versus 2.1*
Bleyer et al. 2005[a]	60	Minocycline-EDTA	Heparin	8.3% versus 0%[c]
Weijmer et al. 2005[a]	291	Trisodium citrate	Heparin	1.1 versus 4.1[‡]
Saxena et al. 2006	119	Cefotaxime/heparin	Heparin	1.67 versus 3.60[†]
Nori 2006	62	Minocycline-EDTA	Heparin	0.4 versus 4*
		Gentamicin/tricitrate	Heparin	0 versus 4[†]

Note: EDTA = ethylenediaminetetraacetic acid, [a] these studies included both cuffed and uncuffed catheters, [b] rates of catheter-related bacteraemia per 1000 catheter days, [c] rates not stated, * $p < 0.05$, [†] $p < 0.01$, [‡] $p < 0.001$.

Question 8

Regarding bacterial biofilms within catheter lumens, which of the following statements is/are true?

(a) Biofilms form rapidly within the catheter lumen after insertion.
(b) Biofilms within central venous catheters can be cleared by the administration of intraluminal antimicrobials.
(c) Bacteria growing within biofilms commonly have reduced antimicrobial sensitivity.
(d) Negative blood cultures taken from the catheter excludes the presence of a biofilm within the catheter lumen.
(e) Silver impregnated catheters are associated with reduced bacteraemia rates through a reduction in biofilm formation.

Answer
A and C

Explanation

The formation of a biofilm is a process by which micro-organisms irreversibly attach to and grow on a surface, be it a central venous catheter lumen or another medical device such as a prosthetic heart value. The micro-organisms produce extracellular polymers that facilitate attachment and matrix formation which results in an altered phenotype of the organisms with respect to growth rate and gene transcription. Biofilms can form rapidly after the insertion of a central venous catheter. It has been well documented that the altered biofilm mode of growth confers a measurable decrease in antimicrobial susceptibility and biofilms within catheters cannot usually be cleared by antimicrobial agents. Due to the decreased antimicrobial susceptibility, organisms might be absent from blood cultures taken from the catheter but still survive within the biofilm in the catheter lumen.

Given that bacteria in a biofilm coating the inner lumen of the dialysis catheter are an important source of catheter-related bacteraemia, efforts have been directed at the prevention of biofilm formation using antibiotic lock solutions (see Question 7) or applying different coatings to the catheters. Standard triple lumen and untunnelled dialysis catheters have been coated in antibiotics such as rifampicin and monocycline but this approach has not yet been tested in tunnelled dialysis catheters. Silver has antimicrobial activity, with in vitro studies demonstrating suppression of catheter colonisation when silver ions were applied directly to the catheter. However, a RCT performed by Trerotola et al. (1998) found no difference in frequency of catheter-related bacteraemia between patients with silver-coated tunnelled dialysis catheters and those with untreated catheters (1.8 infections per 1000 catheter days versus 1.1 per 1000 catheter days respectively, non-significant).

 Clinical pearls

- Bacterial biofilms are an important source of infection in central venous catheters.
- Negative blood cultures taken from a central venous catheter do not exclude the presence of a biofilm formation within catheter lumen and bacteria growing within biofilms have reduced antimicrobial sensitivity.

Bibliography

Level A
1. Allon, M. (2004) Dialysis catheter-related bacteraemia: treatment and prophylaxis. Am J Kidney Dis. 44, 779–91.
2. National Kidney Foundation. (2006) KDOQI Clinical practice guidelines and clinical practice recommendations for 2006 updates: hemodialysis adequacy, peritoneal dialysis adequacy and vascular access. Am J Kidney Dis. 48, S1–322.

Level B
3. Allon, M. (2004) Dialysis catheter-related bacteraemia: treatment and prophylaxis. Am J Kidney Dis. 44, 779–91.

4. Gosbell, I.B. (2005) Diagnosis and management of catheter-related bloodstream infections due to *Staphylococcus aureus*. Intern Med J. 35(Supp. 2), S45–62.

Level C

5. Allon, M. (2004) Dialysis catheter-related bacteraemia: treatment and prophylaxis. Am J Kidney Dis. 44, 779–91.
6. Betjes, M.G. & van Agteren, M. (2004) Prevention of dialysis catheter-related sepsis with a citrate-taurolidine-containing lock solution. Nephrol Dial Transplant. 19, 1546–51.
7. Bleyer, A.J., Mason, L., Russell, G., Raad, I.I. & Sherertz, R.J. (2005) A randomized, controlled trial of a new vascular catheter flush solution (minocycline-EDTA) in temporary hemodialysis access. Infect Control Hosp Epidemiol. 26, 520–4.
8. Dogra, G.K., Herson, H., Hutchison, B., Irish, A.B., Heath, C.H., Golledge, C., Luxton, G. & Moody, H. (2002) Prevention of tunneled hemodialysis catheter-related infections using catheter-restricted filling with gentamicin and citrate: a randomized controlled study. J Am Soc Nephrol. 13, 2133–9.
9. Dogra, G.K. (2006) Preventing catheter-related infections with antibiotic lock solutions: are we spoilt for choice? Nephrology. 11, 297–8.
10. Donlan, R.M. (2001) Biofilm formation: a clinically relevant microbiological process. Clin Infect Dis. 33, 1387–92.
11. McIntyre, C.W., Hulme, L.J., Taal, M. & Fluck, R.J. (2004) Locking of tunneled hemodialysis catheters with gentamicin and heparin. Kidney Int. 66, 801–5.
12. Saxena, A.K., Panhotra, B.R., Sundaram, D.S., Naguib, M., Morsy, F. & Al-Arabi Al-Ghamdi, A.M. (2006) Enhancing the survival of tunneled haemodialysis catheters using an antibiotic lock in the elderly: a randomised, double blind clinical trial. Nephrology. 11, 299–305.
13. Nori, U.S., Manoharan, A., Yee, J. & Besarab, A. (2006) Comparison of low-dose gentamicin with minocycline as catheter lock solutions in the prevention of catheter-related bacteremia. Am J Kidney Dis. Oct., 48(4), 596–605.
14. Weijmer, M.C., van den Dorpel, M.A., Van de Ven, P.J., ter Wee, P.M., van Geelen, J.A., Groeneveld, J.O., van Jaarsveld, B.C., Koopmans, M.G., le Poole, C.Y., Schrander-Van der Meer, A.M., Siegert, C.E. & Stas, K.J. (2005) Randomized, clinical trial comparison of trisodium citrate 30% and heparin as catheter-locking solution in hemodialysis patients. J Am Soc Nephrol. 16, 2769–77.
15. Johnson, D.W., MacGinley, R., Kay, T.D., Hawley, C.M., Campbell, S.B., Isbel, N.M. & Hollett, P. (2002) A randomized controlled trial of topical exit site mupirocin application in patients with tunnelled, cuffed haemodialysis catheters. Nephrol Dial Transplant. 17, 1802–7.
16. Johnson, D.W., van Eps, C., Mudge, D.W., Wiggins, K.J., Armstrong, K., Hawley, C.M., Campbell, S.B., Isbel, N.M., Nimmo, G.R. & Gibbs, H. (2005) Randomized, controlled trial of topical exit-site application of honey (Medihoney) versus mupirocin for the prevention of catheter-associated infections in hemodialysis patients. J Am Soc Nephrol. 16, 1456–62.
17. Lok, C.E., Stanley, K.E., Hux, J.E., Richardson, R., Tobe, S.W. & Conly, J. (2003) Hemodialysis infection prevention with polysporin ointment. J Am Soc Nephrol. 14, 169–79.
18. Trerotola, S.O., Johnson, M.S., Shah, H., Kraus, M.A., McKusky, M.A., Ambrosius, W.T., Harris, V.J. & Snidow, J.J. (1998) Tunneled hemodialysis catheters: use of a silver-coated catheter for prevention of infection—a randomized study. Radiology. 207, 491–6.

Part D
Peritoneal dialysis

Case 23
Peritoneal dialysis adequacy

FIONA BROWN

LEVEL A

Case history

A 52-year-old woman with end-stage kidney failure due to non-insulin dependent diabetes mellitus commenced peritoneal dialysis 4 weeks ago. Her medications at that time were frusemide 80 mg daily, irbesartan 150 mg daily, Caltrate 600 mg three times a day, sodium bicarbonate 840 mg twice daily and calcitriol 0.25 mcg three times weekly. On review at 4 weeks, she is feeling well. On examination her blood pressure (BP) is 140/80 mmHg supine and 130/80 mmHg erect with her jugular venous pressure (JVP) 2 cm above the clavicle, a clear chest and no evidence of peripheral oedema. Investigations reveal the following results.

Laboratory data

	Results	Reference range
Serum potassium	5.9 mmol/L	(3.7–5.3)
Serum bicarbonate	22 mmol/L	(20–32)
Serum urea	18 mmol/L	(2.5–8.0)
Serum creatinine	642 µmol/L	(60–110)
Random blood glucose	12 mmol/L	(4.0–7.8)

The patient is currently receiving continuous ambulatory peritoneal dialysis (CAPD) with 4 × 2 L 2.5% glucose dialysis fluid exchanges per day.

Question 1

The most likely cause/s of her hyperkalaemia is/are:

(a) inadequate dialysis
(b) metabolic acidosis
(c) dietary intake
(d) unstable diabetes due to increased glucose absorption from the glucose-based dialysis solution
(e) volume depletion.

Answer

C

Explanation

Excessive intake of dietary potassium is a common cause of hyperkalaemia. Her serum urea and creatinine suggest she is dialysing adequately although there has been no formal assessment of adequacy. This can be done with a peritoneal equilibration test (PET) and Adequest. The PET involves the infusion of a 2 L 2.5% dextrose dialysis solution which is then drained 4 hours later. Dialysate and a blood sample are collected at the time of infusion, at 2 hours and at the time of drainage at 4 hours. The dialysate to plasma creatinine ratio can then be calculated, giving information on the transport characteristic of the peritoneal membrane documenting whether the patient is a rapid (high) or slow (low) transporter. The Adequest program determines how well the patient is dialysing by measuring Kt/V and creatinine clearance. Kt/V is a measure of urea clearance as defined by the calculated peritoneal and renal urea clearance (Kt) corrected for total body water (V). This is measured using 24-hour drained dialysate and urine volumes in addition to blood samples.

The serum bicarbonate is normal in this patient at 22 mmol/L; therefore, she does not have metabolic acidosis. Dietary and fluid restrictions are very important for peritoneal dialysis patients although they are often less hyper-kalaemic than patients on haemodialysis due to the continuous (versus inter-mittent) nature of peritoneal dialysis. Glucose is absorbed systemically from the glucose-based dialysis solution resulting in hyperglycaemia in diabetic patients. However, hyperglycaemia is not a cause of hyperkalaemia unless the patient develops ketoacidosis (insulin-dependent diabetes mellitus). Examination findings do not support volume depletion with a raised JVP at 2 cm and no postural hypotension.

Clinical pearl

- Dietary and fluid restrictions are important for peritoneal dialysis patients although they are often less hyperkalaemic than patients on haemodialysis.

Question 2

The change/s in her medication that may have caused hyperkalaemia include:

(a) cessation of irbesartan

(b) cessation of frusemide

(c) commencement of glipizide due to poor glucose control

(d) cessation of sodium bicarbonate

(e) commencement of erythropoietin.

Answer

B

Explanation

Cessation of irbesartan may lower the serum potassium as angiotensin II receptor antagonists can cause hyperkalaemia in patients with renal impairment. Cessation of frusemide may result in hyperkalaemia, as she still has residual renal function; so in addition to increasing the urine volume, frusemide may result in increased urine potassium excretion. Diuretics may also be beneficial in patients on peritoneal dialysis as they may increase urine volumes and thus less peritoneal removal of fluid by peritoneal dialysis is required. This means that dialysis solution of a lower glucose concentration is used, which results in a lower cumulative glucose exposure and may result in less peritoneal membrane damage and peritoneal dialysis technique failure. Commencement of glipizide and erythropoietin should not affect potassium levels. Cessation of sodium bicarbonate may result in acidosis that could cause hyperkalaemia but as she is on peritoneal dialysis, the acidosis should be corrected and her serum bicarbonate is normal at 22 mmol/L.

 Clinical pearls

- Continuation of diuretics in patients on peritoneal dialysis is recommended to maintain urine volumes and may also help control hyperkalaemia.
- In addition, the maintenance of significant urine volume means less peritoneal removal of fluid is required, allowing dialysis solution of lower glucose concentration to be used, which may result in less peritoneal membrane damage.

Case history continued ...

Three months later, the patient presents with fluid overload. She has not altered her dialysis regimen, she is voiding 800 mL urine/day and her daily peritoneal ultrafiltration is 1.2 L.

Question 3

The most likely cause of her fluid overload is:

(a) poor compliance with fluid intake restrictions

(b) reduced urine volumes

(c) use of inappropriate dialysis solutions (4 × 2 L exchanges of 1.5% glucose-based dialysis fluid)

(d) inadequate peritoneal ultrafiltration (removal of fluid)

(e) hyperglycaemia.

Answer

A

Explanation

Poor compliance is the most likely cause of her fluid overload as she is losing a total of 2.5 L daily with a urine volume of 800 mL, peritoneal ultrafiltration 1.2 L and insensible losses of 0.5 L. Therefore, a residual urine volume of 800 mL is more than adequate to maintain a euvolaemic state provided she adheres to a fluid restriction of 2.5 L daily. As she is ultrafiltrating an average of 300 mL per 1.5% bag of dialysis solution, she should not need to increase the glucose concentration. Peritoneal ultrafiltration failure is defined as a drained volume of less than 400 mL on a 2 L 4.25% dialysis solution exchange and less than 200 mL on a 2 L 2.5% dialysis solution exchange over 4 hours. She is ultrafiltrating 300 mL on a 2 L 1.5% dialysis solution exchange and although it has not been formally tested with a 2 L 2.5% or 4.25% dialysis solution exchange over 4 hours, it is unlikely she has peritoneal ultrafiltration failure. Hyperglycaemia can contribute to reduced peritoneal ultrafiltration as there is loss of the osmotic gradient between dialysate and blood but she does not have ultrafiltration failure. Thus, poor compliance with excessive fluid intake is the most likely cause of her fluid overload.

 Clinical pearl

- Peritoneal ultrafiltration failure is defined as an ultrafiltration volume of less than 400 mL on a 2 L 4.25% dialysis solution exchange and less than 200 mL on a 2 L 2.5% dialysis solution exchange over 4 hours.

LEVEL B

Case history continued ...

On review 6 months later, the patient complains of significant lethargy. Examination shows she is normotensive, her weight is stable and she is euvolaemic. Investigations show her serum urea is 30 mmol/L (normal 2.5 to 8 mmol/L), creatinine 960 µmol/L (normal 60 to 110 µmol/L) and albumin 32 g/L (normal

36 to 48 g/L). Her peritoneal equilibration test (PET) and Adequest demonstrates a dialysate/plasma creatinine (D/P Cr) of 0.68, total Kt/V 2.2 (peritoneal Kt/V 1.8 and residual renal function Kt/V 0.4) and total creatinine clearance (CrCl) 65 mL/min (peritoneal CrCl 50 mL/min and residual renal CrCl 15 mL/min).

Question 4

Given these results, which of the following statement/s is/are true?
- **(a)** She will not clear urea well across the peritoneal membrane.
- **(b)** She will not clear creatinine well across the peritoneal membrane.
- **(c)** She will not clear sodium well across the peritoneal membrane.
- **(d)** She will ultrafiltrate well across the peritoneal membrane.
- **(e)** She will not ultrafiltrate well across the peritoneal membrane.

Answer
E

Explanation

D/P Cr as measured by the peritoneal equilibration test (PET) determines the peritoneal transport of creatinine across the peritoneal membrane. This determines the patient's transport status: the mean D/P Cr is 0.65, with low transporters <0.5, low average 0.5 to 0.64, high average 0.66 to 0.81 and high >0.81. High transporters (high-average and high) are more likely to develop peritoneal ultrafiltration failure and thus have a reduced time on peritoneal dialysis; some studies suggest increased mortality. High transporters will dialyse reasonably well with high D/P creatinine, D/P urea and D/P sodium as there is a rapid equilibration across the peritoneal membrane, but they may not ultrafiltrate well as there is a rapid loss of the osmotic gradient. Her D/P Cr is 0.68, meaning she is a high average transporter and she will clear urea, creatinine and sodium well but as a result she will lose her osmotic gradient and will not ultrafiltrate well across the peritoneal membrane.

Clinical pearls

- D/P Cr as determined by the peritoneal equilibration test (PET) determines peritoneal transport status. The mean D/P Cr is 0.65, with low (L) transporters <0.5, low average (LA) 0.5 to 0.64, high average (HA) 0.66 to 0.81 and high (H) >0.81.
- High transporters (high-average and high) are more likely to develop peritoneal ultrafiltration failure and thus have reduced peritoneal dialysis technique survival and increased mortality.

Question 5

Which of the following statements is/are true?

(a) In determining peritoneal dialysis adequacy, the Kt/V is more useful than the CrCl.

(b) Residual renal function contributes significantly more to Kt/V than CrCl.

(c) Peritoneal dialysis contributes significantly more to CrCl than Kt/V.

(d) Her total creatinine clearance suggests adequate dialysis.

(e) Her total Kt/V suggests adequate dialysis.

Answer

D and E

Explanation

Kt/V measures the clearance of urea in comparison to the creatinine clearance but both are important measures of peritoneal dialysis adequacy. Peritoneal dialysis contributes more to Kt/V than creatinine clearance in comparison to residual renal function, which contributes more to creatinine clearance. A large randomised controlled trial, ADEMEX, suggested a minimum Kt/V of 1.84 represents adequate dialysis. There are different minimum targets for creatinine clearance depending on the peritoneal membrane transport status as measured by PET. The Caring for Australasians with Renal Impairment (CARI) guidelines recommend a minimum creatinine clearance of 60 mL/min for H/HA and 50 mL/min for LA/L transporters.

 Clinical pearls

- Kt/V measures the clearance of urea; both it and creatinine clearance are important measures of peritoneal dialysis adequacy.
- Peritoneal dialysis contributes more to Kt/V than creatinine clearance in comparison to residual renal function, which contributes more to creatinine clearance.
- A large randomised controlled trial, ADEMEX, suggested a minimum Kt/V of 1.84 is adequate. CARI guidelines recommend a minimum creatinine clearance of 60 mL/min for H/HA and 50 mL/min for LA/L transporters.

Question 6

The ideal peritoneal dialysis regimen for this patient would be:

(a) CAPD with 4 × 2 L dialysis solution exchanges per day

(b) CAPD with 4 × 2.5 L dialysis solution exchanges per day

(c) CAPD with 5 × 2 L dialysis solution exchanges per day

(d) automated peritoneal dialysis (APD) with 6 × 2 L dialysis solution exchanges overnight with a dry day (no dialysis)

(e) APD with 6 × 2 L dialysis solution exchanges overnight with a long day dwell with icodextrin.

Answer

E

Explanation

Her D/P Cr is 0.68, meaning that she is a high average transporter. High transporters dialyse better with frequent short exchanges because there is rapid loss of the osmotic gradient that reduces ultrafiltration. Thus, increasing the dialysis exchange volumes may not increase dialysis adequacy and may result in reduced peritoneal ultrafiltration. APD with frequent short exchanges overnight would be the recommended peritoneal dialysis regimen. A dry day may be suitable but would not allow for any dialysis or ultrafiltration during this time. In addition, some peritoneal dialysis patients may experience abdominal pain with a long dry day. Icodextrin, a hyperosmolar glucose polymer, can be used for the long day dwell as it allows for ultrafiltration over a 12- to 14-hour dwell. Low transporters should have longer dwell times and may benefit from larger dialysis fluid volumes as glucose is slowly transported across the peritoneal membrane and thus the clearance of other solutes such as creatinine and urea is slower.

Clinical pearls

- High transporters dialyse better with frequent short exchanges and icodextrin for the long dwell.
- Low transporters should have longer dwell times with larger volumes to improve dialysis adequacy.

LEVEL C

Case history continued ...

The patient is well for the next 2 years with the only complication being an episode of *Staphylococcus aureus* peritonitis. She now presents with fluid overload and a low serum albumin of 28 g/L.

Her current regimen is APD with 6 × 2 L exchanges of 1.5% glucose dialysis solution and 2.5 L icodextrin for the long day dwell. A repeat PET reveals her

D/P Cr has increased to 0.78 with total Kt/V 1.95, total creatinine clearance 60 mL/min and a 4-hour 2 L 4.25% dialysis solution exchange drained volume of 2.2 L. The mass transfer area coefficients (MTAC) for urea and creatinine are measured at urea 20 mL/min and creatinine 12 mL/min. The peritoneal protein loss is 6 g/d. Her 24-hour urine volume is 150 mL with a spot urine protein/creatinine ratio of 130 mg/mmol. Her normalised protein equivalent of protein appearance (nPNA) is low at 0.7 g/kg/day and her C-reactive protein (CRP) is 35 mg/L (normal <10 mg/L).

Question 7

What factor/s is/are important when assessing whether a patient is adequately dialysed?
(a) Kt/V
(b) Creatinine clearance
(c) Serum albumin
(d) Fluid status
(e) Serum pre-albumin

Answer
All are correct

Explanation

Adequacy of dialysis is not just measured by Kt/V and creatinine clearance. The patient's fluid status and nutritional status are also crucial elements. Serum albumin is a very important prognostic factor with a low serum albumin correlating with an increased mortality in peritoneal dialysis patients. A low serum albumin could indicate malnutrition but may also indicate systemic inflammation such as infection, cardiac failure, increased protein losses (both peritoneal and renal) or chronic liver disease. The serum pre-albumin may be a more specific marker of poor nutrition as it has a shorter half-life than albumin (2 to 3 days compared to 14 to 20 days); however, it is often increased in patients with renal failure and may be reduced in acute catabolic states.

 Clinical pearl

- Adequacy of peritoneal dialysis is determined by assessing Kt/V, creatinine clearance, fluid status, nutritional status and presence or not of uraemic symptoms.

Question 8

The most likely cause/s of her low serum albumin is/are:
(a) inadequate dialysis
(b) inadequate dietary intake
(c) peritoneal protein loss
(d) renal protein loss
(e) inflammation.

Answer
B, C and E

Explanation

Malnutrition is very common in peritoneal dialysis patients, with studies suggesting that up to 35% of peritoneal dialysis patients are malnourished. There are multiple contributing factors to poor nutrition, including inadequate dietary protein intake, peritoneal and renal protein losses, inadequate dialysis and systemic inflammation with increased protein catabolism. She is dialysing adequately by ADEMEX and CARI criteria with a Kt/V of 1.95 and creatinine clearance of 60 mL/min. The nPNA is low with a recommended target of 1.2 g/kg/day, suggesting inadequate dietary protein intake. Normal peritoneal protein loss on peritoneal dialysis is between 5 and 10 g/day, so at 6 g/day her peritoneal protein loss is in the expected range but will contribute significantly to the low serum albumin. She has persistent proteinuria but given her small urine volumes, this is unlikely to be a major contributing factor. Her CRP is elevated suggesting systemic inflammation and thus a catabolic state requiring an increased dietary protein intake.

 Clinical pearl

- Malnutrition is common in peritoneal dialysis patients and there are multiple contributing factors: inadequate dietary protein intake (recommended minimum 0.8 g/kg/day), peritoneal and renal protein losses, inadequate dialysis and systemic inflammation with increased protein catabolism.

Question 9

After 2 years on peritoneal dialysis, the patient's Adequest is repeated. Compared to the assessment made at 6 months, her total Kt/V has fallen from 2.2 to 1.95, her MTAC is measured at urea 20 mL/min and creatinine 12 mL/min. Which of the following statement/s is/are true?

(a) A single episode of *Staphylococcus aureus* peritonitis does not reduce Kt/V.
(b) Reduced urine volumes do not affect Kt/V.
(c) APD results in a more rapid decline in Kt/V than CAPD.
(d) The MTACs for urea and creatinine suggest inadequate dialysis.
(e) Cumulative dialysis glucose exposure may cause a decline in Kt/V.

Answer
E

Explanation

Peritonitis, even a single episode, may damage the peritoneal membrane and result in a reduced peritoneal and total Kt/V. Reduced urine volumes may reduce the renal Kt/V and renal creatinine clearance. Loss of residual renal function on peritoneal dialysis is an important cause of inadequate dialysis. There is no good evidence that APD results in a more rapid decline in Kt/V, although patients on APD may have a higher total dialysis glucose exposure, which may damage the peritoneal membrane. MTACs are used to measure the clearance of a solute such as urea or creatinine across the peritoneal membrane per unit of time assuming that the dialysate flow is infinitely high. Typical MTAC values are 17 mL/min for urea and 10 mL/min for creatinine. Her MTAC readings are slightly elevated with urea 20 mL/min and creatinine 12 mL/min. The MTAC for individual solutes such as creatinine may increase if there is an increase in the peritoneal surface area such as with increased peritoneal capillaries as a result of neovascularisation secondary to glucose dialysis fluid exposure. The MTAC is not routinely measured in peritoneal dialysis patients as a measure of dialysis adequacy but can be useful in determining the diffusion capacity of the peritoneal membrane. There is evidence that cumulative glucose dialysis exposure damages the peritoneal membrane resulting in peritoneal fibrosis and neovascularisation, which results in a decline in peritoneal adequacy as measured by Kt/V and loss of ultrafiltration.

 Clinical pearl

- Cumulative dialysis glucose exposure damages the peritoneal membrane and may result in a decline in dialysis adequacy as measured by Kt/V and/or creatinine clearance.

Question 10

A peritoneal equilibration test shows that compared to the assessment made at 6 months, her D/P Cr has increased from 0.68 to 0.78. What manoeuvre/s would prevent a further increase in her D/P Cr?

(a) Reduce the glucose concentration of standard dialysis solution.
(b) Replace the long day dwell icodextrin with a more hypertonic glucose-based dialysis solution.
(c) Change all dialysis fluid to low glucose degradation product (GDP) dialysis solutions.
(d) Replace one dialysis exchange with amino acid based dialysis solution (Nutrineal).
(e) None of the above.

Answer
E

Explanation

The D/P Cr has increased after 2 years on peritoneal dialysis suggesting there has been damage to the peritoneal membrane, which could be from the episode of peritonitis and/or cumulative exposure to glucose-based dialysis fluids. Potential ways to reduce glucose and glucose degradation products exposure include the use of less hypertonic standard glucose dialysis solutions or the use of alternative dialysis solutions such as icodextrin, low GDP solutions or Nutrineal. However, at this stage there is no definitive evidence that changing dialysis solutions would prevent a further increase in the D/P Cr.

 Clinical pearls

- D/P Cr increases with time on peritoneal dialysis, resulting in a higher membrane transport status.
- The increase in D/P Cr correlates with cumulative glucose exposure.

Question 11

Which of the following dialysis modification/s would improve the patient's dialysis adequacy and fluid status?
(a) Increase the strength of her glucose-based dialysis solution.
(b) Change to low GDP dialysis solution.
(c) Increase to two icodextrin exchanges daily.
(d) Change her to haemodialysis temporarily.
(e) Change her to haemodialysis permanently.

Answer
D and E

Explanation

The patient has peritoneal ultrafiltration failure with only 2.2 L drained from a 2 L 4-hour 4.25% dialysis solution exchange. Increasing the strength of her glucose dialysis solution may result in increased peritoneal ultrafiltration (which may improve her fluid status) but this is only a temporary measure and the increased glucose exposure may cause further peritoneal membrane damage with further loss of ultrafiltration. At this stage, there is no evidence that changing her to a low GDP dialysis solution will improve ultrafiltration. Icodextrin ultrafiltrates best in a long dwell of 12 to 14 hours and thus it is not practical to increase to two exchanges daily as she will not receive adequate dialysis. In addition, she may begin to accumulate maltose, a metabolic breakdown product of icodextrin with an extra exchange. There are some studies that suggest peritoneal rest may improve ultrafiltration; however, in general if patients have peritoneal ultrafiltration failure on the optimal peritoneal dialysis regimen and there are no contraindications to haemodialysis then they should be changed permanently.

 Clinical pearl

- Temporary cessation of peritoneal dialysis may improve peritoneal ultrafiltration; however, in general if patients have ultrafiltration failure on the optimal regimen for their membrane transporter status, and there are no contraindications to haemodialysis, then they should be permanently changed.

Bibliography

Level B

1. Council of the Australian and New Zealand Society of Nephrology (ANZSN) & the Board of Kidney Health Australia (KHA). (2005) Caring for Australasians with Renal Impairment (CARI) guidelines on peritoneal dialysis adequacy. Nephrology. Oct.
2. Daugirdas, J., Blake, P. and Ing, T. (2001) *Handbook of Dialysis*, 3rd edn. Philadelphia: Lippincott Williams & Wilkins.
3. Paniagua, R., Amato, D., Vonesh, E., Correa-Rotter, R., Ramos, A., Moran, J. and Mujais, S; Mexican Nephrology Collaborative Study Group. (2002) Effects of increased peritoneal clearances on mortality rates in peritoneal dialysis: ADEMEX, a prospective, randomized, controlled trial. J Am Soc Nephrol. May, 13(5), 1307–20.
4. Rumpsfeld, M., McDonald, S.P. and Johnson, D.W. (2006) Higher peritoneal transport status is associated with higher mortality and technique failure in the Australian and New Zealand peritoneal dialysis patient populations. J Am Soc Nephrol. Jan., 17(1), 271–8.

Level C

5. Davies, S.J. (2004) Longitudinal relationship between solute transport and ultrafiltration capacity in peritoneal dialysis patients. Kidney Int. Dec., 66(6), 2437–45.

Case 24
Cloudy bag

KAMAL SUD

LEVEL A

Case history

A 65-year-old diabetic man with stage 5 chronic kidney disease is brought to his general practitioner by his family, with abdominal pain and constipation. He was started on continuous ambulatory peritoneal dialysis (CAPD) 9 months ago. On examination, his blood pressure is 140/85 mmHg, pulse is 90 beats/min, temperature is 37.2°C and his abdomen is diffusely tender with audible bowel sounds.

Question 1

The possible causes of abdominal pain in a patient on CAPD include:
(a) diverticulitis
(b) peritonitis related to peritoneal dialysis
(c) pancreatitis
(d) mesenteric ischaemia.

Answer
All are correct

Explanation

Due to innovations in connection techniques, the incidence of peritonitis has steadily reduced over the last three decades (current rates of peritonitis are <0.3 per patient year or 1 episode every 36 months on peritoneal dialysis). Peritonitis related to peritoneal dialysis (PD) should be excluded in all PD patients presenting with abdominal pain. Abdominal pain in patients with peritonitis is usually severe; however, some episodes may be associated with mild or even no pain. Other causes of abdominal pain should be considered only once PD-related peritonitis has been excluded. Urgency and high index of suspicion is required for making this diagnosis, as a delay in diagnosis can lead to significant morbidity including hospitalisation, peritoneal membrane failure and sometimes death.

Clinical pearls

- Peritonitis must be excluded in all patients on PD presenting with abdominal pain.
- All other causes of abdominal pain should also be considered once peritonitis has been excluded.

Question 2

Which investigation would be the most appropriate to make a diagnosis of CAPD-related peritonitis in this patient?

(a) Plain abdominal X-ray

(b) Ultrasound of abdomen

(c) Computerised tomography (CT) scan of abdomen with oral and intravenous (IV) contrast

(d) Peritoneal dialysis effluent cytology and culture

Answer

D

Explanation

Peritonitis can easily be diagnosed in PD patients by inspecting the PD effluent and sending this fluid for cytology and culture. A cloudy effluent supports the diagnosis of peritonitis, but a clear effluent does not exclude this possibility. The PD effluent cell count with white blood cells >100/μL with at least 50% neutrophils indicates acute peritoneal inflammation. Presence of two of the following three criteria is essential to make a diagnosis of CAPD peritonitis:

1. abdominal pain
2. cloudy effluent with evidence of acute inflammation on cytology
3. detection of organisms on gram stain/culture of PD fluid.

An erect plain film of the abdomen may show free air under the diaphragm in PD patients; this does not always indicate bowel perforation as air may have been inadvertently infused with the PD fluid by the patient during a recent exchange. Other investigations such as ultrasound abdomen and CT scan may be required if a complication of PD-related peritonitis or bowel perforation is suspected or other causes of abdominal pain are being looked for.

 Clinical pearls

- Examination of PD effluent is the initial investigation of choice for diagnosis of peritonitis in a patient on PD.

- PD effluent white cell count (WCC) of > 100/μL with >50% neutrophils indicates acute peritoneal inflammation.
- Other investigations are done if complications of PD-related peritonitis are suspected or to look for other causes, once peritonitis has been excluded.

Question 3

What would be the most appropriate initial line of treatment in this patient with PD-related peritonitis?

(a) Laparotomy without removal of CAPD catheter
(b) Laparotomy with removal of CAPD catheter
(c) Antibiotic administration and stopping CAPD
(d) Antibiotic administration and continuation of CAPD

Answer
D

Explanation

Antibiotic administration is the mainstay of treatment of PD-associated peritonitis. Antibiotics can be administered systemically or intraperitoneally. An intraperitoneal route is preferred in patients without signs of systemic sepsis as this route is associated with increased local concentration of the drug where it is required. All attempts are made to continue peritoneal dialysis, as dialysis may help to lavage the infected peritoneal cavity, along with helping in controlling the ongoing azotaemia in a hypercatabolic setting. Laparotomy with or without catheter removal is not indicated as the initial modality of treatment, unless bowel perforation is strongly suspected by demonstration of polymicrobial growth on PD fluid cultures or there is an inadequate response to administration of antibiotics.

Clinical pearl

- Unlike surgical causes of peritonitis, PD-related peritonitis is best managed medically with intraperitoneal antibiotics and continuation of PD.

Question 4

A cloudy PD effluent may also be seen in which of the following conditions?

(a) Haemoperitoneum
(b) Chemical peritonitis

(c) Chylous ascites
(d) Eosinophilic peritonitis

Answer
All are correct

Explanation

Presence of a cloudy effluent almost always represents infection-related peritonitis and to prevent delays, treatment should be initiated while awaiting results of cell counts, gram stains and cultures from the laboratory. If the PD effluent does not demonstrate >100/µL WBC with >50% neutrophils and the cultures are sterile, then other causes such as those listed above should be considered. However, these conditions are rare and usually associated with a benign outcome. Occurrence of haemoperitoneum can easily be confirmed on cytology and will need appropriate investigation to delineate the cause. Menstruating females may develop episodes of haemoperitoneum with their menstrual cycles as a result of blood refluxing from the fallopian tubes into the peritoneal cavity. Chemical peritonitis may be seen in patients receiving intraperitoneal agents or antibiotics, or as a result of the constituents of the PD fluid bag such as icodextrin or acetaldehyde. PD effluent cytology generally reveals an abundance of macrophages and the peritonitis is usually transient, but requires exclusion of the inciting agent from the PD fluid. Eosinophilic peritonitis is diagnosed if eosinophils constitute more than 10% of cells in the effluent. This form of peritonitis is usually seen in the initial two weeks of starting PD, is thought to be related to hypersensitivity to one of the constituents of the PD fluid, is relatively asymptomatic and is generally self limiting. Patients may be treated with a short course of steroids once infection has been definitely excluded and diagnosis confirmed by demonstrating eosinophilia in the PD effluent. Chylous ascites may be associated with tubercular infection or lymphoma, although benign and recurrent forms of chylous ascites complicating PD have also been reported.

 Clinical pearl
- Other non-infective causes of a cloudy effluent should be considered once PD-related peritonitis has been excluded.

LEVEL B

Case history continued ...

The PD effluent from the cloudy bag is sent for cytology, gram staining and cultures. The cytology and gram stains are obtained, showing a WCC of 350 cells/µL with 60% polymorphonuclear cells, but negative gram stain.

Question 5

Which of the following organisms are commonly isolated from the PD fluid in a patient suspected of having peritonitis?

(a) Coagulase-negative staphylococcus
(b) *Staphylococcus aureus*
(c) Enterococci
(d) Gram-negative bacteria

Answer

All are correct

Explanation

The epidemiology and microbiology of peritonitis among PD patients varies by location. Although the incidence of coagulase-negative staphylococcus (*Staphylococcus epidermidis*) peritonitis, which occurs primarily from touch contamination, has reduced with the introduction of better connection techniques, this and *Staphylococcus aureus* continue to be the most common organisms responsible for PD-related peritonitis. *Staphylococcus epidermidis* generally produces a mild form of peritonitis that responds readily to antibiotics. *Staphylococcus aureus* usually causes a more severe infection and is frequently associated with exit site or tunnel infection. Streptococcal and enterococcal infections also tend to be more severe as compared to coagulase-negative staphylococcus infections. Gram-negative peritonitis from *E. coli*, *Klebsiella* and *Proteus* is likely to occur from transmural migration of these enteric bacteria in patients with constipation or colitis. *Pseudomonas aeruginosa* peritonitis is also frequently associated with catheter infections. Only about 10% episodes of peritonitis are culture negative if proper culture techniques are followed. Potential reasons for negative cultures include culturing too little effluent, not culturing the sediment after centrifuging the PD effluent, not inoculating the fluid into blood culture bottles or sending off the effluent after starting antibiotics. Other causes of 'sterile' peritonitis include occurrence of tubercular/fungal/chemical or eosinophilic peritonitis or a sealed-off intra-abdominal abscess.

 Clinical pearls

- Epidemiology of organisms causing peritonitis differs by location.
- If the correct techniques are employed to culture the PD effluent, only 10% of PD-related peritonitis may be culture negative.

Question 6

Which of the following statements is/are true regarding antibiotic treatment of peritonitis?
(a) Empiric antibiotics should cover organisms likely to cause peritonitis based on the clinical picture.
(b) Choice of antibiotics should be based on sensitivities of organisms causing peritonitis in that area/centre.
(c) Intravenous administration is not the preferred route of administration of antibiotics in patients on CAPD.
(d) In patients on automated peritoneal dialysis (APD), intraperitoneal route of administration is contraindicated because of concerns regarding bioavailability.

Answer
B and C

Explanation

In most cases the organism causing the peritonitis cannot be suspected reliably on clinical grounds. Therefore, empiric antibiotics must cover both gram-positive and gram-negative organisms. The choice of antibiotics to be started should be based on the sensitivity patterns of organisms causing peritonitis at that particular centre. Most centres would employ first-generation cephalosporin or vancomycin to cover gram-positive organisms and third-generation cephalosporins or amino-glycoside antibiotics to cover gram-negative organisms. Many units, however, avoid the empirical use of vancomycin because of the risk of increasing the incidence of vancomycin-resistant organisms (VRE). Short-term use of aminoglycoside antibiotics appears to be safe and not associated with a high risk of vestibular toxicity/ototoxicity or deleterious effects on residual renal function (Baker et al. 2003). In patients with previous known peritonitis/exit site infection by organisms such as MRSA or *Pseudomonas*, the choice of initial empiric antibiotics must cover these organisms based on their known sensitivity patterns.

Patients without evidence of systemic sepsis are best treated via the intraperi-toneal route of administration, as this provides ease of administration as well as the high local concentrations of antibiotics. Intraperitoneal administration of antibiotics can be intermittent or continuous (depending on the pharmacokinet-ics of the antibiotic) and there is no difference in response rates between the two protocols, provided at least a 6-hour dwell can be ensured with the intermittent regimens. Vancomycin, aminoglycoside and cephalosporin antibiotics can be mixed in the same dialysis solution bag without loss of bioactivity, thereby mak-ing the intermittent dosing regimens easy and possible. Providing a minimum 6-hour dwell for antibiotic administration can be an issue in patients on APD, who usually undergo rapid exchanges at night, with either 1 or 2 exchanges and are often 'dry' through the day. In these patients, the antibiotics can be administered intraperitoneally, just before coming off the machine in patients who are 'dry', or infused into the long day exchange in patients doing a day exchange. Many patients are converted to CAPD temporarily for treatment of peritonitis. As both vancomycin and aminoglycoside accumulate in patients with renal failure, subsequent dosing should be based on drug levels.

 Clinical pearls

- The exact organism/s responsible for PD-related peritonitis can not be reliably predicted by the clinical presentation.
- Empiric antibiotics should cover both gram-positive and gram-negative organisms and be based on local sensitivity patterns.
- Short-term use of aminoglycoside antibiotics with blood level monitoring is safe.
- In the absence of severe systemic sepsis, intraperitoneal route of administration is preferred for treating PD-related peritonitis.

Question 7

Which of the following statements is/are correct regarding duration of antibiotic treatment?
- **(a)** Patients with peritonitis from gram-positive (non MRSA) bacteria should receive treatment for 7 days.
- **(b)** Patients with peritonitis from MRSA should receive antibiotics for 2 weeks.
- **(c)** Patients with peritonitis from gram-negative bacteria should receive antibiotics for 3 weeks.
- **(d)** Patients with culture-negative peritonitis should receive antibiotics for 2 weeks.

Answer
C and D

Explanation

Once sensitivity results are available, the empiric antibiotic regimen should be adjusted based on the organism isolated and its sensitivity pattern. The International Society of Peritoneal Dialysis (ISPD) Guidelines 2005 recommend that gram-positive peritonitis be treated for 2 weeks, MRSA peritonitis for 3 weeks, gram negative peritonitis for 3 weeks, *pseudomonas* peritonitis for 3 weeks and culture-negative peritonitis for 2 weeks. The addition of rifampicin (for 1 week) to vancomycin for MRSA peritonitis is recommended, as is the use of two antibiotics (with different mechanisms of activity) for *pseudomonas* peritonitis, for their synergistic effects. If culture results demonstrate a polymicrobial infection from gram enteric organisms, intra-abdominal disease such as diverticulitis or ischaemic bowel should be considered, metronidazole should be added to the therapeutic regimen, and removal of catheter considered.

Clinical pearls

- Duration of antibiotic treatment varies according to the organism causing peritonitis.
- MRSA and gram-negative peritonitis, including that due to *pseudomonas*, requires 3 weeks of antibiotic treatment.

LEVEL C

Case history continued ...

The PD fluid culture comes back with growth of *Pseudomonas aeruginosa* and antibiotics are changed to ceftazidime and amikacin (based on sensitivity results) and given for a total of 3 weeks. Repeat PD fluid cytology done after 4 days of starting antibiotics show a WCC of 40 cells/µL with 80% lymphomononuclear cells. The patient comes back 3 weeks after stopping antibiotics with recurrence of cloudy bags.

Question 8

Which of the following statements is/are correct?
- **(a)** This patient has refractory peritonitis.
- **(b)** The patient should be investigated for bowel perforation.
- **(c)** The exit site should be closely examined for a possible exit site infection.
- **(d)** Treatment of choice is medical management including restarting antibiotics with anti-pseudomonal cover.

Answer
C

Explanation

Patients are said to have a relapse if peritonitis recurs from the same organism or after a sterile culture, within 4 weeks of stopping antibiotics. Repeat peritonitis is an episode with the same organism that occurs after 4 weeks of stopping antibiotics. Peritonitis is said to be recurrent if it occurs from a different organism within 4 weeks of stopping antibiotics. Refractory peritonitis is defined as failure of effluent to clear after 5 days of appropriate antibiotics. Catheter-related peritonitis is defined as peritonitis occurring in conjunction with an exit-site or tunnel infection, with the same organism. The exit site and catheter tunnel should be closely examined in every patient presenting with peritonitis, as presence of these is associated with a different therapeutic strategy. Relapsing peritonitis is thought to occur because of production of a bio-film in the catheter lumen, where antibiotics are unable to reach in adequate concentrations.

 Clinical pearls

- Clinical evidence of tunnel and exit site infections should be looked for in every patient presenting with PD-related peritonitis.
- Relapses occur due to catheter-related infections or production of bio-film in the catheter lumen.

Question 9

The patient has an exit site infection from *Pseudomonas aeruginosa* and the PD effluent also grows the same organism. The patient is restarted on antibiotics. Which of the following statements is/are correct?

(a) Antibiotics should be given for at least 6 weeks.

(b) The patient should be started on IV antibiotics in addition to local antibiotic creams for the exit site infection.

(c) The patient should undergo removal of PD catheter and antibiotics continued for 2 weeks while on haemodialysis.

(d) The patient should undergo surgical replacement of the PD catheter followed by 2 weeks of intraperitoneal anti-pseudomonal antibiotics.

Answer

C

Explanation

Indications for catheter removal in patients with PD-related infections are refractory peritonitis, relapsing peritonitis, catheter-related peritonitis, and patients with refractory exit site or tunnel infections. Other indications for catheter removal include patients with fungal or multiple enteric organism peritonitis. Early removal of the catheter in patients with refractory peritonitis has been shown to reduce morbidity and mortality as well as to preserve the peritoneal membrane for future PD. In treating patients for peritonitis, the focus should be on patient morbidity and mortality in addition to preserving the peritoneal membrane, not saving the catheter. Simultaneous catheter removal and new catheter replacement is usually successful in non-infectious indications of catheter removal. In addition, this could be considered in patients with a refractory exit site/tunnel infection where the new PD catheter is inserted under antibiotic cover, away from the infected site. The PD catheter can also be replaced in selected patients with relapsing peritonitis once the PD effluent has first been cleared with appropriate antibiotics.

The above approach is not recommended in patients with *pseudomonas* infection, as it often results in recurrence of infection in the new PD catheter. This procedure should also not be considered in patients with refractory peritonitis or those with fungal peritonitis and a minimum period of 2 to 3 weeks (twice as long for fungal peritonitis) between catheter removal and reinsertion is recommended.

 Clinical pearls

- When treating peritonitis, the focus should be on patient morbidity and mortality, in addition to preserving the peritoneal membrane for future PD, and not preserving the catheter.
- PD catheter should be removed early in patients with refractory peritonitis.
- Patients with relapsing peritonitis or those with catheter-related peritonitis can be treated with simultaneous insertion of a new catheter provided the PD effluent is cleared with appropriate antibiotics.

Question 10

Which of the following statements is/are true for fungal peritonitis in PD patients?
- **(a)** A prior episode of bacterial peritonitis in the last 30 days predisposes to fungal peritonitis.
- **(b)** Oral nystatin has been found to be effective in preventing fungal peritonitis in patients receiving antibiotics for prolonged periods.
- **(c)** Fungal peritonitis is associated with mortality rates that are higher than those associated with bacterial peritonitis.
- **(d)** Intraperitoneal amphotericin is used as an adjunctive treatment for fungal peritonitis.

Answer
A, B and C

Explanation

Sixty-five per cent of patients with fungal peritonitis have a history of exposure to antibiotics in the last 30 days and in the majority, the antibiotics are given to treat an episode of bacterial peritonitis. Recent exposure to antibiotics may predispose to fungal peritonitis by shifting the balance of the patient's endogenous skin and bowel flora towards yeast species, thereby increasing the chances of contamination during catheter manipulation. Other risk factors include HIV infection, recent abdominal surgery and concomitant fungal infection elsewhere in the body. Oral nystatin 50 000 units four times a day was found to be effective in preventing fungal peritonitis in patients being treated with antibiotics for bacterial peritonitis. Lo et al. (1996) randomised 397 patients with bacterial peritonitis at a single centre at Hong Kong to receive either oral nystatin or no treatment during the duration of antibiotic prescription for bacterial peritonitis. Although not all the episodes of *Candida* peritonitis were temporally related to antibiotics, patients on the antifungal prophylaxis had a significantly higher probability of being free of *Candida* peritonitis at 2 years as compared to those not receiving the prophylaxis.

Other possible preventive strategies include use of nystatin vaginal pessaries 100 000 units twice a day or oral fluconazole 100 mg daily. Mortality rates of patients with fungal peritonitis are higher as compared to those with bacterial peritonitis and range between 15 and 45% (as compared to 1 to 3% for bacterial peritonitis). Treatment revolves around early removal of PD catheter and use of oral antifungal agents such as fluconazole, itraconazole and voriconazole. IV amphotericin can be considered in highly immuno-compromised sick patients or in those with history of recent treatment with azoles. Amphotericin is not recommended for intraperitoneal administration because of associated pain during instillation, and the risk of adhesion formation and subsequent loss of peritoneal membrane for future PD. Removal of PD catheter is recommended as retained catheters may serve as a nidus for persistent infection. In addition, catheter retention has been associated with increased mortality. After the catheter has been removed a new catheter may be replaced after an interval of 4 to 6 weeks, provided the patient is well and there is not thought to be permanent damage to the peritoneal membrane.

Clinical pearls

- Recent antibiotic usage, abdominal surgery and immuno-compromised status are risk factors for occurrence of fungal peritonitis.
- Antifungal prophylaxis with nystatin may be used in conjunction with antibiotics in 'at risk' PD patients detailed above.
- Fungal peritonitis is associated with a high mortality rate that can be reduced with early removal of PD catheter.
- An interval of 4 to 6 weeks is recommended before a new catheter can be re-inserted after fungal peritonitis.

Bibliography

Level A

1. Tzamaloukas, A.H. & Fox, L. (2004) Infections in patients on peritoneal dialysis, *Principles and Practice of Dialysis*, Henrich, W.L. (ed). New York: Lippincott Williams and Wilkins, Chapter 41.

Level B

2. Piraino, B., Bailie, G.R., Bernardini, J., Boeschoten, E., Gupta, A., Holmes, C., Kuijper, E.J., Li, P.K., Lye, W.C., Mujais, S., Paterson, D.L., Fontan, M.P., Ramos, A., Schaefer, F. & Uttley, L. (2005) ISPD Ad Hoc Advisory Committee ISPD guidelines/ recommendations. Peritoneal dialysis-related infections recommendations: 2005 update. Perit Dial Int. 25, 107.
3. Tintillier, M., Pochet, J.M., Christophe, J.L., Scheiff, J.M. & Goffiri, E. (2002) Transient sterile chemical peritonitis with iodextrin: clinical presentation, prevalence and literature review. Perit Dial Int. 22(4), 534–37.
4. Kim, D.K., Yoo, T.H., Ryu, D.R., Xu, Z.G., Kim, H.J., Choi, K.H., Lee, H.Y., Han, D.S. & Kang, S.W. (2004) Changes in causative organisms and their antimicrobial susceptibilities in CAPD peritonitis: a single center's experience over one decade. Perit Dial Int. 24, 424.
5. Baker, R.J., Senior, H., Clemienger, M. & Brown, E.A. (2003) Empirical aminoglycosides for peritonitis do not affect residual renal function. Am J Kidney Dis. 41, 670.

Level C

6. Singhal, M.K., Vas, S.I. & Oreopoulos, D.G. (1998) Treatment of peritoneal dialysis catheter-related infections by simultaneous catheter removal and replacement. Is it safe? Perit Dial Int. Nov.–Dec. 18(6), 565–7.
7. Prasad, N. & Gupta, A. (2005) Fungal peritonitis in peritoneal dialysis patients. Perit Dial Int. 25, 207.
8. Lo, W.K., Chan, C.Y., Cheng, S.W., Poon, J.F., Chan, D.T. & Cheng, I.K. (1996) A prospective randomized control study of oral nystatin prophylaxis for Candida peritonitis complicating continuous ambulatory peritoneal dialysis. Am J Kidney Dis. Oct., 28(4), 549–52.

Case 25
Ultrafiltration failure

KAMAL SUD

LEVEL A

Case history

A 63-year-old female with type 2 diabetes mellitus and end-stage kidney failure from diabetic nephropathy on chronic ambulatory peritoneal dialysis (CAPD) presents with resistant hypertension. Her previous medical history includes coronary artery disease, hypertension requiring three antihypertensive medications for control, previous abdominal hernia repairs and a laparotomy for bowel perforation from ischaemic bowel. The blood pressure (BP) recordings have been consistently above 180/110 mmHg while on amlodipine 10 mg daily, atenolol 100 mg daily and prazosin 10 mg twice daily.

Question 1

What physical sign/s should be looked for?
(a) Weight gain
(b) Elevated jugular venous pressure (JVP)
(c) Vascular bruits
(d) All of the above

Answer
D

Explanation

In patients with diabetes and/or renal disease, resistant hypertension is defined as BP above 130/80 mmHg (140/90 mmHg in patients without diabetes or renal disease) despite adherence to an appropriate three-drug regimen. Diabetic patients with end-stage kidney failure could have resistant hypertension from a number of causes and these include presence of renal failure per se, salt and water retention (causing weight gain and signs of fluid overload), reno-vascular disease, and all other causes, including essential hypertension, seen in the general population. Fluid overload from salt and water retention is the most common cause for difficult-to-control BP in patients on dialysis.

Clinical pearls

- Patients with end-stage kidney failure can have difficult-to-control BP from causes that are related to kidney failure as well as from other causes seen in the general population.
- Fluid overload from salt and water retention is the most common cause for difficult-to-control BP in patients on dialysis.

Case history continued ...

The patient's JVP is raised and there is moderate pedal oedema with a history of weight gain over the past 6 weeks. There are audible bruits over both carotid arteries and dorsalis pedis and posterior tibial arterial pulsations in both legs are difficult to palpate.

Question 2

What would be the most pertinent next step/s in evaluation?
(a) Assess residual renal function by asking about daily urine volume.
(b) Order a computerised tomography (CT) angiogram to look for evidence of renal artery stenosis.
(c) Check peritoneal dialysis (PD) records to review daily ultrafiltration volume.
(d) Assess daily fluid intake.

Answer
A, C and D

Explanation

Ultrafiltration forms an important component of any dialysis modality and this, along with solute clearance, constitutes the two most important parameters against which adequacy of PD is assessed. Ultrafiltration refers to the removal of plasma water by means of pressure or osmotic gradient and *net* ultrafiltration is determined by the amount of water that is removed with the PD fluid and the amount of water that is reabsorbed into the capillaries and the lymphatics in the peritoneal cavity. The average surface area of the peritoneal membrane is between 1.0 and 1.3 m^2 in adults. Since only a third of the visceral peritoneum is in contact with dialysis solution, it is primarily the parietal peritoneum that participates in peritoneal transport.

Inadequate solute clearance manifests with increasing blood urea and serum creatinine levels, or the appearance of uraemic symptoms (despite seemingly successful PD), and can be assessed by measuring small solute clearances by the peritoneal equilibration test (PET). Patients with inadequate ultrafiltration present with weight gain due to fluid retention, hypertension and clinical features of heart failure. Residual renal function forms an important contributor not only for solute clearance but also for maintaining fluid balance in PD patients. Although loss of residual renal function may be slower in PD patients as compared to patients on haemodialysis (HD), this could be an important factor in patients presenting with fluid retention. Other causes of fluid retention include non-compliance with fluid restriction or peritoneal dialysis regimen. These can be assessed by reviewing PD records for daily ultrafiltration volume and assessment of daily fluid intake by history. Renovascular disease as a cause of resistant hypertension is not the first consideration in PD patients, but could be considered in patients presenting with flash pulmonary oedema.

 Clinical pearls

- Ultrafiltration is an important component of PD adequacy.
- Important causes of weight gain from fluid retention on PD include non-compliance with fluid restriction and/or PD regimen, and loss of residual renal function.
- Patients with renovascular disease can present with episodes of flash pulmonary oedema.

Question 3

How would you assess this patient further once you have decided that there is fluid overload?

(a) Reassess the patient's dry weight.
(b) Examine the patient for hernias or for evidence of localised retention of fluid.
(c) Conduct a supervised PD exchange.
(d) Perform an abdominal X-ray to check the position of PD catheter.

Answer
All are correct

Explanation

All patients should be assessed for their dry weight and prescribed a PD regimen accordingly. Inaccurate assessment of a dialysis patient's dry weight can lead to fluid overload. Quite often, the dry weight requires reassessment and may need to be reduced if the patient has lost lean body mass for any reason, such as recent hospitalisation for a major illness, malignancy or malnutrition associated with inadequate dialysis.

Weight gain from fluid retention can be either localised or generalised. Patients can present, soon after initiation of PD, with localised fluid retention resulting from leak of dialysate into subcutaneous tissues of the abdominal wall or into a defect in the peritoneum at the site of catheter insertion. In addition, fluid can leak into the scrotum if the inguinal canal communicates with the peritoneal cavity. Fluid can also leak into the pleural cavity from a pleuroperitoneal communication. The resulting pleural effusion can often be quite large, leading to respiratory compromise. To help confirm the diagnosis and delineate the anatomy of a peritoneal fluid leak, peritoneal scintigraphy or CT scanning after infusion of dialysate containing contrast material is usually performed. Management involves measures aimed at reducing intra-abdominal pressures by decreasing dialysate volumes or performing the exchanges in supine position with the use of cyclers; or temporary discontinuation of PD. Most patients, however, usually need surgical correction of the leak.

Problems with fluid drainage may be detected by conducting a supervised PD exchange. In the 'fill and drain test', one should ascertain whether there are any mechanical or anatomical reasons for the poor drainage, such as concomitant difficulty with inflow, fibrin clots partially occluding catheter lumen or fluid drainage that is position dependent. Causes of outflow failure, defined as incomplete recovery of instilled dialysate, include constipation, catheter malposition, intraluminal catheter occlusion (by fibrin/thrombus), extraluminal catheter occlusion (usually by omentum or adhesions) or catheter kinking. Most patients with outflow failure usually respond to laxatives, which not only correct constipation, but the intense bowel movements may also correct minor degrees of catheter malposition or kinking. Where outflow failure persists, an anteroposterior X-ray of the abdomen (including pelvis) is useful for diagnosing catheter malposition and kinking. For optimal function, the tip of the PD catheter should be seen in the most dependent part of the pelvis on the X-ray. Although malpositioned or kinked catheters frequently require replacement (particularly for long-term patency), they can sometimes be managed with stiff wire manipulation using fluoroscopy. Extraluminal causes can be diagnosed on peritoneal scintigraphy or CT scanning after infusion of dialysate containing contrast material through the catheter. Conversely, many surgeons proceed to a peritoneoscopy/laparoscopy, which allows direct visualisation of the catheter, enabling omentectomy/adhesiolysis or catheter redirection/replacement as required.

Clinical pearls

- Effective management of fluid overload is based on accurate diagnosis of the underlying problem.
- Fluid overload can be localised in patients with defects in the peritoneal membrane resulting in fluid leak into the subcutaneous tissues of the abdominal wall, pleural cavity or scrotum.

- A supervised PD exchange by an experienced nurse can give valuable information on the presence or absence of mechanical or anatomical conditions impairing fluid drainage.
- Radiological investigations can assist in making the diagnosis and guide further management.

LEVEL B

Case history continued ...

The fill and drain test was negative and there was no clinical evidence of localised leaks. On reviewing the PD charts, the patient was using three 2.5% dextrose bags and one 1.5% dextrose bag per 24 hours to achieve a net ultrafiltration of 400 to 500 mL/day. The daily urinary output was approximately 600 mL/day and the patient claimed to be compliant with a daily 1500 mL fluid restriction.

Question 4

What recommendations should be made to manage the fluid overload?
- **(a)** The patient should be asked to further reduce fluid intake to less than 1200 mL per day.
- **(b)** The patient should be prescribed frusemide 250 mg twice daily.
- **(c)** Antihypertensive therapy should be increased to control BP.
- **(d)** All the above.

Answer
D

Explanation

Once it is clear that the most likely cause of resistant hypertension and weight gain is fluid retention, dietary fluid restriction (particularly if intake is excessive) would be the obvious first step in management. However, fluid restrictions are difficult to sustain over prolonged periods and adversely impact quality of life on dialysis. Diuretics can be used to augment urinary output, but are generally ineffective if the residual urinary output is less than 500 mL/day. Further, as very high doses of loop diuretics (e.g. frusemide 250 mg twice daily) are required to make any appreciable impact on urinary output, patients run the risk of developing ototoxicity. It is important to remember that augmentation of urine output with diuretics does not have any effect on the residual creatinine clearance from the diseased kidneys and therefore improvements in urinary output with diuretics should not be construed to suggest that residual renal function has improved. Antihypertensive medications may also need to be increased to reduce the short- and long-term effects of uncontrolled hypertension on morbidity and mortality.

Clinical pearls

- Fluid restriction is difficult to sustain over long periods of time and adversely affects quality of life on dialysis.
- High dose loop diuretics can augment urinary output in patients with good residual renal function.
- Loop diuretics only augment free water excretion and have no effect on residual creatinine clearance.

Case history continued ...

The patient's fluid overload resolves with the outlined management but 18 months later she again presents with fluid overload and difficult to control BP. The urine output has fallen to less than 250 mL/day on frusemide 500 mg twice daily and the BP is consistently above 180/100 mmHg despite treatment with amlodipine 20 mg daily, atenolol 100 mg daily and prazosin 10 mg twice daily. Ultrafiltration volume with PD has remained unchanged at 400 to 500 mL/day despite the replacement of the 1.5% dextrose PD bag with a 4.25% dextrose bag.

Question 5

What management strategies should be considered in this situation?
(a) Use more 4.25% dextrose PD bags
(b) Reduce the dwell time
(c) Use icodextrin containing PD solution
(d) Increase the volume of PD bags

Answer
A, B and C

Explanation

The ultrafiltration volumes are inversely proportional to peritoneal transport characteristics for solutes, except in conditions where there is loss of surface area of the peritoneal membrane from scarring or adhesions. Therefore, patients with low rates of transport of the solutes across the peritoneal membrane have good ultrafiltration, because the osmotic gradient produced by the osmotic agent (i.e. dextrose) is maintained throughout the entire dwell. Conversely, patients with high rates of transport of solutes rapidly absorb the osmotic agent into peritoneal capillaries. This diminishes the osmotic stimulus for ultrafiltration within a few hours of dwell, providing opportunity for reabsorption of fluid in the peritoneal cavity through the rest of the dwell.

There is as yet no accepted definition of ultrafiltration failure (UFF), but a practical rule-of-thumb is an inability to achieve adequate fluid balance despite the use of two or more hypertonic (4.25%) exchanges per day. In patients who have had a PET, UFF can be defined as net UF <400 mL after a 4-hour dwell with a 4.25% dextrose solution or UF of <200 mL after a 4-hour dwell with a 2.5% dextrose solution. The cumulative risk of UFF increases with time on PD and has been documented to be in excess of 30% in patients on PD for 6 years or longer and is the cause of technique failure in 10% of patients.

UFF due to high peritoneal transport status may be transient or sustained. An episode of acute peritonitis is the classical cause of transient increase in peritoneal transport, due to inflammation. Repeated episodes of peritonitis can, however, lead to sustained increase in solute transport and persistent (and permanent) loss of ultrafiltration. Other causes of UFF include inadequate provision of ultrafiltration conditions, such as long dwell times, mismatched prescription of PD with PET status, occult leakage or catheter malposition/migration.

Initial management of poor ultrafiltration leading to fluid overload revolves around ensuring that there is adequate osmotic stimulus for ultrafiltration to occur (by the use of hypertonic PD solutions), attempting to provide suitable conditions for the peritoneal membrane to respond to the osmotic stimulus (by shortening the dwell time, so as to drain the PD fluid from the peritoneal cavity before the osmotic stimulus dissipates and the fluid is reabsorbed by the peritoneal membrane lymphatics) and looking for and managing mechanical or anatomical problems preventing ultrafiltration. Increasing the volume of PD fluid has a negative impact on ultrafiltration volumes, as the resultant increase in intraperitoneal hydrostatic pressure reduces net movement of fluid from the blood compartment to the dialysate compartment and also enhances lymphatic reabsorption of fluid from the peritoneal cavity.

Regular and frequent use of hypertonic dextrose containing PD fluids can lead to several metabolic complications, such as hyperinsulinaemia, hyperglycaemia, hyperlipidaemia and weight gain from glucose absorption. Further, exposure of the peritoneal membrane to high glucose concentrations, low pH and glucose degradation products can also enhance bio-incompatibility and affect peritoneal host defence mechanisms by inhibiting phagocytosis and bactericidal activity. Occurrence of hyperglycaemia from glucose absorption (especially in patients with high peritoneal transport status using hypertonic dextrose containing PD fluids) also reduces ultrafiltration volume by reducing the transmembrane osmotic gradient that facilitates movement of fluid into the dialysate compartment.

These potential side effects have prompted the use of non-glucose-based PD solutions with high molecular weight osmotic agents, such as those containing icodextrin or amino acids. Icodextrin is a relatively inert glucose polymer that is less permeable than dextrose, thereby offering the advantage of decreased absorption and increased ultrafiltration for a longer period of time. The 7.5% icodextrin-containing PD solution provides roughly equivalent UF volume as a 4.25% dextrose-containing PD solution, but has the additional advantage that it can be used in a long dwell. Therefore, the substitution of one daily exchange of hypertonic dextrose with 7.5% icodextrin is particularly appealing in diabetics and in those patients where PD regimen includes a long dwell whose ultra-filtration capacity needs to be enhanced. The reduced carbohydrate load with icodextrin also has the potential advantage of reducing the long-term metabolic complications associated with hypertonic dextrose containing PD fluids. Amino acid-based PD solutions may be considered for use in patients with protein malnutrition as, like glucose, amino acids are ready absorbed and may help in achieving a positive nitrogen balance in this subset of patients. However, their long-term effects on patient survival are yet to be determined in clinical trials. These solutions can be used in short dwells, but their routine prescription is limited by cost considerations at present.

 Clinical pearls

- Ultrafiltration volumes on PD are dependent on individual peritoneal membrane characteristics.
- Shortening dwell times and use of hypertonic PD fluids can have a positive impact of ultrafiltration volumes.
- Frequent use of hypertonic dextrose-containing PD fluids to enhance ultrafiltration can lead to several metabolic complications.
- Replacing one daily exchange of hypertonic dextrose with 7.5% icodextrin enhances ultrafiltration over long dwells and avoids the metabolic complications associated with use of hypertonic dextrose.

Question 6

The patient undergoes a PET to assess peritoneal membrane characteristics. Which of the following peritoneal membrane characteristics on PET may be associated with UFF?

(a) High transport status

(b) High–average transport status

(c) Low–average transport status

(d) Low transport status

Answer

All are correct

Explanation

PET is a standardised test used to assess peritoneal membrane transport characteristics and involves a 4-hour exchange with a 2 L 2.5% dextrose PD fluid. On the basis of ultrafiltration volume, the effluent dialysate glucose level and most importantly the effluent dialysate/plasma (D/P) creatinine ratio, patients can be subdivided into the four groups shown in Table 25.1.

Table 25.1 Classification of peritoneal membrane transport characteristics based on PET

Transport classification	D/P creatinine	Dialysate Glucose (mg/dL)	Drainage Volume (mL)	Net ultrafiltration (mL)
High	0.82–1.03	230–501	1580–2084	–470–35
High–average	0.66–0.81	502–722	2085–2367	35–320
Low–average	0.50–0.64	724–944	2369–2650	320–600
Low	0.34–0.49	945–1214	2651–3326	600–1276

This test can be used not only for peritoneal membrane transport classification, but also as a guide to predict dialysis dose, choose a PD regimen, monitor peritoneal membrane function and diagnose causes of inadequate ultrafiltration or solute clearance. Based on the PET test, patients with a high transport status (due to increased peritoneal membrane permeability or vascularity) either have inherently high membrane transport characteristics or have acquired this after being on long-term PD or transiently (and reversibly) following an episode of peritonitis. The influence of glucose load on alterations in membrane transport characteristics has been supported by the observation that patients who develop an increase in D/P creatinine over time have had greater cumulative glucose exposure than time-matched controls.

UFF can occur in patients with even low or average peritoneal membrane transport characteristics (vide infra), but is more commonly seen in patients with high transport status. Patients with a high solute transport status are associated with higher mortality rates as well as higher rates of technique failure, as compared to those with a low transport status. High transporters are best managed either by using poorly absorbed osmotic agents (i.e. icodextrin) for the long night dwells, or by avoiding long dwells with dextrose-containing PD fluids (by keeping the nights 'dry' or performing automated night exchanges).

The dwell times can also be shortened by switching patients to automated PD at night with either a 'dry' day or using short daytime dwells. Rarely, resting the membrane for a few weeks by switching to haemodialysis or using adjunctive haemodialysis for fluid removal can be tried.

Clinical pearls

- PET is a standardised test to assess peritoneal membrane characteristics.
- UFF can be associated with high, low or average peritoneal membrane transport characteristics, but is more commonly seen in high transporters.
- Patients with high transport status have higher mortality rates and rates of technique failure as compared to those with low transport status.
- Patients classified as high/high–average transporters are best treated with use of PD fluids with poorly absorbable osmotic agents (i.e. icodextrin) in long dwells or by shortening the dwell time.

LEVEL C

Question 7

The PET shows that the patient has a low average peritoneal transport status. What is/are the possible cause/s for UFF in this situation?

(a) PD catheter malfunction
(b) Dialysate leak
(c) Enhanced lymphatic absorption
(d) Sclerosing encapsulating peritonitis

Answer
All are correct

Explanation

Some patients with UFF may have reduced solute transport and low drain volumes on the PET. Although peritoneal catheter malfunction or extraperitoneal dialysate leakage can be seen in patients with any type of peritoneal membrane solute transport, these conditions should be specifically excluded as it is unusual to develop UFF in patients with low transport status. In addition, enhanced lymphatic absorption as a cause of UFF can occur in association with any peritoneal membrane transport status. Lymphatic absorption of peritoneal fluid not only negatively influences net ultrafiltration, but also reduces net solute removal by partially negating the effect of diffusive and convective solute transport, without altering the concentration of solutes in the dialysate or the D/P ratios despite significant reductions in ultrafiltration volumes.

Although not part of routine clinical practice, some PD centres perform the peritoneal lymphatic flow test, a manoeuvre that involves the instillation of macromolecules into the peritoneal cavity. This is followed by measurement of the subsequent rate of their disappearance from the peritoneal cavity to assess lymphatic absorption. Normal rates of peritoneal lymphatic absorption have been estimated to be 1 mL/min in upright position and 1.5 mL/min in supine position. Measurement of lymphatic flow is uncommon in clinical practice because of the complexity of the procedure and UFF from increased lymphatic absorption generally becomes a diagnosis of exclusion.

Since transcapillary ultrafiltration is normal in patients with increased lymphatic absorption, osmotically mediated water transport into the intraperitoneal cavity results in a dilution of sodium concentration of the dialysate. This is because the sieving coefficient of sodium is 0.5; that is, the sodium concentration in ultrafiltrate is 50% that of serum, leading to a relative increase in intraperitoneal-free water that dilutes the initial dialysate sodium concentration. A decrease in dialysate sodium (sodium sieving) of >5 mmol/L is normally observed within 1 hour of a 2-L 4.25% dextrose dialysate dwell and has been used as indirect evidence of normal transcapillary ultrafiltration. In patients with reduced net ultrafiltration secondary to increased lymphatic absorption, the normal decline in sodium concentration is maintained. This is markedly diminished in patients with rapid decline in osmotic gradient, such as seen in patients with high solute transport status.

Although patients with increased lymphatic absorption have been documented to have reduced dialysate content of phosphatidylcholine, and intraperitoneal administration of this compound was documented to increase ultrafiltration, this approach is clinically impractical. Oral supplementation of this compound was not effective in improving ultrafiltration, although oral administration of lecithin, which contains phosphatidylcholine in addition to other lipids, was shown to improve ultrafiltration. Oral administration of bethanechol chloride (which has similar cholinergic properties to phosphatidylcholine) before each exchange was also shown to increase ultrafiltration by 18%. The cholinergic agent works by contracting the subdiaphragmatic lymphatic stoma, reducing lymphatic flows.

Other therapeutic measures that can be tried include use of high doses of diuretics in patients with preserved residual renal functions, exposing the peritoneal membrane to hypertonic dextrose exchanges with their potential long-term deleterious effects or trying small-volume exchanges (to reduce intraabdominal pressure) using automated peritoneal dialysis (APD).

Clinical pearls

- UFF due to enhanced lymphatic absorption can occur in patients with any peritoneal membrane status.
- As transcapillary ultrafiltration is normal, sodium sieving is maintained in patients with UFF from enhanced lymphatic absorption.
- Small volume dwells using APD can also be tried in patients with UFF due to enhanced peritoneal lymphatic absorption.
- Cholinergic compounds have been shown to increase ultrafiltration by contracting the subdiaphragmatic lymphatic stoma, thereby reducing lymphatic absorption.

Question 8

This patient's lymphatic absorption studies showed normal lymphatic absorption rates. The change in D/P Na$^+$ after a 1-hour exchange with 2-L 4.25% dextrose PD solution is 3.4 mmol/L. Which of the following statements is/are true with respect to the cause of UFF?

(a) The cause of UFF is still not apparent from the results of the above investigations.

(b) The patient has abnormal transcapillary ultrafiltration.

(c) Patients with this condition are likely to present early after starting PD.

(d) Advanced glycosylation end-products have been implicated in the pathogenesis of UFF associated with this condition.

Answer

B and D

Explanation

A group of patients with UFF with no associated increase in solute transport (for creatinine or glucose) or lymphatic absorption rate have been identified; their UFF can be explained by loss of transcapillary ultrafiltration as evidenced by loss of sodium sieving. Patients with this condition usually present late after starting PD. In a recent study evaluating the causes of UFF (Smith et al. 2005) in patients with early (less than 2 years on PD) and late (more than 4 years on PD) onset UFF, patients with loss of transcapillary ultrafiltration were more likely to present late after starting PD (see Table 25.2). High transporters were equally distributed in both the groups. However, patients in the early onset UFF group were more likely to have enhanced effective lymphatic absorption rates. Patients with mechanical causes such as catheter malposition and leaks were excluded from this analysis.

Table 25.2 Causes of UFF based on time of presentation

	Early UFF (*n* = 25)	Late UFF (*n* = 23)
High transporters	44	61
High effective lymphatic absorption rate	68	30*
Low ▲D/P Na$^+$	8	43*

Note: * p<0.01. Values refer to % of patients.
Source: Smith et al. 2005

According to the three-pore model of solute transport, the capillary wall consists of a system of three types of pores that are size-selective in restricting solute transport. The abundant small pores (radius 40 to 50 Å) mediate transport of low molecular weight solutes and the numbers of these pores limit transport of these solutes. The large pores (radius 200 to 300 Å) constitute less than 0.1% of the total number of pores, whereas the ultra small pores (radius 4 to 5 Å) or aquaporin-1 are the channels that are permeable only to water (thereby explaining the sodium sieving). The latter are distinct to the aquaporin-2 channels in the collecting tubules, as they are not sensitive to the actions of antidiuretic hormone. These channels are responsible for transcellular water transport induced by the osmotic gradient created by the hypertonic dialysate in the peritoneal cavity. On average they account for approximately 40% of total ultrafiltration, with the remainder occurring via the paracellular route. The aetiology of this selective defect in transcapillary ultrafiltration is largely unknown and is best explained to result from changes to aquaporin-1 permeability associated with formation of advanced glycosylation end-products (from prolonged use of dextrose containing PD fluids) within the peritoneal membrane vasculature.

In the early stages, either icodextrin or other glucose-free PD solutions can be used to manage these patients. However, once this condition develops, the likelihood of continuing PD is poor and most patients will require adjunctive haemodialysis or conversion permanently to haemodialysis for volume control. Some patients may have a temporary and partial recovery of peritoneal function after resting the peritoneal membrane with a short (6- to 12-week) interval of haemodialysis. The types of UFF based on pathophysiology are shown in Table 25.3.

 Clinical pearls

- Patients with loss of transcapillary ultrafiltration have loss of sodium sieving.
- UFF from this cause usually occurs after many years of PD.
- Aetiology is likely to be related to changes in aquaporin-1 permeability associated with formation of advanced glycosylation end-products (from prolonged use of dextrose containing PD fluids).
- Adjunctive haemodialysis or permanent transfer to haemodialysis is generally required for volume control.

Table 25.3 Types of ultrafiltration failure

Cause of UFF*	Pathophysiology	Comments
Associated with high transport status	Rapid loss of osmotic gradient due to absorption of dextrose from PD fluid	Most common cause of UFF. Patients best treated with use of PD fluids with poorly absorbable osmotic agents (i.e. icodextrin) in long dwells or by shortening the dwell time (by using a cycler). Excessive utilisation of hypertonic (2.5 or 4.25% dextrose) PD fluids is another option, but can lead to several metabolic complications and peritoneal membrane failure.
Associated with low transport status	Inadequate peritoneal surface area or sclerosis/fibrosis of peritoneal membrane (Sclerosing Encapsulating Peritonitis)	Suspect in patients with UFF and low peritoneal membrane transport status, after excluding mechanical causes* of UFF. Adjunctive haemodialysis or permanent transfer to haemodialysis is usually required, as PD is generally ineffective.
Enhanced lymphatic absorption	Enhanced reabsorption of ultrafiltrate from the peritoneal cavity by lymphatics	Patients usually present early after starting PD and can occur in association with any type of peritoneal membrane transport status. Sodium sieving† is normal, indicating normal transcapillary UF. Lymphatic reabsorption can be reduced by decreasing intra-peritoneal hydrostatic pressure (by reducing dwell volumes) and by using cholinergic agents that stimulate contraction of subdiaphragmatic lymphatic stoma.
Deficient aquaporin function	Loss of transcapillary ultrafiltration due to changes in aquaporin permeability from prolonged use of dextrose-containing PD fluids	Patients usually present late after starting PD and can occur in association with any type of peritoneal membrane transport status. Sodium sieving† is lost, indicating reduced transcapillary ultrafiltration. Although partial recovery may occur with temporary discontinuation of PD, most patients would require either adjunctive or permanent haemodialysis.

Note: *After excluding mechanical causes of UFF, such as hernias, leaks and catheter malposition/kink. † Sodium concentration in dialysates normally falls by more than 5 mmol/L within 1 hour of a 2 litre 4.25% dextrose dwell (sodium sieving) due to osmotically mediated ultrafiltration, since the sodium concentration in ultrafiltrate is 50% that of serum. Loss of sodium sieving denotes reduced transcapillary ultrafiltration.

Question 9

Which of the following statements is/are true regarding sclerosing encapsulating peritonitis (SEP)?

(a) It is associated with high transport status on the PET.
(b) Prolonged exposure to PD is a risk factor for its development.
(c) The majority of patients with SEP are symptomatic.
(d) Total parenteral nutrition is the mainstay of treatment.

Answer

B

Explanation

SEP is fortunately a rare cause of reduced solute transport and drain volumes due to decrease in the peritoneal ultrafiltration coefficient. SEP is characterised by extensive intraperitoneal fibrosis and encasement of bowel loops and should not be confused with the generally benign and subclinical peritoneal fibrosis that occurs in most patients on CAPD. The peritoneal fibrosis of SEP may be induced by episodes of peritonitis (particularly if these are severe) or may simply be a consequence of a prolonged duration of CAPD. A study in Japanese patients on PD reported an incidence of 0, 0.7, 2.1, 5.9, 5.8 and 17.2% for those who had undergone PD for 3, 5, 8, 10, 15 and greater than 15 years, respectively. Other factors implicated in its pathogenesis include use of acetate as a dialysate buffer, beta-blockers and possible reaction to plasticisers from catheters. Although frequently asymptomatic, patients may present with a multitude of abdominal symptoms including abdominal pain, constipation, diarrhoea or with symptoms related to progressive loss of UF. An abdominal computerised tomography (CT) scan shows thickening of the peritoneal membrane with or without calcification, loculated ascites, adherent bowel loops or bowel luminal narrowing. PD is generally ineffective and adjunctive haemodialysis or permanent transfer to haemodialysis is the only option available. For patients with abdominal symptoms related to SEP, steroids with or without enterolysis (surgical division/removal of intestinal adhesions) or total parenteral nutrition (TPN) have been tried. A Japanese group reported a 39% success rate with use of steroids and 58% success with total enterolysis in relief of obstructive symptoms. None of the patients treated with bowel rest and TPN, without steroids or surgery, recovered.

 Clinical pearls

- The incidence of sclerosing encapsulating peritonitis (SEP) increases with duration on PD and with repeated episodes of peritonitis.
- In the absence of active infective peritonitis, SEP is associated with low peritoneal membrane transport characteristics.

- Clinical features range from patients being asymptomatic to non-specific abdominal symptoms and frank bowel obstruction.
- Adjunctive haemodialysis or permanent transfer to haemodialysis is required, as PD is generally ineffective.
- Total enterolysis and steroids offer better therapeutic options as compared to conservative measures including total parenteral nutrition.

Bibliography

Level A

1. Harris, D., Elder, G., Kairaitis, L. & Rangan, G. (eds) (2005) *Basic Clinical Dialysis.* Sydney: McGraw-Hill. 165–230.

Level B

2. Boudville, N. & Blake, P.G. (2007) Volume status and fluid overload in peritoneal dialysis. *Handbook of Dialysis*, 4th edn, Daugirdas, J.T., Blake, P.G. & Ing, T.S. (eds). Philadelphia: Wolters Kluwer Lippincott Williams & Wilkins. 410–16.
3. Korbet, S.M. & Rodby, R.A. (2004) Causes, diagnosis, and treatment of peritoneal membrane failure. *Principles and Practice of Dialysis*, 3rd edn, Henrich, W.L. (ed.). Philadelphia: Lippincott Williams and Wilkins, Philadelphia. 206–26.

Level C

4. Heimburger, O., Waniewski, J., Werynski, A., Tranaeus, A. & Lindholm, B. (1990) Peritoneal transport in CAPD patients with permanent loss of ultrafiltration capacity. Kidney Int. Sep., 38(3), 495–506.
5. Kawanishi, H., Kawaguchi, Y., Fukui, H., Hara, S., Imada, A., Kubo, H., Kin, M., Nakamoto, M., Ohira, S. & Shoji, T. (2004) Encapsulating peritoneal sclerosis in Japan: a prospective, controlled, multicenter study. Am J Kidney Dis. 44, 729.
6. Baranowska-Daca, E., Torneli, J., Popovich, R.P. & Moncrief, J.W. (1995) Use of bethnechol chloride to increase available ultrafiltration in CAPD. Adv Perit Dial. 11, 69–72.
7. Smith, W., Parikova, A., Struijk, D.G. & Krediet, R.T. (2005) The difference in causes of early and late ultrafiltration failure in peritoneal dialysis. Perit Dial Int. Feb., 25(Supp 3), S41–5.

Part E
Transplantation

Case 26
Live kidney donation

NIKKY ISBEL

LEVEL A

Case history

A 40-year-old male, Jim, is approaching end-stage kidney disease (ESKD) secondary to IgA nephropathy (serum creatinine 463 µmol/L, estimated glomerular filtration rate, eGFR, 20 mL/min/1.73 m²). He is in good health, with controlled hypertension and no other medical problems. He is married with two young children and works as a geologist for a large mining company. His work often necessitates long periods in remote locations and he is concerned that he will not be able to continue when he starts dialysis. Until 2 years ago, his work commitments had made it difficult to keep his medical appointments but the severity of his medical problem has now become apparent to him and his compliance is good. His 38-year-old brother (blood group A), 44-year-old wife (blood group O) and 62-year-old father (blood group O) have all offered to 'give him a kidney'. All the potential donors have normal renal function on routine biochemistry. Jim is blood group O and has a panel reactive antibody screen (anti-HLA antibodies) of 15%.

Question 1

In relation to live donor (LD) transplantation, which of the following statements is/are true?
(a) Transplants from live donors provide better recipient outcomes.
(b) Live kidney donation is increasing as a source of donor organs.
(c) Transplantation should only occur after Jim starts dialysis.
(d) It is unlikely that Jim will be able to return to work after the transplant.

Answer
A and B

Explanation

Live donor kidney transplantation has been performed for more than 50 years and is an extremely successful form of renal replacement therapy. Patients who receive LD transplants, when compared to deceased donor (DD) recipients, enjoy better patient (96 versus 85% 5-year survival) and graft (86 versus 73% 5-year survival) outcomes. There are many reasons for this: avoidance of the renal injury associated with brain death, shorter cold ischaemia times and more thorough assessment of quality of the donor kidney.

In current times, live donors are particularly important due to the disparity between the increasing number of dialysis patients (7952 Australian patients on dialysis in 2004) and the relatively static number of deceased donor kidneys available for transplant (406 DD transplants performed in 2004). This has resulted in much longer waiting times for deceased donor kidneys; greater than 5 years in many cases. In response to the shortage of deceased donor organs, there has been a steady increase in live donor operations performed over the last decade, now accounting for 37% of all renal transplants performed in Australia.

There are many other benefits for the recipient in live donor transplantation. The transplant can occur as a planned procedure before the patient starts on dialysis (pre-emptive). The difficulties related to creating dialysis access and the restrictions to lifestyle and diet and the progression of co-morbidities such as cardiovascular disease associated with dialysis, can be avoided. Patients who receive pre-emptive live donor transplants are more likely to return to work. There is also good evidence that pre-emptive transplantation is associated with better patient and graft outcomes. In the past, a period of dialysis was thought to be useful as a way of increasing the recognition by the recipient of the value of a transplant and enhancing compliance. However, this approach is no longer justified and alternative approaches to motivate compliance are required. From a health economic perspective, transplantation is more cost effective than dialysis.

 Clinical pearls

- Live donor transplantation is an accepted practice and associated with excellent patient and graft survival.
- Pre-emptive live donor transplantation is the goal if feasible.

Question 2

In relation to selecting a potential donor, which of the following statements is/are true?

(a) His brother would not be a suitable donor.

(b) The presence of anti-HLA antibodies reduces the chances of finding a compatible donor.

(c) His wife would not be a suitable donor as she is not a 'blood relative'.

(d) His father is too old to be a donor.

Answer

A and B

Explanation

Transplantation of organs requires that the donor and recipient be compatible in terms of blood group and cross matching. The cross match determines if the recipient has any preformed antibodies to the donor tissue (human leucocyte antigens, HLA). Transplantation of organs follows the same compatibility rules as blood transfusion. ABO antigens are found on epithelial and endothelial cells as well as red blood cells and lymphocytes. Transplantation across ABO blood groups does occur, particularly in countries where deceased donor transplantation is limited. The protocol for achieving a successful outcome is more complex and is still an experimental procedure.

All patients being considered for a renal transplant have their serum tested for the presence of anti-HLA antibodies and are cross-matched against donor lymphocytes. Patients become 'sensitised' to HLA by pregnancy, blood transfusion or previous transplant. Highly sensitised patients have a higher likelihood of having a positive cross-match with the potential donor. The presence of anti-HLA antibodies is also associated with an increased risk of rejection and graft loss. Careful thought is required before transfusing patients with chronic kidney disease who might one day be transplant candidates. If transfusion is required, a white cell filter should be used and consideration of a short period of immunosuppression (cyclosporine) to reduce the chance of developing anti-HLA antibodies.

In the early days of transplantation, benefits accrued due to the better HLA matching associated with genetically related donors. Currently parents and siblings account for 57% of donors. There is also a steady increase in the number of adult children donating to their parents, as transplantation of the older patients with ESKD becomes a more accepted practice. The efficacy of modern immunosuppressive regimens has meant that HLA matching now provides a lesser benefit than previously (considered a bonus rather than a prerequisite). This has opened the way for genetically unrelated but emotionally related donors. The incidence of early rejection is slightly higher, but short- and long-term outcomes are similar to related live donor transplants. In 2004, 20% of donors (to adult recipients) were the spouse of the patient.

Older donor age per se does not preclude live kidney donation. However, as age increases, the likelihood of finding a co-morbid condition which excludes the donation also increases. Healthy older donors with normal kidney function can provide excellent quality kidneys and the results for the recipients are comparable to that of younger donors. Conversely, very young donors raise some ethical concerns. Legally donors must be greater than 18 years old. Long-term follow-up of young donors showed no increase in risk of kidney disease and although the data are limited, there appears to be no increased risk associated in pregnancy following nephrectomy. Careful consideration of all potential future risks to renal function needs to be undertaken.

Clinical pearls

- Blood transfusion should be considered very carefully in patients with chronic kidney disease who may require a future kidney transplant. White cell filters should be used and a short course of immunosuppression considered.
- Live kidney donors do not need to be genetically related to the recipient.
- The younger the donor, the greater the focus should be on assessing potential future risks to kidney function.

Question 3

In relation to benefits and risks associated with donor nephrectomy, which of the following statements is/are true?

(a) Live kidney donation may improve the donor's quality of life.

(b) The estimated risk of death from live donor nephrectomy is 3 per 10 000 procedures.

(c) Following nephrectomy the GFR of the donor will be reduced by 50% at 1 year.

(d) There is a small increase in proteinuria over time in live kidney donors.

Answer

A, B and D

Explanation

The majority of donors experience an increased feeling of wellbeing and an increase in self-esteem following donation. Donors who are closely involved in the patient's life may have an improvement in their own quality of life. For example, following donation to a child, in addition to the psychological benefit of seeing an improvement in the health of their child, the parent may no longer have to spend time doing the dialysis. Donation to a spouse may allow couples freedom to pursue other activities such as travel that are not possible when one partner is on dialysis. There are, however, a small number of donors who experience a negative outcome. These donors tend to be more remotely related to the recipient, have donated to a patient who dies or has a poor outcome, or have themselves experienced significant perioperative pain.

The risks to donors can be divided into short term (associated predominantly with the perioperative risk) and long term (associated with the risk of developing future kidney disease). The estimate of perioperative mortality is taken from large cohorts of patients from Iran and the United States and has been stable at between approximately 0.02 and 0.03%. Deaths are related to pulmonary emboli, anaesthetic accidents and coronary events. Potential donors are evaluated to assess cardiac risk (e.g. a cardiac stress procedure may be performed in at-risk groups such as those aged over 40 years or smokers). Minimisation of pulmonary embolus risk with deep venous thrombosis prophylaxis is standard practice. Smoking increases the risk of thromboembolism and postoperative chest and wound infections, and should be strongly discouraged.

The long-term follow-up (up to 45 years) of patients who have a nephrectomy due to trauma or as kidney donors has shown excellent long-term renal outcomes. Patients who have normal kidney function at the time of nephrectomy have no increase in the prevalence of renal dysfunction compared to normal controls, but there is a small increase in mild proteinuria and in systolic blood pressure (BP) (2.4 mmHg, then 1.1 mmHg per decade). A meta-analysis (Kasiske et al. 1995) of 48 studies and 3124 patients demonstrated that a unilateral nephrectomy was associated with a decline in GFR by 17.1 mL/min following donation and GFR remained stable or improved with subsequent follow-up. Analysis of living donors from Sweden showed a significantly lower mortality rate than the general population; this is reassuring although not surprising given the selection bias towards the healthiest of the population being used as donors.

There are, however, patients who have been previous donors who have themselves developed ESKD. This is rare, but must be discussed with the potential donor. The causes for ESKD include development of glomerulonephritis, diabetic nephropathy, trauma or cancer in the remaining kidney. It is recommended that donors should maintain a healthy lifestyle, normal weight, not smoke and have regular follow-ups of kidney function and BP.

Clinical pearls

- Donation may result in an improvement in quality of life for the donor.
- For patients who start with two normal kidneys, the long-term renal outcomes are excellent.
- Lifelong follow-up of donors is advised.
- A thorough knowledge by the donor, of the risks and benefits of donor nephrectomy, is a crucial part of the informed consent process.

LEVEL B

Case history continued ...

Following preliminary discussion, Jim's father comes forward as the potential donor. He is a 62-year-old Vietnam veteran and a recently retired dairy farmer. He describes his health as 'excellent' and sees his general practitioner infrequently. He has had no history or symptoms of kidney or cardiac disease. He has had hypertension for 5 years that has been well controlled. His exercise tolerance is good and he walks 5 km regularly. He has had a hernia repair and removal of several basal cell and squamous cell carcinomas. He is under regular dermatology review. There is no family history of diabetes, but his two brothers have had coronary bypass grafting in their 60s. He stopped smoking 5 years ago and is on atenolol 50 mg daily. He has previously been treated for post-traumatic stress disorder, but reports that his mood has been stable for the last 15 years. On examination, his BP is 130/80 mmHg, body mass index (BMI) is 23.5 kg/m^2 and apart from extensively sun-damaged skin, his examination is normal. He has no proteinuria (75 mg/day) and urine microscopy is unremarkable. His serum creatinine is 78 μmol/L and EDTA-GFR is 97 mL/min. He is negative for HIV, hepatitis B and C and serologically positive for cytomegalovirus (CMV) and Epstein-Barr virus (EBV). The cardiac stress test is normal at high workload. Ultrasound demonstrates two kidneys of 10 cm, one of which contains a small (3 mm) calculus in the lower pole of the left kidney. The computerised tomography (CT) angiogram demonstrates minor atheroma and single arteries and veins to both kidneys.

Question 4

In relation to live donor transplantation, which of the following statements is/are true?

(a) It is possible to transmit hepatitis B via organ transplantation.
(b) A history of basal and squamous cell carcinomas in the donor is a contraindication to donation.
(c) Treated hypertension may be acceptable in a donor.
(d) The finding of the renal calculus is a relative contraindication to donation.
(e) Past psychiatric history is a contraindication to transplant donation.
(f) Laparoscopic nephrectomy is associated with an earlier return to work for donors.

Answer

A, C, D and F

Explanation

The workup of the donor involves a detailed medical history, thorough clinical examination and specific investigations directed at determining the short- and long-term risks to the donor. Also assessed are risks that relate to transmission of disease (infective or malignant) from the donor to the recipient. An essential part of the donor workup is the education of the donor on the implications of donation in their particular circumstances. This includes information on the likelihood of a successful outcome for the recipient. It is important that there is opportunity for the prospective donor to ask for clarification of risk, to reflect on the issues involved and to be able to withdraw from the process if they are ambivalent or there is evidence of coercion. As part of this process, donors are assessed by a multidisciplinary team which includes physicians, surgeons, nurses, psychiatrists/psychologists and social workers. It is important that the donor is assessed by a physician who is not the treating doctor of the recipient. This avoids the problem of competing interests in complex cases.

Variability exists as to criteria considered to be absolute contraindications to live donor nephrectomy. Donor co-morbidities that increase operative risk (e.g. ischaemic heart disease, chronic liver disease) or associated with risk of future kidney disease (diabetes, severe hypertension, bilateral renal calculi) are considered to be absolute contraindications by most transplant units. Evidence of kidney disease in the donor includes significant proteinuria or impaired kidney function (defined as GFR <80 mL/min, but caution if GFR <90 mL/min in younger patients). There is considerable debate as to the best method of determining kidney function in donors. The formulas for eGFR are not reliable in patients with near-normal kidney function. Twenty-four hour creatinine clearance is useful within the limitations of the test (collection errors, over-estimation of GFR). Calculation of GFR by clearance of labelled isotopes (iothalamate, technetium etc.) is generally used as the 'gold standard'.

Prospective donors with persistent microscopic haematuria require a thorough urological assessment to exclude urological malignancy. If the haematuria is of glomerular origin, a kidney biopsy may be considered to exclude glomerular pathology. On occasion, structural renal abnormalities are found that may prevent donation of a kidney. Complex vascular anatomy may also be identified which may increase the potential complications as reconstruction of multiple renal arteries and veins is then required as part of the transplant procedure which increases the risk of graft thrombosis. Chronic active viral infection (hepatitis B, C or HIV) is a contraindication to transplantation as infection of the recipient may occur. A history of malignancy with a high metastatic potential (e.g. melanoma, lung, breast, lymphoma) in a donor is also unsuitable.

Hypertension is a relative contraindication to living kidney donation. Meta-analysis of follow-up studies of donors suggests that the prevalence of hypertension does not increase following nephrectomy but that a small rise in systolic BP (mean 2.4 mmHg) does occur. The clinical impact of a rise in BP of this magnitude on patients who are already hypertensive is unclear. One short-term, small study (Textor et al. 2004) showed that in the year following donation, the BP of hypertensive Caucasian donors improved due to better medical care. Post-nephrectomy kidney function was slightly lower in the hypertensive donors than in normotensive donors (61 versus 68 mL/min) and microalbuminuria was equivalent between groups. In a second study (Ghods 2002), with follow-up to 7 years, there was no difference in kidney function between normotensive and donors with controlled hypertension. Longer studies are required to determine if there is any progressive loss of function in donors with controlled hypertension. The risk for donors with a family history of hypertension is also unknown.

Twenty-four-hour ambulatory monitoring has been shown to be more specific than clinic BP in determining significant hypertension in potential donors and correlates more closely with end-organ damage. Currently, if the BP is well controlled on a single agent, there is no evidence of end-organ damage and the balance of risk versus benefit is reasonable, donors with mild hypertension may be cautiously considered.

The history of a kidney stone has previously been considered to be a contraindication to donation. Patients with a history of stones have a high rate of recurrent stone formation (probably greater than 30%) and there is a risk of the recurrent stones causing scarring or obstruction to a single kidney. The availability of minimally invasive techniques for stone management including flexible ureteroscopy and extracorporeal shock wave lithotripsy, has slightly liberalised this criterion and patients with a single, uncomplicated calculus may be considered as donors after appropriate counselling regarding additional potential risks and exclusion of metabolic abnormalities that place the patient at risk of recurrent stone formation.

Psychological assessment is a valuable part of the workup. The motivation of an individual to donate an organ is often complex and the decision often has psychological and social impacts on the donor and their wider family. Past psychiatric history is not a contraindication to donation; however, knowledge of previous events such as depression is often helpful in providing additional assistance post-donation for those at risk. Patients must be mentally competent to give informed consent and the presence of active psychosis is a contraindication.

Laparoscopic nephrectomy is now an established technique in most transplant units. The mortality risk of the procedure appears similar to that of open nephrectomy and has the advantage of smaller surgical incisions, reduced (but not absence of) pain, shorter hospital stays and earlier return to normal activities. Not all patients are suitable for the procedure on technical grounds and on occasion the laparoscopic procedure needs to be converted to an open incision.

Clinical pearls

- The overall purpose of the donor evaluation is to undertake a thorough medical, surgical and psychosocial evaluation of the donor to ensure that there are no predictable risks of short- or long-term harm to donor or recipient.
- Absolute contraindications to donor nephrectomy include evidence of donor renal disease, ischaemic heart disease, diabetes, severe hypertension, active infection, uncontrolled malignancy and psychosis.

Question 5

In relation to live donor transplantation, which of the following statements is/are true?
(a) It is unlikely that the original disease (IgA disease) will recur in the transplant kidney.
(b) EBV-naïve recipients have an increased risk of lymphoma following a transplant from an EBV-positive donor.

Answer
B

Explanation

Recurrent glomerulonephritis is an important cause of graft loss (irrespective of the source of the donor kidney). Recurrence of IgA disease in the graft is usually manifest in the second decade of the transplant with recurrence of haematuria, proteinuria and progressive loss of function. There are some reports that the risk of recurrence is higher in well-matched live donor kidneys. It is important for the donor and recipient to be aware of the risk of graft loss from the outset to avoid feelings of guilt, anger and so on in the future, but it does not preclude transplantation.

Some types of glomerulonephritis are associated with greater risks of recurrence and more-rapid graft dysfunction. Primary focal and segmental glomerulosclerosis (FSGS), particularly if the original disease was aggressive, associated with heavy proteinuria and a rapid progression to ESKD, has a high rate of recurrence. The recurrence can occur early (within minutes of anastomosis of the transplant vessels) and can cause rapid graft dysfunction. Haemolytic uraemic syndrome is another condition with a risk of recurrence and premature graft loss. Potential donors to recipients with a high risk of recurrent disease need to be very well informed as to the possible graft outcomes.

CMV and EBV can remain dormant in the kidney following the primary infection in the donor and are therefore transmitted to the recipient. The recipient who is naïve to these viruses is at risk of developing *de novo* infection following transplantation. The advent of effective antiviral prophylaxis and treatment has rendered primary CMV in the recipient a less severe disease. There is no proven therapy to reduce the risk of primary EBV infection and the clinical syndromes may vary from mononucleosis syndrome to a post-transplant lymphoproliferative disorder. In the absence of a live donor who is EBV-negative, the benefits of live donor transplantation generally outweigh the risk of EBV associated disease.

Clinical pearl

- Information regarding the likely success rate of the proposed transplant must be given to the donor prior to donation.

LEVEL C

Case history continued ...

Unfortunately the dermatology review reveals that Jim's father has a level 3 melanoma on his shoulder and is therefore not a suitable donor. Jim's wife, Jane, now presents for evaluation. She is 44 years old and is in good current health. She has had two pregnancies, the second of which was complicated by gestational diabetes. Following the birth of her second child her blood sugars have been normal. With the worry over Jim's illness she has put on weight in the past couple of years and is currently 78 kg and 163 cm tall (BMI 29.4). Her mother has type 2 diabetes diagnosed in her 60s and is well controlled on oral hypoglycaemic medication. Jane is of Aboriginal heritage and her paternal aunt is on dialysis.

Her BP is 125/85 mmHg and apart from anxiety and central obesity, her physical examination is normal. Her preliminary investigations demonstrate that she has two normal kidneys on ultrasound, her renal function is normal (EDTA-GFR 105 mL/min) and the absence of microalbuminuria. Jane is distraught over the impact that her husband's illness is having on the family unit and is very keen to donate.

Question 6

Regarding future risk to the donor, which of the following statements is/are true?

(a) If the oral glucose tolerance test is normal, Jane is at low risk of future diabetic kidney disease.

(b) Obesity is a risk factor for progression of renal impairment following nephrectomy.

(c) A family history of renal disease is a risk factor for future CKD.

(d) If Jane is fully informed of the risks of donation and demands to proceed, the transplant unit should accede to her wishes.

Answer

C (the answers to B and D are unknown)

Explanation

Diabetes is a contraindication to live kidney donation. This relates partly to the increase in perioperative morbidity and mortality, but predominantly to the unknown impact that nephrectomy may have on the development or progression of diabetic nephropathy. Animal models suggest that unilateral nephrectomy increases the rate of progression of diabetic nephropathy. Human data are very limited. Silveiro et al. (1998) investigated the impact of having a single kidney on urine albumin excretion and GFR in patients with type 2 diabetes. Patients, who mostly had a unilateral nephrectomy undertaken for medical reasons, were studied in a small retrospective study. The diabetic patients with a single kidney had a twofold increase in risk of microalbuminuria when compared to non-diabetic patients with a single kidney or diabetic patients with two kidneys. Microalbuminuria occurred earlier in the diabetic patients with a single kidney versus non-diabetic single kidney (23 versus 43.5 years post donation). Renal function was not different between groups.

Increasing numbers of patients at risk for diabetes are coming forward as potential kidney donors. Well-established risk factors for type 2 diabetes include obesity, family history of diabetes and indigenous background. Women with a history of gestational diabetes have a 30 to 50% risk of developing diabetes within 10 years. The safety of nephrectomy in this group of patients is unknown. In addition, it is unclear if lifestyle modification or the use of renoprotective agents, such as renin angiotensin blockers, will alter the risk of renal disease. Important factors to consider in assessing patients with the risk of future diabetes or impaired glucose tolerance include the closeness of the relationship with the recipient and the age of the donor. A 40-year-old female with impaired glucose tolerance has a projected life expectancy of 45 years and thus a greater lifetime risk of developing diabetic nephropathy when compared to a 65-year-old male.

Obesity is reaching epidemic proportions in the community and is strongly linked with the exponential rise in type 2 diabetes and cardiovascular disease. In addition, it is likely that obesity via the association with hypertension and also hyperfiltration injury promotes the progression of chronic kidney diseases. There are few published data regarding the impact of nephrectomy for renal donation in obese patients. Praga et al. (2000) retrospectively studied seventy-three patients undergoing unilateral nephrectomy for medical indication who had normal baseline kidney function, no proteinuria or diabetes. The probability of proteinuria or renal insufficiency was 92% in obese patients (BMI >30) versus 12% in non-obese patients at 10 years. The study is limited in that it was small, retrospective and the nephrectomy was not performed for purposes of donation, but it does raise concerns. Obese patients should be encouraged to lose weight prior to donation and advised not to donate if there are other co-morbid conditions.

The risk of kidney disease in first-degree relatives of patients with ESKD has repeatedly been shown to be increased above the background rate for the population studied. As this is the very group who is most likely to come forward as potential donors, it is important that they are evaluated very carefully in cases where there is a genetic component to the cause of ESKD in the recipient. This is relatively straightforward in patients with adult polycystic kidney disease (APKD). The specificity and sensitivity of ultrasound in determining the risk of APKD is 100% in donors greater than 30 years old. In the absence of specific genetic testing, donors less than 30 years old should be discouraged. Other types of kidney disease may cluster in families, but the genetics and best method to exclude disease may not be fully determined. For example, primary focal and segmental glomerulosclerosis may be a familial disease. There have been numerous reports of live donors who were completely asymptomatic at time of donation going on to develop FSGS. In a report of donors who have themselves been listed for transplantation, FSGS as a cause for ESKD is over-represented.

The degree of medical risk that a donor should be sanctioned to accept is controversial and widely debated. Risks are often ill-defined due to lack of adequate data and represent potential for future harm rather than the more obvious and immediate benefits derived from allowing the transplant to proceed. Opinions range widely and vary from paternalistic determination as to what constitutes 'acceptable' risk versus allowing complete patient autonomy to self-determine risk. Most transplant units balance the risk assumed by the donor against the direct benefits to the donor, such that the risk assumed by a partner donating to a spouse may be greater than that for an altruistic donor in whom any significant increase in medical risk would be unacceptable.

Clinical pearls

- Relative contraindications to donor nephrectomy include obesity, family history of kidney disease or diabetes, and controlled hypertension.
- Screening for and careful assessment of future risk of diabetes is a crucial part of donor workup. Diabetic nephropathy is the commonest cause for ESKD in past donors.
- Long-term registry follow-up is required to determine the outcomes of marginal donors (ANZDATA live donor registry commenced 2005).

Question 7

What is the best option for Jim?

(a) Proceed with his wife as a donor.

(b) Evaluate the brother for an ABO-incompatible transplant.

(c) Enter a paired donor kidney exchange program.

(d) Perform a xenotransplant from a genetically modified pig.

(e) Be placed on the deceased donor transplant list.

Answer

A, B or E

Explanation

This case illustrates the difficulty that arises when there is no one best option. Clearly the wife, who has much to gain from a successful transplant in her husband, has many risk factors that increase the possibility of future kidney disease (diabetes, obesity, indigenous background and family history), but no absolute contraindication at present. Following detailed discussion with Jim and his wife, Jim declined the offer of her kidney, not wishing to put her at increased risk.

Other options to be considered include waiting for a deceased donor transplant or consideration of ABO-incompatible transplantation. ABO-incompatible transplantation has been shown to have good short- and medium-term results when compared with ABO-compatible donors and has been practised extensively in Japan, the United States and Scandinavia. Recipients require peritransplant treatment (with plasma exchange, intravenous immunoglobulin and/or immunoadsorption columns) to remove the anti-blood-group antibody, a modest increase in immunosuppression compared with standard regimens and careful post transplant surveillance for antibody mediated rejection. It is anticipated that this procedure will become more widely available over the next few years.

Donor exchange programs are now being established in the United States and Europe as a further option for patients who are incompatible with their donor due to ABO group or a positive cross match. Donor/recipient pairs who are incompatible with each other but compatible with other mismatched pairs are entered into a matching system and sorted according to a computer-generated algorithm. There are legal issues in terms of traffic in organs to be considered, issues of patient privacy when simultaneous transplants are done in the one institution, ethical issues in terms of equity in the exchange and probably a critical size to allow a reasonable chance of success. This proposal is currently under review and not currently practised in Australia.

Bibliography

Level A

1. Delmonico F; Council of the Transplantation Society. (2005) A report of the Amsterdam forum on the care of the live kidney donor: data and medical guidelines. Transplantation. 79, S53–66.
2. Caring for Australasians with Renal Impairment, www.cari.org.au
3. Kasiske, B.L., Ma, J.Z., Louis, T.A. & Swan, S.K. (1995) Long-term effects of reduced renal mass in humans. Kidney Int. 48(3), 814–19.

Level B

4. Textor, S.C., Taler, S.J., Driscoll, N., Larson, T.S., Gloor, J., Griffin, M., Cosio, F., Schwab, T., Prieto, M., Nyberg, S., Ishitani, M. & Stegall, M. (2004) Blood pressure and renal function after kidney donation from hypertensive living donors. Transplantation. 78(2), 276–82.
5. Ghods, A. J. (2002) Renal transplantation in Iran. Nephrol Dial Transplant. 17(2), 222–8.
6. Praga, M., Hernández, E., Herrero, J.C., Morales, E., Revilla, Y., Díaz-González, R. & Rodicio, J.L. (2000) Influence of obesity on the appearance of proteinuria and renal insufficiency after unilateral nephrectomy. Kidney Int. 58(5), 2111–18.

Level C

7. Silveiro, S. P., da Costa, L.A., Beck, M.O. & Gross, J.L. (1998) Urinary albumin excretion rate and glomerular filtration rate in single-kidney type 2 diabetic patients. Diabetes Care. 21(9), 1521–4.

Case 27
Acute transplant dysfunction

NICK CROSS

LEVEL A

Case history

A 45-year-old male presents with one week of vomiting, diarrhoea and cramping abdominal pain. On the day of presentation, he developed a central chest ache with no radiation. There are no other symptoms.

The patient received a deceased donor kidney transplant 8 months ago after 5 years of haemodialysis following end-stage kidney failure secondary to glomerulonephritis. He has longstanding well-controlled hypertension. Gout and type 2 diabetes mellitus have developed since the transplant. His medications are:

- cyclosporine 125 mg twice daily
- prednisone 10 mg daily
- azathioprine 125 mg daily
- ibuprofen 400 mg three times daily
- metformin 1 g three times daily
- ramipril 10 mg daily
- diltiazem SR 180 mg twice daily
- atenolol 100 mg twice daily.

On examination, the patient appears unwell with a heart rate of 45 beats/min regular, blood pressure (BP) 100/44 mmHg, poor peripheral perfusion, but otherwise normal cardiovascular and respiratory examination. His temperature is 35.5°C. He is tender over the kidney transplant. There is no guarding.

Blood test results are available for the current presentation and the last clinic visit.

Laboratory data

	Clinic	Emergency department	Reference range
Na$^+$	143	120	(136–146 mmol/L)
K$^-$	5.6	6.5	(3.2–5.5 mmol/L)
HCO$_3^-$	22	16	(24–31 mmol/L)
Creatinine	160	685	(60–125 µmol/L)

Urea	15.8	39.5	(2.5–6.5 mmol/L)
Glucose	9.4	15.0	(4.0–7.0 mmol/L)
Total cholesterol	5.6	Not measured	(3.5–5.5 mmol/L)
Troponin T	Not measured	0.13	(0.01–0.1 ng/mL)
Haemoglobin	145	175	(135–175 g/L)
Total white cell count	6.5	8.6	(4.0–11.0 × 10⁹/L)
Cyclosporine trough	45	To follow	(100–150 mg/L)

An electrocardiogram (ECG) is recorded (see Fig. 27.1).

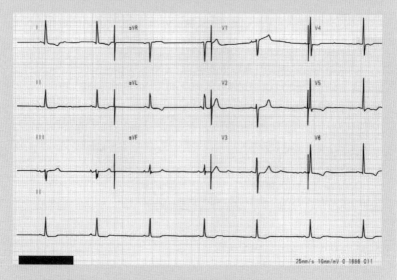

Figure 27.1 Patient's electrocardiograph

Question 1

Which of the following statements is/are true?

(a) The patient has severe dysfunction of his transplant and requires urgent dialysis.

(b) Myocardial infarction with cardiogenic shock is the most likely diagnosis.

(c) Acute transplant rejection is likely and he should be treated with intravenous steroids.

(d) Sepsis is unlikely because of normal temperature, white cell count and lack of tachycardia.

(e) Aggressive fluid resuscitation is indicated.

Answer
E

Explanation

The patient presents with shock. Following a kidney transplant, most patients take immunosuppressive medication for life and have chronic kidney disease. This combination may result in altered presentation of common clinical entities. Sepsis may present with normal temperature, normal neutrophil count and poorly localised symptoms (answer D incorrect). His beta-blocker may prevent tachycardia.

There is no ECG evidence of acute myocardial infarction and the history is atypical. Myocardial infarction causing cardiogenic shock is not the most likely scenario (answer B incorrect). Acute rejection is usually proven by kidney biopsy before commencing intravenous steroids. Steroid replacement is indicated because of steroid dependence rather than at high dose for treatment of rejection (answer C incorrect).

Fluid resuscitation and further investigations are indicated (answer E correct). While it may be required, dialysis could be safely delayed, at least until response to fluid resuscitation is observed (answer A incorrect).

Clinical pearls

- Sepsis in kidney transplant recipients is common and should be considered in all unwell patients.
- Sepsis may present without typical signs as a result of immunosuppression.
- Indications for acute dialysis in transplant dysfunction are the same as in acute renal failure: pulmonary oedema, hyperkalaemia or metabolic acidosis refractory to medical treatment, or uraemic pericarditis.

Question 2

With respect to the hyperkalaemia, which of the following statements is/are correct?
(a) Intravenous calcium gluconate is indicated to rapidly lower the serum potassium.
(b) An insulin infusion should be given to increase potassium excretion.
(c) Medications, including atenolol, cyclosporine and ramipril may contribute to hyperkalaemia.
(d) If the serum potassium were 7.0 or higher, dialysis should be commenced immediately.
(e) Because the ECG does not show signs of hyperkalaemia, no treatment is required.

Answer
C

Explanation

The ECG is reassuring (lack of peaked T waves, normal P waves, normal QRS duration) but the hyperkalaemia may progress to a life-threatening level if left untreated (answer E incorrect).

The ECG, not the potassium concentration per se, is the key to interpreting the significance of hyperkalaemia. Dialysis takes time to arrange acutely. There is a small associated risk of morbidity associated with the access procedure. If the acute renal impairment and hyperkalaemia can be corrected using other methods within a short time and the precipitant avoided/removed, dialysis may be avoided (answer D incorrect).

Many medications may cause hyperkalaemia including beta-blockers, angiotensin-converting enzyme inhibitors (ACEis), cyclosporine and ibuprofen (answer C correct).

The management of hyperkalaemia has three components. The first is calcium to reduce the risk of cardiac arrhythmias (it does not affect the serum potassium concentration, answer A incorrect). The second is measures that act rapidly to reduce extracellular potassium, but which do not remove it from the body. They include dilution by rehydration in the dehydrated patient and redistribution of potassium intracellularly. Glucose and insulin infusion cause intracellular movement of potassium not excretion (answer B incorrect); beta-agonists and treatment of acidaemia with bicarbonate also accomplish this. The third component is to enhance potassium excretion by improvement in kidney function, the use of potassium exchange resins enterically and dialysis.

 Clinical pearl

- Treatment of hyperkalaemia involves three approaches:
  — protect the heart with calcium gluconate or carbonate
  — reduce extracellular K^+ with hydration, insulin/dextrose, beta-agonists and HCO_3^-
  — enhance excretion by improving kidney function, resins and dialysis.

Question 3

Regarding the patient's medications, which one of the following statements is *most correct*?

(a) His diabetes is inadequately controlled and additional oral hypoglycaemic agents should be added.

(b) He has kidney disease and diabetes so ACEis should be continued while he is in hospital.

(c) Stopping diltiazem would mean that the patient will require an increased dose of cyclosporine.

(d) Ibuprofen is potentially contributing to his kidney impairment and should be replaced by a COX2 specific agent.

(e) His gout should be treated with the addition of allopurinol to his current regimen.

Answer

C

Explanation

The raised blood glucose could reflect a response to acute illness and is a single observation. Alterations to his regular diabetes medication should be deferred until he is well, although insulin will be required while he is ill (answer A incorrect). Metformin should be stopped while he is acutely unwell with possible sepsis and kidney failure, as there is an increased risk of metformin induced lactic acidosis.

ACEis slow the rate of decline in kidney function in proteinuric glomerular diseases. The BP-independent component is not firmly established in kidney transplant recipients. ACEis are effective and safe antihypertensive agents in transplant recipients, but should be withheld while the patient has acute kidney failure, hypotension and hyperkalaemia (answer B incorrect).

Diltiazem is an inhibitor of cytochrome P450 3A4 isoenzyme, which metabolises cyclosporine. Combining diltiazem and cyclosporine leads to increased half-life of cyclosporine, resulting in reduced dose requirement to maintain any given serum cyclosporine concentration. Stopping diltiazem will lead to a fall in cyclosporine concentration unless accompanied by an increase in dose (answer C correct).

While non-steroidal anti-inflammatory drugs (NSAIDs) inhibit prostaglandin-mediated pain and inflammation, they may also counteract prostaglandin-induced glomerular afferent arteriolar vasodilation. Thus, NSAIDs may precipitate acute kidney failure, especially in combination with other causes of reduced perfusion, such as ACEis, diuretics and hypotension. Ibuprofen should be stopped immediately. The newer COX2 selective anti-inflammatory drugs have similar effects and should be avoided also (answer D incorrect).

Allopurinol is a xanthine oxidase inhibitor, reducing production of uric acid and acute gout attacks. Active metabolites of azathioprine are inactivated by xanthine oxidase. Continuing normal doses of azathioprine with allopurinol may lead to life-threatening bone marrow suppression (see Case 31, Other complications of immune suppression; answer E incorrect).

 Clinical pearls

- Cytochrome P450 3A4 metabolises cyclosporin and tacrolimus; they have narrow therapeutic windows and changes in chronically co-administered 3A4 inhibitors (e.g. diltiazem) or inducers

(e.g. rifampicin) may lead to rejection or toxicity. Monitor concentrations and adjust.
- Avoid NSAIDs including COX2 selective agents in patients with kidney transplants and others at risk of renal failure.

LEVEL B

Case history continued …

A chest radiograph is normal except for mildly enlarged cardiac silhouette. Urine is sent for microscopy and culture:

WCC	100/µL
RCC	10/µL
Squamous Epithelial cells	++
Protein	+++
Casts	Hyaline + Granular +
Bacteria	+++
Culture	pending

One hundred mL of concentrated urine drains following insertion of a catheter.

Question 4

Which one of the following is *most correct* with respect to management *at this point*?

(a) The urine sample is contaminated and must be recollected before administration of antibiotics.

(b) A kidney biopsy should be performed to establish the cause of the kidney failure.

(c) Aminoglycosides in combination with beta-lactams are first-choice empiric treatment for sepsis as there is evidence of greater efficacy compared to beta-lactams alone.

(d) If ceftriaxone is used, dose reduction is not required in kidney failure.

(e) Fluid resuscitation should continue until urine output is greater than 30 mL/hour.

Answer

D

Explanation

Urinary tract infections are common in kidney transplant recipients (Trzeciak et al. 2004). While the presence of squamous epithelial cells increases the probability of a false-positive culture result and a repeat specimen is desirable, due to the severity of the illness, antibiotics are indicated following blood cultures. Treatment should not be delayed until production of further urine, which may be delayed depending on the degree of acute renal injury (answer A incorrect).

At this stage, the most likely causes of reduced transplant function are prerenal with probable progression to acute tubular necrosis. A biopsy would confirm this, but is not necessary for treatment, and may delay management (answer B incorrect).

A Cochrane systematic review of treatment of sepsis with broad spectrum beta-lactam antibiotics found no reduction in all cause mortality (RR 1.01, 95% CI 0.75 to 1.35) or microbiologic failure (RR 1.11, 95% CI 0.95 to 1.29) with addition of gentamicin. There was also no benefit in immunocompromised patients analysed separately. There was significantly less kidney failure with beta-lactams alone (RR 0.30, 95% CI 0.23 to 0.39) (Paul et al. 2006). Gentamicin should not be used empirically (answer C incorrect). Most beta-lactam antibiotics are excreted in the urine. Ceftriaxone is unusual in that it is only partially excreted unchanged by the kidneys, so dose reduction is not required in renal failure (answer D correct).

Fluid resuscitation is urgently required. Oliguria will not resolve immediately if acute tubular necrosis has supervened. If the patient is adequately resuscitated as assessed by other measures (e.g. BP, central venous pressure) and remains oliguric, then fluid loading may lead to pulmonary oedema (answer E incorrect).

Clinical pearls

- Adding gentamicin increases nephrotoxicity with no improvement in efficacy compared to beta-lactams alone and should be avoided in empiric treatment for community acquired sepsis.
- Recovery of urine output may not occur for days to weeks in established acute tubular necrosis. Do not rely on urine output alone to assess volume status.

Case history continued ...

The patient has a further episode of vomiting and chest discomfort. An ECG is unchanged.

Question 5

Regarding ischaemic heart disease, which of the following is *most correct*?

(a) The patient is young and has few risk factors, so ischaemic heart disease is a very unlikely cause of his chest pain.

(b) Kidney dysfunction may cause elevated troponin T and this test is not useful in this setting.

(c) The patient's risk of ischaemic heart disease death has been reduced by having a kidney transplant compared to remaining on dialysis.

(d) A coronary angiogram should be performed as soon as possible to exclude important coronary artery disease.

(e) Statin treatment has been shown in randomised controlled trials to reduce the risk of death in kidney transplant recipients with hypercholesterolaemia.

Answer

C

Explanation

The incidence of myocardial infarction (MI) at three years post-transplant was 11% in one study. This was lower than the incidence of MI in patients waiting for a transplant (16.7%), but six- to tenfold higher than in the general population (answer A incorrect, answer C correct) (Lentine, Brennan & Schnitzler 2005).

There is no evidence for overall mortality reduction with statins in transplant patients. In the only large-scale randomised trial, the ALERT study (Assessment of LEscol in Renal Transplantation), cardiac events and cardiac mortality were reduced, but all cause mortality was similar in treatment and control arms (RR 1.02, 95% CI 0.81 to 1.30) (Holdass et al. 2003) (answer E incorrect).

Cardiac troponins may be increased in kidney dysfunction in the absence of an acute myocardial ischaemic event, reducing the test specificity (patients without acute ischaemia may have mildly elevated troponin T). Repeat testing is still useful at ruling in an acute myocardial event if the concentration rises (answer B incorrect). An emergent coronary angiogram is not indicated, as there is no convincing evidence of acute myocardial infarction (answer D incorrect).

 Clinical pearls

- Myocardial infarction risk is reduced in patients who receive a kidney transplant compared to patients who remain on dialysis, but is higher than the general population.
- The use of statins to treat hypercholesterolaemia in kidney transplant recipients has not been shown to reduce total mortality, though they do reduce the incidence of acute coronary events and cardiac mortality.

LEVEL C

Case history continued …

Blood and urine cultures grow *E. coli* sensitive to ceftriaxone. Ceftriaxone is continued, but ampicillin and metronidazole, which were started empirically, are stopped. Troponin T levels at 6 and 12 hours are unchanged. His cardiovascular status improves and urine output increases to 300 mL/hour.

On the fifth day his serum creatinine, which had been falling, rises. His cardiovascular status is now normal, and he looks much improved, but his diarrhoea persists. An urgent transplant ultrasound is normal. His temperature is 37.8°C. Cyclosporine concentration from day 1 is 110 ng/mL. A full blood count reveals total white count 3.0×10^9/L, with lymphocytes 0.3.

	Clinic	Admission	Day 2	Day 4	Day 5
Creatinine (60–125 µmol/L)	160	685	550	280	350

Blood and urine cultures are repeated, stool cultures are collected and additional tests considered.

Question 6

Which of the following is *most correct*?

(a) N-acetylcysteine should be given prior to computerised tomography (CT) of the abdomen as it reduces the risk of dialysis because of contrast nephropathy in patients with chronic kidney disease.

(b) There is an increased likelihood of rejection following pyelonephritis and a kidney biopsy should be considered.

(c) The four-variable modification of diet in renal disease (MDRD) equation should be used to calculate his glomerular filtration rate (GFR) to adjust renally excreted drugs.

(d) Cytomegalovirus (CMV) polymerase chain reaction (PCR) on blood is a highly specific test for CMV colitis and should be undertaken in this patient.

(e) The current deterioration in renal function is likely to be due to partially treated urosepsis and antibiotic therapy should be broadened.

Answer

B

Explanation

The patient appears to have partially responded to treatment for sepsis. Ultrasound excludes transplant associated collection, so imaging of other internal abdominal structures with CT is indicated. While his shock is controlled and there is no new information from repeated blood cultures there is no indication to change therapy (answer E incorrect).

Cytomegalovirus disease should be considered. This disease peaks at 6 to 12 months post-transplant, and may cause gastrointestinal symptoms, low-grade fever, reduced lymphocyte count and graft dysfunction. PCR for CMV DNA on blood is a highly sensitive test. Unfortunately it is not specific for CMV-mediated disease; CMV DNA may be present in the blood without CMV colitis being the cause of his symptoms (answer D incorrect).

Contrast nephropathy is more common in patients with pre-existing renal impairment, heart failure, diabetes or volume depletion. It is more likely to occur in patients taking diuretics or ACEis, or with high administered contrast volume. Prehydration is effective to reduce the risk of contrast nephropathy.

N-acetylcysteine (NAC) has been the subject of more than fifteen published randomised controlled trials since 2000. There is considerable variability in the reported benefit of adding NAC to saline prehydration. NAC is often recommended by nephrologists in the absence of conclusive evidence as it has few side effects. Dialysis requirement is rare in trials and no trial has been able to show a benefit at reducing this outcome. Endpoints in trials are surrogates, such as serum creatinine concentration 48 hours post-contrast (answer A incorrect).

A transplant biopsy should now be considered, as there is unexplained transplant dysfunction. There is an association between pyelonephritis and acute rejection (Kamath et al. 2006) (answer B correct). Glomerular filtrate estimating equations are not accurate in the presence of changing renal function, and will overestimate GFR when there is acute renal failure with rising creatinine (answer C incorrect).

 ### Clinical pearls

- Estimated GFR equations should not be used where renal function is not stable.
- Rejection is more likely to occur after infections in renal transplant recipients due to production of pro-inflammatory cytokines.

Case history continued ...

A biopsy is performed revealing acute cellular rejection, Banff grade 1A. There is no evidence of vascular rejection.

A CT of the abdomen shows diffuse colonic thickening with no evidence of focal collections. The *Clostridium difficile* stool toxin test is negative. PCR on blood reveals 3.6 log copies of CMV per mL of blood.

Question 7

Which one of the following statements is *most correct* regarding management at this stage?
- **(a)** Treatment for rejection with intravenous steroids should be deferred until the fever has settled.
- **(b)** Azathioprine should be stopped and mycophenolate mofetil commenced.
- **(c)** Colonoscopy with biopsy is not required as CMV disease is very likely and treatment should commence.
- **(d)** Intravenous ganciclovir is the treatment of choice for invasive CMV disease.
- **(e)** Valganciclovir is preferable to oral ganciclovir for prophylaxis as it has greater efficacy at preventing CMV disease.

Answer
D

Explanation

The CT appearance is consistent with CMV colitis. CMV viral load, although supportive, could occur in viral replication without invasive disease. A colonoscopy with biopsy would aid management, as intravenous ganciclovir is the treatment of choice (answer D correct), but may cause lymphopenia. Treating without confirmation makes it difficult to continue if the white count falls further with initiation of ganciclovir (answer C incorrect). Valganciclovir may be considered for less severe infections and has better bioavailability than oral ganciclovir. It has also not been associated with ganciclovir resistance which may occur with oral ganciclovir. It is easier to use for prophylaxis, with patients requiring one or two capsules per day compared with six or more. Despite this, there is no clear evidence that it is superior at preventing disease (Hodson et al. 2005) (answer E incorrect).

The patient has cell-mediated rejection in the setting of recent sepsis and active CMV replication. There is no septic focus on the CT and deferring increased immunosuppression would lead to increased risk of graft loss. As long as antibiotics are continued and further cultures are taken with any fever spikes, steroid treatment should commence, along with CMV treatment or prophylaxis depending on the result of the colonoscopy (answer A incorrect).

Increased baseline immunosuppression should be considered. Substituting mycophenolate mofetil for azathioprine would be an option, but in the setting of diarrhoeal illness and lymphopenia this will be poorly tolerated. This change should be deferred until the symptoms settle (answer B incorrect). A further option to consider would be changing from cyclosporine to tacrolimus.

Clinical pearls

- Treating rejection soon after sepsis is possible but it is important to ensure that the infection is controlled and to continue effective antibiotics.
- When rejection occurs in the presence of good compliance consider increasing baseline immunosuppression but weigh side-effects and risks.
- Intravenous ganciclovir is the treatment of choice for invasive CMV disease.

Question 8

Regarding CMV disease in kidney transplant recipients, which *one* of the following statements is *most correct*?

(a) Prophylaxis reduces the incidence of disease in CMV antibody negative recipients, but not CMV antibody positive recipients.

(b) Patients who have CMV disease are at increased risk of rejection, but patients with rejection are not at increased risk of CMV disease.

(c) Induction with interleukin-2 receptor antagonists is not associated with increased risk of CMV disease.

(d) While the incidence of CMV disease is decreased with antiviral prophylaxis, no effect on mortality has been observed.

(e) CMV resistance to ganciclovir has not been described.

Answer

C

Explanation

Patients with acute rejection are at increased risk of subsequent CMV disease and vice versa (answer B incorrect). Rejection associated inflammatory mediators such as tumour necrosis factor stimulate intracellular viral reactivation and replication. Treatment of rejection episodes with increased immunosuppression also increases viral reactivation and replication. CMV disease may necessitate reduced immunosuppression increasing the likelihood of rejection. Inflammatory mediators associated with CMV disease also increase endothelial display of MHC class II, which may increase the risk of rejection (Fishman & Rubin 1998).

A Cochrane systematic review showed that there is no increase in risk of CMV disease at 1 year in patients receiving IL-2 receptor antagonists in addition to usual immunosuppression (Webster et al. 2004) (answer C correct).

Prophylaxis with antiviral drugs is effective at preventing invasive CMV disease in solid organ recipients irrespective of recipient antibody status at the time of transplantation (answer A incorrect). Prophylaxis reduces all cause mortality

(RR 0.63, 95% CI 0.43 to 0.92) due to reduction in CMV-related mortality (answer D incorrect) (Hodson et al. 2005).

Unfortunately, CMV resistance to ganciclovir has been described. Treatment is with alternative agents including foscarnet (Fishman & Rubin 1998) (answer E incorrect).

Clinical pearls

- CMV disease prophylaxis is universally beneficial to transplant recipients, with less CMV disease and reduced mortality in patients receiving antiviral therapy.
- CMV disease incidence is increased following bacterial infections or rejection.
- CMV disease increases the incidence of rejection and other infections.

Bibliography

Level B

1. Trzeciak, S., Sharer, R., Piper, D., Chan, T., Kessler, C., Dellinger, R. & Pursell, K. (2004) Infections and severe sepsis in solid-organ transplant patients admitted from a university-based ED. Am J Emerg Med. 22(7), 530–3.
2. Paul, M., Silbiger, I., Grozinsky, S., Soares-Weiser, K. & Leibovici, L. (2006) Beta lactam antibiotic monotherapy versus beta lactam-aminoglycoside antibiotic combination therapy for sepsis. Cochrane Database of Systematic Reviews (1).
3. Lentine, K.L., Brennan, D.C. & Schnitzler, M.A. (2005) Incidence and predictors of myocardial infarction after kidney transplantation. J Am Soc Nephrol. 16(2), 496–506.
4. Holdaas, H., Fellström, B., Jardine, A.G., Holme, I., Nyberg, G., Fauchald, P., Grönhagen-Riska, C., Madsen, S., Neumayer, H.H., Cole, E., Maes, B., Ambühl, P., Olsson, A.G., Hartmann, A., Solbu, D.O. & Pedersen, T.R.; Assessment of LEscol in Renal Transplantation (ALERT) Study Investigators. (2003) Effect of fluvastatin on cardiac outcomes in renal transplant recipients: a multicentre, randomised, placebo-controlled trial. Lancet. 361(9374), 2024–31.

Level C

5. Kamath, N.S., John, G.T., Neelakantan, N., Kirubakaran, M.G. & Jacob, C.K. (2006) Acute graft pyelonephritis following renal transplantation. Transpl Infect Dis. 8(3), 140–7.
6. Hodson, E.M., Jones, C.A., Webster, A., Strippoli, G., Barclary, P.G., Kable, K., Vimalachandra, D. & Craig, J.C. (2005) Antiviral medications to prevent cytomegalovirus disease and early death in recipients of solid-organ transplants: a systematic review of randomised controlled trials. Lancet. 365(9477), 2105–15.
7. Fishman, J.A. & Rubin, R.H. (1998) Infection in organ-transplant recipients. N Engl J Med. 338(24), 1741–51.
8. Webster, A.C., Playford, E.G., Higgins, G., Chapman, J.R. & Craig J. (2004) Interleukin 2 receptor antagonists for kidney transplant recipients. Cochrane Database of Systematic Reviews (1).

Case 28
HLA sensitisation and anti-HLA antibodies

SHLOMO COHNEY

Case history

A 32-year-old woman with end-stage renal failure presents to the dialysis clinic for review. She has been on continuous ambulatory peritoneal dialysis (CAPD) for a year having developed renal failure as a result of lupus nephritis. She has had no other manifestations of systemic lupus erythematosus (SLE) or antiphospholipid syndrome. She has been coping well with dialysis, and remained free of peritonitis. She lives with her husband and two teenage children and works part-time as a museum curator.

On clinic review, her blood pressure (BP) is 125/80 mmHg, haemoglobin is 119 g/L, with satisfactory phosphate control. As she is about to leave, she enquires about her prospects for transplantation and position on the 'transplant waiting list'. She is blood group AB, and has been on the waiting list since shortly after commencing dialysis.

Question 1

The patient is managing well on dialysis. Should her nephrologist be concerned about the time she is waiting for transplantation?

(a) Yes, she will tire of dialysis with a risk of depression.
(b) No, she is young, managing well and will eventually receive a transplant.
(c) Yes, her peritoneal membrane will fail and she will no longer be able to perform peritoneal dialysis.
(d) Yes, transplantation is the optimal form of renal replacement therapy.

Answer

D

Explanation

A successful transplant improves quality of life. The impositions of dialysis, the dietary and lifestyle restrictions may all impact on the individual, and those around them. Patients may require financial, practical and psychological support.

Total 'renal' clearance in patients on peritoneal dialysis depends on residual renal function as well as the clearance contributed by dialysis. Residual renal function generally persists longer in patients undergoing peritoneal dialysis in comparison to those performing haemodialysis. Residual function is eventually lost, and clearance from peritoneal dialysis may decline over time, eventually becoming inadequate. Nevertheless, the patient has the option of changing to haemodialysis.

The principal reason for concern over transplant 'status' is the disparity in lifespan between patients on dialysis and those with a functioning transplant. Studies from Australia and elsewhere show greater survival for patients transplanted compared to those remaining on the waiting list (i.e. comparing outcomes of transplant recipients with patients who were 'equally fit' to begin with: deemed fit enough to receive a transplant but who have not yet received one). Furthermore, patient and graft survival following transplantation diminish with lengthening waiting time.

Clinical pearls

- Renal transplantation provides a substantial survival advantage over dialysis.
- Longer 'waiting times' impact adversely on both patient and graft survival following transplantation.
- Transplant options should be considered prior to commencement of dialysis where possible.

Question 2

The nephrologist confirms that the patient is on the waiting list. He should:

(a) reassure her that she will receive a kidney within the next 3 years as the average waiting time for kidney transplantation is 4 years

(b) inform her that she has a long wait because she is blood group AB, and this is the least-common blood group

(c) make specific enquiries to the tissue-typing laboratory.

Answer

C

Explanation

The average waiting time for a deceased donor kidney in Australia is between 3 and 6 years. This average is comprised of patients waiting longer periods (up to 10 years), and some more fortunate patients who receive a transplant in a relatively short time. The 'waiting time' to receive a transplant depends on human leucocyte agent (HLA) typing/matching and blood group, and varies among states of Australia.

If HLA matching were the only determinant of kidney allocation, individuals with uncommon/rare HLA typing would wait inordinately long periods and some would never receive a transplant. Various algorithms have been devised to allocate kidneys utilising a combination of HLA matching, and the period the individual has been on dialysis. (The 'waiting time' is the length of time from commencement of dialysis, even if this date is long before the patient's name is entered onto the list.) As O is the most common blood group, there are more patients 'competing' for O kidneys and waiting time is in fact longest for group O patients.

This patient, being blood group AB, can safely receive a kidney transplant from a donor of any blood group (A, B, AB and O) as she will have no A or B isoagglutinins (antibodies) in her serum. In transplantation, as with blood transfusion blood group, compatibility is very important with unsuspected incompatibility having the capacity to cause hyperacute rejection and graft loss. O is the universal donor group but O recipients can only accept from O donors, while A can receive from A or O, B from B or O; AB is the universal recipient. Although AB is a rare blood group and there are few AB donors, there are only a small number of AB patients on the waiting list. Thus in Australia, AB patients have the shortest waiting time. However, the small pool of AB donors results in AB patients rarely receiving a well (HLA) matched graft.

In view of the variables determining kidney allocation and 'waiting time' for a deceased donor kidney, it is often advisable to make a specific enquiry to obtain an accurate idea of an individual's prospects for transplantation. This may impact on choice of dialysis modality, and consideration of potential live donors.

Clinical pearls

- Blood group compatibility in transplantation is similar to compatibility in transfusion medicine.
- Transplant waiting time is blood-group specific.
- Allocation of cadaveric kidneys and transplant 'waiting time' depends on a combination of HLA matching and length of time on dialysis.
- There is a small degree of regional variation in algorithms for allocation of deceased donor kidneys.

- Specific information should be sought to establish each patient's prospects for transplantation. This should be conveyed to the patient.

Case history continued ...

The nephrologist contacts the tissue-typing laboratory and enquires as to the patient's position on the waiting list. Her HLA typing is A1, A3; B7, B8; DR3, DR15.

This is one of the more common Caucasian HLA genotypes and one might have expected a kidney to have been offered (based on matching) by this time. The tissue typing service informs the nephrologist that the computer matching system had on one occasion allocated a kidney to her on matching, but the kidney was not offered to her because of a positive T-cell cross match.

Question 3

The positive T-cell cross match detects:
(a) compatibility of T-cells between individuals
(b) antibodies against HLA antigens on T-cells
(c) poor HLA matching.

Answer
B

Explanation

The cross match assay examines the reactivity of recipient blood to donor T lymphocytes. The donor lymphocytes act as a source of class I HLA antigen and thus detect antibodies to Class I (though T-cells express many other epitopes on their surface). A positive cross match arises when recipient anti-HLA antibodies bind to class I antigens on the T lymphocyte cell surface causing cell lysis in a cytotoxicity assay. As T lymphocytes do not express class II antigen, a positive T lymphocyte cross match is associated with donor-specific class I sensitisation in the recipient.

The role of cross matching in renal transplantation was established in the 1960s when a strong correlation was noted between a positive lymphocytotoxic cross match, the occurrence of acute rejection, and poor transplant outcome (Patel & Terasaki 1969). Since then, the cross match has been used to determine whether a transplant can proceed; a positive cross match being a contraindication to transplantation. It later became apparent that the positive cross match, associated rejection/s and premature graft failure were attributable to the presence of preformed anti-HLA antibodies. The use of the cross match (in conjunction with the avoidance of blood group incompatibility) has led to near complete prevention of hyperacute rejection as a cause of graft loss.

In order to detect donor specific class II antibodies a cross match is performed with B lymphocytes. In addition to expressing class I molecules, B-cells display class II molecules on their surface. The clinical implication of a positive B-cell cross match has long been a source of contention, with a number of publications reporting a poor correlation between a positive B-cell cross match and graft loss. This uncertainty and the time constraints associated with kidney allocation have led to cross matching for deceased donor kidneys being largely restricted to T-cell. B-cell cross matching has been incorporated into assessments for live donor transplantation for some time with the same concerns about interpretation; however, more sensitive assays for anti-HLA antibodies have largely clarified this. It is now generally accepted that a positive B-cell cross match in the presence of a donor-specific anti-HLA antibody is of a similar significance to a positive T-cell cross match.

There are generally six HLA alleles involved in HLA matching (two each of HLA-A, -B and -DR); a 'haplotype' is inherited from each parent (one HLA-A, -B and -DR). In general, better HLA matching between donor and recipient is associated with improved long-term graft outcome. It is actually the degree of mismatching that is important (i.e. the number of HLA antigens that are foreign to the recipient). A large difference in graft outcome is only seen when comparing a complete match (six antigens) with a complete mismatch, where 5-year transplant survival can differ by up to 10%. However, HLA matching has no direct impact on cross matching (though a patient will not make antibodies against one of their own HLA antigens).

Clinical pearls

- A negative T-cell cross match is a prerequisite for renal transplantation to proceed.
- Cross matching requires donor cells and recipient serum.
- T-cells express class I HLA antigens and the T-cell cross match is designed to detect antibodies against class I HLA antigens.
- HLA matching improves transplant outcome, but has no direct bearing on the cross match or the likelihood of donor-specific anti-HLA antibodies.

LEVEL B

Case history continued ...

At a clinic review 6 months later, the patient again asks about her transplant prospects. The nephrologist is also puzzled, expecting that the shorter waiting time for blood group AB patients should have led to an offer by now. A call to the tissue typing service reveals that a further kidney had been allocated, but again a weak positive T-cell cross match prevented the kidney being offered to her.

Question 4

The nephrologist should:

(a) ascertain if there is a problem with the laboratory assays, and whether any patients are achieving negative cross matches

(b) tell the patient that the repeated positive cross matches mean she will never receive a kidney transplant

(c) suspect that the positive result may be due to non-HLA antibodies, and alternative assays may clarify the situation.

Answer
C

Explanation

The donor HLA typing was: A1, A2; B7, B8; DR3, DR4 indicating a single mismatch with the recipient at the A locus. However, specific (solid phase) assays for both class I and II antibodies were consistently negative, suggesting that the weak positive T-cell cross match was not due to antibodies against donor HLA.

The patient had developed an autoantibody, which in the absence of detectable anti-HLA antibodies appears to be the cause of the positive cross match. This is more common in patients with SLE. The autoantibody was demonstrated by testing the patient's serum against autologous T and B lymphocytes using a conventional cytotoxicity assay. The patient's own serum is aliquoted into a microlymphocytotoxicity tray and incubated with the patient's own B- and T-cells (these are already separated into distinct populations using specific monoclonal antibodies bound to magnetic beads). After incubating serum and cells, rabbit serum is added as a source of complement so that bound antibody can trigger cell lysis. In this case the T- and B-cell cross matches were positive, indicating the presence of cytotoxic autoantibodies. These antibodies of unknown specificity are not associated with rejection, and have no known clinical significance. These antibodies bind at 22 degrees C in vitro and binding is often abolished at 37 degrees C.

As nearly all lymphocytotoxic autoantibodies are IgM in origin, final confirmation of the autoantibody as the source of this patient's positive cross match was achieved by treating the serum with dithiothreitol (DTT). The latter is a reducing agent that destroys IgM structure by reducing di-sulphide bonds. DTT treatment in this case caused both the auto and (retrospective) donor cross match to revert to negative.

Thus, the 'falsely' positive T-cell cross match prevented the patient from receiving a well-matched kidney. Unfortunately, this phenomenon has resulted in a number of patients not receiving offers for kidneys for which they would have been suitable recipients.

A major advance in overcoming the potentially misleading results of cross matching has been the advent of 'solid phase assays': enzyme-linked immunosorbent assay (ELISA) and Luminex (using fluorescent beads). These not only detect HLA antibodies but also provide information regarding antibody specificities.

The ELISA test utilises HLA molecules bound to the bottom of microwells that are available for binding antibody contained in patient sera. The bound antibody is detected by addition of an enzyme labelled antihuman IgG antibody, followed by the addition of a substrate that results in a colour change. The latter is detected and quantitated by a colorimeter.

The Luminex assay employs 100 beads, each containing a unique dye and an HLA molecule attached to the surface. A second anti-human IgG antibody with a fluorescent molecule attached is used to detect the binding of the primary antibody. The detection system identifies both the fluorescent molecule and the specific bead dye, enabling detection of antibody positivity and HLA specificity. The Luminex system is the most sensitive of antibody testing methods, while ELISA is still significantly more sensitive than the cell-based cytotoxicity assays.

 Clinical pearls

- A positive cross match is not always due to anti-HLA antibodies.
- The clinical significance of a positive cross match may need clarification using solid phase assays. This can determine the presence and specificity of anti-HLA antibodies.

Question 5

If a further donor becomes available and the T-cell cross match is positive the transplant team should:

(a) decline the offer, as the positive cross match predicts a high likelihood of severe rejection

(b) proceed, and administer DTT to the patient to counteract the autoantibodies

(c) proceed without any special intervention

(d) ensure that cross matching takes place with DTT

(e) disregard or dispense with cross matches in future.

Answer

D

Explanation

It has been established that this patient has autoantibodies, and these are likely to persist. However, the patient may still develop antibodies that will not be 'auto' and that may be directed against antigens on a donor kidney; thus cross matching remains necessary. To minimise the chance of 'false' positive cross matches, patients known to have autoantibodies require cross matching samples to be tested in the presence of DTT. Following this episode, the patient's serum was included on a DTT cross matching tray for testing in the event of a kidney becoming available for transplantation.

Clinical pearl

- In patients known to have autoantibodies, all cross matches should be performed in the presence of DTT.

Case history continued ...

Two months later the patient is on a month-long holiday at a friend's rural property. By the end of the second week, she is complaining of increasing fatigue, and exertional dyspnoea. She presents to the local hospital where she is found to be slightly volume overloaded with haemoglobin of 80 g/L and associated iron deficiency. Upper-gastrointestinal endoscopy reveals a *Helicobacter pylori* positive duodenal ulcer. She is given omeprazole, and receives a single unit of blood and an iron infusion.

She makes a prompt recovery and after 36 hours returns to the farm and completes the prescribed *Helicobacter pylori* eradication therapy. A few days later she is contacted with the offer of a kidney from a deceased donor. The donor is a 50-year-old male with a history of hypertension who suffered brain death following a subarachnoid haemorrhage. He maintained good urine output throughout his stay in intensive care and the 'terminal' creatinine is 85 µmol/L. Donor HLA typing is: A1, A11; B8, B13; DR3, DR12.

The operation is uncomplicated though some atheroma is noted in the transplant renal artery; cold ischaemic time is 18 hours. The patient receives antirejection prophylaxis consisting of cyclosporine A, prednisolone and mycophenolate mofetil. There are no major postoperative problems, though the patient is anuric, and continues to require dialysis. A MAG3 renal scan supports the diagnosis of acute tubular necrosis (ATN) and the initial poor function seems consistent with the cold ischaemic time, atheroma and the donor-related vascular disease visible on the implantation biopsy.

After 5 days, urine output is 20 mL per hour, and the patient remains dependent on dialysis. A renal ultrasound shows a small collection around the kidney and a renal scan suggests minor impairment of perfusion. A renal biopsy is performed after the administration of DDAVP (to correct uraemic platelet dysfunction). The biopsy shows moderate ATN, and the pathologist notes that some of the peri-tubular capillaries are a little dilated. There is a cellular infiltrate near the cortex, but in the absence of tubulitis it is not thought to indicate cellular rejection. The patient remains well, but after 12 days is still oliguric and dialysis dependent.

Question 6

The transplant team should:
(a) perform another renal scan and not repeat the biopsy, as it is known that the patient has ATN.
(b) stop the calcineurin inhibitor (cyclosporine), as the associated nephrotoxicity is aggravating the ATN.
(c) perform another renal biopsy after imaging the kidney.
(d) remove the kidney as it is clear the kidney is not going to work.

Answer
C

Explanation

It is important to consider all potential causes of transplant dysfunction including volume depletion, obstruction, ureteric leak, calcineurin toxicity, but definitive assessment usually requires a renal biopsy. The original biopsy was consistent with ATN; however, the cause of renal dysfunction may change (e.g. initially ATN and later rejection) and multiple causes may be present. Therefore, another renal biopsy is appropriate.

If calcineurin toxicity is confirmed, the dose of calcineurin inhibitor (CNI) should be reduced. In the case of ATN, some physicians maintain CNI at normal levels, fearing the combined effects of delayed graft function and rejection; others reduce CNI levels or adopt 'CNI-sparing' strategies using anti-T-cell antibodies or anti-CD25 monoclonal antibodies. Drug levels are only a guide to the likelihood of toxicity, and a biopsy is needed to confirm whether there is CNI toxicity, rejection or both.

It would be inappropriate to remove the kidney even though it is not yet functioning well. ATN can persist for weeks with eventual recovery and attainment of adequate renal function.

Case history continued ...

Consideration is given to a further biopsy; however, being a Friday the ultrasound suite is overbooked, and it is decided to see whether renal function will improve over the weekend. Unfortunately on Monday the patient remains anuric, and a further renal biopsy is performed after DDAVP. The biopsy shows glomerulitis, marked peritubular capillary dilatation and severe arteritis, with circumferential C4d staining of peritubular capillaries. There is minimal interstitial inflammation and no tubulitis.

Question 7

Optimal management at this stage is:
(a) removal of the transplant kidney.
(b) OKT3.
(c) plasma exchange and intravenous immunoglobulin (IVIG).
(d) pulse methylprednisolone alone, as the rejection has not yet proved 'steroid resistant'.

Answer
C

Explanation

The biopsy has features typical of severe antibody mediated rejection (AbMR), supported by characteristic staining for the complement breakdown product C4d. The patient should receive treatment for AbMR.

The earliest changes of AbMR may include an appearance indistinguishable from ATN, but will usually be accompanied by C4d staining of the peritubular capillaries. The latter has a relatively high degree of sensitivity and specificity for AbMR; however, C4d staining in the absence of histological changes is insufficient for a diagnosis of AbMR.

Similarly, C4d is not always present. Other histological features of AbMR include peritubular capillary (PTC) dilatation and infiltration with mononuclear cells in both PTC and glomeruli (glomerulitis). Arteritis and interstitial haemorrhage are more advanced features.

Diagnostic criteria for AbMR include detection of donor-specific antibody (DSAb), though this information is often not available at the time of biopsy. The histological features seen on the day-5 biopsy probably indicated early AbMR, and C4d staining at the time may have been helpful. Clinically significant AbMR may occur without all diagnostic criteria being met. As AbMR can cause rapid graft destruction, early diagnosis and intervention is important and clinical suspicion should be raised if the patient has risk factors for sensitisation.

While the changes on the second biopsy are quite severe, the process is potentially reversible. Historically, the treatment for 'severe/steroid-resistant rejection' consisted of antibodies directed against T-cells (OKT3 or ATG);

these agents were often ineffective, and associated with significant morbidity. The recognition of distinct histopathology, and response to high dose IVIG (~2 g/kg), or more commonly plasma exchange with low dose IVIG (~0.1 g/kg), have dramatically improved short- and medium-term outcomes following AbMR.

Steroids alone will be ineffective, though most clinicians will use some steroid in association with IVIG and plasma exchange. OKT3 targets only T-cells, and while these may have a role in AbMR, anti-T-cell antibodies are unlikely to be effective (alone) and have significant toxicity. OKT3 is effective in steroid-resistant cellular rejection (as is IVIG), but in this patient there is no tubulitis or cellular infiltrate to suggest cellular rejection. Polyclonal anti-T-cell antibodies (e.g. thymoglobulin) have anti-B-cell properties (in vitro) and have been used in AbMR; however, they have also failed in the past. Thymoglobulin has also proven ineffective in preventing AbMR in patients receiving kidney transplants in the presence of preformed antibodies (e.g. sensitised patients with a positive cross match or transplantation across the ABO blood group barrier).

Rituximab is a monoclonal antibody directed against the CD20 molecule on the surface of B-cells, which is being used empirically in AbMR. There are anecdotal reports of success, and its low incidence of side effects (in patients receiving it for B-cell malignancies) makes it an attractive therapy. However, the antibody producing plasma cells do not express CD20, and are not eliminated by rituximab. There are no reports demonstrating efficacy of rituximab in the absence of IVIG or plasma exchange; thus its role remains uncertain, and its use experimental.

 Clinical pearls

- In the event of prolonged renal dysfunction after transplantation, the aetiology may change over time, and multiple causes may coexist.
- AbMR should be considered in patients who have risk factors for sensitisation.
- C4d staining of the peritubular capillaries is helpful in the diagnosis of AbMR, and may increase the suspicion of AbMR even in the absence of florid histological features.
- C4d is not 100% sensitive or specific, and evaluation must take into consideration other histological, clinical and serological features.
- IVIG, usually combined with plasma exchange, is the treatment of choice for AbMR.

LEVEL C

Case history continued ...

Despite steroids, plasma exchange and intravenous immunoglobulin (IVIG) the kidney is lost. As the patient's general condition begins to deteriorate, the kidney is removed. Subsequent testing with donor cells (obtained from stored spleen) and recipient sera (from post-transplant day 7 onwards) yields a positive T-cell cross match. Repeat testing with the pre-transplant sera (which was used for allocation) still shows a negative T-cell cross match. The transplant team are puzzled.

Question 8

The most likely reason/s for AbMR despite a negative cross match include:
(a) the development of antibodies post-transplant
(b) the presence of antibodies at a sublytic level (i.e. present but not detectable by cytotoxicity)
(c) the autoantibody
(d) non-HLA antibodies
(e) pre-existing antibodies to class II HLA.

Answer
B and E

Explanation

As indicated previously the autoantibody is of no significance with respect to the development of rejection. Published literature has reported that in the years following renal transplantation, around 20% of patients develop anti-HLA antibodies; these have been associated with an increased incidence of graft loss and may be part of the immune component of chronic allograft damage. Not all of these antibodies are donor specific, and evidence is awaited to establish the extent to which these antibodies have an initiating role, are a response to tissue damage or both. However, it is unlikely that such *de novo* antibodies would cause acute AbMR so soon after transplantation.

There are a few reports suggesting a role for antibodies to other targets in acute AbMR (e.g. endothelial cells) and for thrombophilia. However, the most common reason for AbMR following a negative cross match is the presence of pre-existing but undetected anti-HLA antibodies to class I, or class II HLA antigens.

In this case, only a T-cell cross match was performed pre-transplant, leaving anti-HLA class II antibodies undetected; these antibodies are capable of causing AbMR in some instances. The prospective use of B-cell cross matching is

C 406   PART E TRANSPLANTATION

increasingly common in allocation algorithms, as is 'solid phase' screening of patient sera for antibodies to class I and II antigens; this enables avoidance of the relevant antigens.

Case history continued ...

Sera from the patient were subjected to solid phase assays, including post-transplant samples, and samples from up to 3 years before the transplant. Both the ELISA and Luminex assays gave clear positive results for A11 in all sera, including those from several years earlier. Luminex detected antibodies to B44 and DR7, but only in sera from day 5 post-transplant and beyond.

Question 9

In relation to the AbMR and the HLA antibodies detected which of the following is correct?
(a) All the detectable anti-HLA antibodies have arisen from previous pregnancies.
(b) The transfusion did not contribute to AbMR, as the new antibodies detected post transfusion (B44 and DR7) are not directed against antigens on the donor kidney.
(c) The antibody directed against A11 is likely to have arisen from a previous pregnancy, but the transfusion may have been an additional source of exposure to this antigen.
(d) Many patients on the transplant waiting list have anti-HLA antibodies that arise spontaneously the longer they are on dialysis.

Answer
C

Explanation

Anti-HLA antibodies do not occur spontaneously but may arise in response to 'sensitising events'; these are pregnancy, blood transfusions and transplant/s. All patients who have a history of a potential sensitising 'event' should be considered 'at risk' of AbMR.

Patients listed for a deceased donor kidney provide serum every 2 months; the sera are screened for HLA antibodies (by cytotoxicity), and used on cross matching trays, when a kidney becomes available. The serum on the cross matching tray used for this patient's pre-transplant cross match was obtained 6 weeks before the transplant and prior to the blood transfusion. Retrospective testing of recipient serum obtained on the day of transplantation revealed a strong A11 antibody by cytotoxicity (titre 1:8), but not in any other sera, including that obtained from the rural hospital prior to transfusion. Subsequent HLA typing of the blood donor was A32, A11; B35, B44; DR1, DR7 suggesting that transfusion was a source of immunisation.

The detection of antibodies to A11 by ELISA and Luminex in pre-transfusion sera indicates previous exposure ('sensitisation') to this antigen, with the response after transfusion and post-transplantation being a secondary or memory response. As the patient had not been transfused prior to the gastrointestinal bleed, the original source of sensitisation to A11 was probably a previous pregnancy. The husband's HLA typing is A1, A11; B38, B62; DR3, DR4, with the presence of A11 consistent with the pregnancy being the primary immunising event. However, as B44 and DR7 are not present in the husband's HLA, it would appear that immunisation to these antigens (detected by Luminex in the post-transplant serum) is transfusion-related. Antibodies to B44 and DR7 were not detected by either ELISA or cytotoxicity, consistent with the known greater sensitivity of Luminex.

Paradoxically, several large studies have shown a positive impact of blood transfusion on transplant survival, even in the era of modern immunosuppression. However, the 'trade-off' is that some individuals become sensitised to HLA antigens, and the consequent development of anti-HLA antibodies can be a major impediment to transplantation. White cell filters and leucocyte-depleted red cells have been used to minimise the risk of sensitisation, though of course the best strategy is to minimise transfusion. Erythropoietic stimulating agents are extremely helpful in this regard.

Clinical pearls

- Patients are at risk of sensitisation to HLA antigens in response to transfusions, pregnancy and transplanted organs, leading to production of anti-HLA antibodies.
- The risk of sensitisation is increased with each sensitising event.
- In every situation, the need for transfusion should be considered, but particularly in end-stage kidney disease (ESKD) patients. Transfusion in ESKD patients can be minimised by appropriate use of erythropoietic stimulating agents.
- Tissue-typing laboratories should be informed of potential sensitising events, and should receive fresh serum 2 weeks or more after each one.
- A transplant recipient with a history of potential sensitising events is at risk of AbMR even in the presence of a negative cross match.

Case history continued ...

Following the failed transplant, the patient continues on CAPD but annual testing reveals that her clearance is falling. She remains reluctant to change to haemodialysis.

The possibility of a living related transplant has been raised previously, but both of her parents are dead, her husband has diabetes mellitus, and her children are too young to be donors. She has a brother in the United Kingdom with whom she has lost contact, but a lifelong female friend now comes forward and offers to donate a kidney.

Her friend is 34 years old, has three children and no intention of further pregnancies. She is assessed by an independent nephrologist, and deemed medically and psychologically suitable to be a kidney donor. Her HLA typing is: A31, A2; B44, B38; DR4, DR11 and both B- and T-cell cross matches with the recipient are negative. However, this donor does carry the B44 antigen against which the patient is immunised (notwithstanding the negative cross match).

The patient's 38-year-old brother returns to Australia and hearing of his sister's plight requests investigation as a potential kidney donor. He is medically suitable and his HLA typing is: A1, A11; B8, B7; DR15, DR3. In addition to sharing a haplotype with his sister, he has an additional matching B and DR specificity on the other haplotype so that there is only a single antigen mismatch. However, the B- and T-cell cross match between the patient and her brother are strongly positive with a titre of 1:4 for the T-cells and 1:32 for the B-cells (even with addition of DTT). It is presumed that the strongly positive cross match is a result of the A11 antibody; sensitisation occurring during pregnancy and boosted through repeat exposure associated with the blood transfusion.

Question 10

Although antibodies to the brother are presumed to be directed against the class I antigen A11, the cross match is stronger with B-cells than T-cells. This reflects:
(a) diminished viability of the T-cells
(b) the presence of undetected non-HLA antibodies and autoantibodies
(c) greater sensitivity of B-cells than T-cells to class I antibodies.

Answer
C

Explanation

It is not unusual to have difficulties with B-cell viability, as B-cells are present in relatively small numbers. Difficulties with T-cell viability are rare and the T-cell cross match was successful but of lower titre than the B-cell cross match.

Although a positive B-cell cross match would be expected to reflect reactivity to class II donor antigen, it can reflect the presence of an antibody to class I antigen, even when the T-cell cross match is negative. B-cells have a greater density of class I on their cell surface, making them more sensitive to antibodies directed against HLA class I. This highlights the benefit of solid phase assays in determining antibody specificities and clarifying results of cytotoxic assays.

 Clinical pearls

- B-cells express both class I and II HLA antigens.
- A positive B-cell cross match may indicate sensitisation to class I and/or class II antigens.

Question 11

Given the choices now before the patient and nephrologist, the patient should:

(a) wait for a kidney from a non-living kidney donor.

(b) accept a kidney from the friend as the cytotoxic cross match is negative.

(c) accept a kidney from her brother with whom there is a high degree of HLA matching.

(d) train for 'nocturnal' haemodialysis (the presence of donor-specific antibodies (DSAb) renders both live donors unsuitable, and the patient's sensitisation predicts a low probability of receiving a deceased donor transplant).

Answer

B

Explanation

An attempt should be made to provide this patient with a transplant option with the greatest chance of success and least risk. The overwhelming survival advantage of transplantation over dialysis has led to a growing reluctance to designate a patient 'not for transplantation' until all options have been explored. The presence of anti-HLA antibodies will make it difficult for this patient to receive a transplant from the deceased donor pool, and as already witnessed places her at risk of developing AbMR. However, the ability to detect and monitor anti-HLA antibodies, and promptly diagnose AbMR, has been accompanied by improved therapy for treating and sometimes preventing AbMR. Experience in the 1990s demonstrated that IVIG could reverse some cases of steroid-resistant rejection and overcome a positive cross match. IVIG has been used for this purpose on an increasingly frequent basis, usually in combination with plasma exchange.

A number of institutions now perform live donor transplantation in patients with DSAb and a positive cross match based on one of two strategies:

1. Administration of high-dose IVIG (~2 g/kg) until the cross match becomes negative.
2. Regular plasma exchanges with low-dose IVIG (0.1 g/kg) till the cross match becomes negative.

While both approaches have been successful, a negative cross match is more likely in protocols employing plasma exchange. As some of the higher risk patients may fail to achieve a negative cross match, high-dose IVIG therapy (without plasma exchange) may select a group of patients at slightly lower risk of AbMR and graft loss.

Published series using these regimens continue to report a 30 to 50% incidence of AbMR necessitating further plasma exchange and IVIG. The anti-CD20 monoclonal antibody rituximab has been used in cases of refractory AbMR and some centres have incorporated it in their induction regimens, though its efficacy remains unproven and requires clinical trials. Despite the high incidence of AbMR, centres using 'desensitisation' protocols are reporting 1-year graft survival of 85 to 95%. The likelihood of AbMR (and graft loss) is related to the strength of the DSAb response.

The combination of assays now available provide greater guide to the risk of AbMR, though are not absolute predictors. Moving from a relatively specific functional test (cytotoxicity) to more sensitive testing (Flow, ELISA, Luminex) can minimise risk, but has the potential to exclude donor/recipient pairs that may not lead to AbMR. Risk is perceived to be greatest when DSAb is accompanied by a positive cytotoxic cross match. Whether a positive B-cell cross match constitutes a lesser risk remains contentious, but consensus guidelines rank them equally. DSAb with a positive cross match by flow cytometry predicts a lesser though still significant risk.

Results obtained with historic sera (especially so-called peak sera, the sera with the highest PRA and antibody presence) are also evaluated. Some consider a positive cross match with historic sera as a contraindication to transplantation. Sera more distant in time may be less relevant to current allocation/outcome, but the presence of memory B-cells and the anamnestic response is well recognised.

A further assessment of risk involves the titreing of cross matches (i.e. diluting recipient serum to determine at what point the cross match remains negative). While there may be some laboratory-dependent variation, titres of greater than 1:64 and certainly greater than 1:128 have a very high incidence of AbMR and graft loss.

This patient has antibodies directed against HLA antigens carried by both donors so that transplantation of either kidney would carry a risk of AbMR. Although the 'friend' is a complete mismatch, and a donor-specific antibody is present, the cytotoxic cross match is negative. A transplant from this donor probably constitutes a lower risk than from the brother, who although well matched has an antigen that is resulting in a positive cytotoxic cross match.

If transplantation were attempted using the brother as a donor, plasma exchange and/or IVIG would be mandatory; in the case of the 'friend' it would still be strongly recommended in view of the DSAb (despite the negative cross match). Extreme vigilance with a low threshold for biopsy of the transplant kidney would be necessary in either case.

Advances in testing and therapy are changing the role of the tissue typing laboratory from one solely determining confirmation/veto of a transplant to one of risk estimation and guidance as to the necessity for desensitisation strategies.

However, there remain sensitised patients for whom a suitable donor is not available, or where donor-specific anti-HLA antibody titre is thought to pose too great a risk. Options available for this group include the following:

1. 'Desensitisation' with IVIG. Patients receive infusions of IVIG on a monthly basis to try and induce sustained change in the B-cell/antibody repertoire. This approach has had some anecdotal success, as well as promising results in an NIH trial where the cadaveric transplant rate was 37% in the IVIG group compared to 18% in the control arm.
2. Paired exchange. Incompatible donor/recipient pairs may be able to enter into an 'exchange' with another donor and recipient in a similar situation. This has been performed in a number of centres around the world on a small scale with success.

Bibliography

Level A

1. McDonald, S.P. & Russ, G.R. (2002) Survival of recipients of cadaveric kidney transplants compared with those receiving dialysis treatment in Australia and New Zealand, 1991–2001. Nephrol Dial Transplant. 17(12), 2212–19.
2. Wolfe, R.A., Ashby, V. B., Milford, E.L., Ojo, A.O., Ettenger, R.E., Agodoa, L.Y.C., Held, P.J. & Port, F.K. (1999) Comparison of mortality in all patients on dialysis, patients on dialysis awaiting transplantation, and recipients of a first cadaveric transplant. N Engl J Med. 341(23), 1725–30.
3. Patel, R. & Terasaki, P.I. (1969) Significance of the positive crossmatch test in kidney transplantation. N Engl J Med. 280, 735–9.
4. Mahoney, R.J., Taranto, S. & Edwards, E. (2002) B-cell crossmatching and kidney allograft outcome in 9031 United States transplant recipients. Hum Immunol. 63, 324–35.

Level B

5. Gebel, H.M., Bray, R.A. & Nickerson, P. (2003) Pre-transplant assessment of donor-reactive, HLA-specific antibodies in renal transplantation: contraindication vs risk. Am J Transplant. 3, 1488–500.
6. Jordan, S., Cunningham-Rundles, C. & McEwan, R. (2003) Utility of intravenous immune globulin in kidney transplantation: efficacy, safety and cost implications. Am J Transplant. 3, 653–64.

7. Takemoto, S.K., Zeevi, A., Feng, S., Colvin, R.B., Jordan, S., Kobashigawa, J., Kupiec-Weglinski, J., Matas, A., Montgomery, R.A., Nickerson, P., Platt, J.L., Rabb, H., Thistlethwaite, R., Tyan, D. & Delmonico, F.L. (2004) National conference to assess antibody-mediated rejection in solid organ transplantation. Am J Transplant. 4, 1033–41.

8. Jordan, S.C., Vo, A.A., Toyoda, M., Tyan, D. & Nast, C.C. (2005) Post-transplant therapy with high-dose intravenous gammaglobulin: applications to treatment of antibody-mediated rejection. Pediatr Transplant. 9, 155–61.

9. Jordan, S.C., Vo, A.A., Tyan, D., Nast, C.C. & Toyoda M. (2005) Current approaches to treatment of antibody-mediated rejection. Pediatr Transplant. 9, 408–15.

Level C

10. Stegall, M.D., Gloor, J., Winters, J.L., Moore, S.B. & Degoey, S. (2006) A comparison of plasmapheresis versus high-dose IVIG desensitization in renal allograft recipients with high levels of donor specific alloantibody. Am J Transplant. 6(2), 346–51.

11. de Klerk, M., Witvliet, M.D., Haase-Kromwijk, B.J., Claas, F.H. & Weimar, W. (2006) A highly efficient living donor kidney exchange program for both blood type and crossmatch incompatible donor-recipient combinations. Transplantation. 27 Dec., 82(12), 1616–20.

12. Segev, D.L., Gentry, S.E., Warren, D.S., Reeb, B. & Montgomery, R.A. (2005) Kidney paired donation and optimizing the use of live donor organs. JAMA. 293, 1883–90.

Case 29
Infection in the immunocompromised host

OMAR KAISAR AND RANDALL FAULL

LEVEL A

Case history

A 34-year-old man presents to the emergency department 2 weeks following a deceased donor renal transplant, with a 1-day history of fever, mild graft discomfort and dysuria. He had end-stage renal failure secondary to type 1 diabetes mellitus and had previously been on haemodialysis via a right brachiocephalic fistula. He was last dialysed on the day of his transplant pre-operatively. He had received a 5 out of 6 human leucocyte antigen (HLA) mismatched kidney and was sensitised with a peak reactive antigen level of 20% secondary to previous blood transfusions. Donor was Cytomegalovirus (CMV) IgG and Epstein-Barr virus (EBV) IgG positive while recipient was CMV IgG negative and EBV IgG positive. He had received mycophenolate mofetil, cyclosporine, prednisolone and daclizumab as induction therapy and his immediate post-transplantation course was uncomplicated apart from hypertension. His post-operative creatinine had fallen to150 µmol/L. His other medications at discharge included atenolol, trimethoprim-sulfamethoxazole (for 6 months), insulin, ranitidine and valganciclovir (for 3 months). A stent was placed in the transplant ureter intraoperatively, and its removal was planned for 4 weeks following surgery.

On review in the emergency department, he looks unwell with a supine blood pressure (BP) of 90/60 mmHg. His pulse is 110 beats/min, weak and regular and his temperature is 39°C. He is peripherally warm and the jugular venous pressure is low. Examination findings are unremarkable apart from mild tenderness over the renal allograft, without obvious overlying cellulitis. The following investigations are undertaken.

Laboratory data

	Results	Reference range
Na$^+$	135 mmol/L	(136–145)
K$^-$	5.6 mmol/L	(3.5–4.9)
HCO$_3^-$	17 mmol/L	(22–32)

Creatinine	200 µmol/L	(50–120)
Urea	17 mmol/L	(2.7–8.0)
Glucose	20 mmol/L	(3.8–5.5)
White cell count (WCC)	22×10^9/L	(4.0–11.0)
Neutrophil	17×10^9/L	(1.8–7.5)

Urinalysis reveals the following:

Glucose	3+
Leucocytes	3+
Red blood count	2+
Ketones	nil

A chest X-ray shows a normal cardiothoracic ratio. It also shows bibasal plate collapse.

Question 1

Based on the above information, the patient's clinical presentation is most consistent with:
(a) severe sepsis/septic shock
(b) acute rejection
(c) dehydration
(d) diabetic ketoacidosis.

Answer
A and C

Explanation

The combination of pyrexia, hypotension, tachycardia and elevated WCC is consistent with sepsis. The low BP in sepsis is due to peripheral vasodilatation secondary to altered metabolic autoregulation by vasoactive mediators produced during sepsis. Severe sepsis responds to intravenous fluids while shock requires ionotropic support. Sepsis is typically associated with warm peripheries on examination due to vasodilatation, though severe shock may be associated with cool peripheries. Dehydration accompanying sepsis, due to increased insensible loss and decreased fluid intake, may also present with hypotension and signs of volume depletion, but not with fever and allograft tenderness. Rejection can rarely present with graft tenderness and fever, but is not typically associated with hypotension. Hyperglycaemia and insulin resistance is common in septic patients, due to a combination of cytokine release and counter-regulatory hormones. Diabetic ketoacidosis is usually associated with dehydration, acidosis and sepsis, but its diagnosis requires the presence of urinary ketones. The rise in creatinine could be explained by sepsis and dehydration, with the acidosis secondary to acute worsening of renal function. Table 29.1 shows factors that affect the net state of immunosuppression in transplant recipients.

Table 29.1 Factors affecting the net state of immunosuppression in transplant recipients

- Immunosuppressive therapy
  — Dose, duration and temporal sequence
- Underlying immune deficiency
- Neutropenia, lymphopenia
- Metabolic conditions
  — Uraemia
  — Diabetes
  — Malnutrition
  — Alcoholism with cirrhosis
- Infection with immunomodulating viruses
  — Cytomegalovirus
  — Epstein-Barr virus
  — Hepatitis B and C
  — Human immunodeficiency virus
- Devitalised tissue and presence of foreign body

Source: Adapted from Fishman and Rubin 1998

Question 2

What is the most likely source of the infection?
(a) Allograft pyelonephritis
(b) Wound infection
(c) Pneumonia
(d) Infection of brachiocephalic fistula

Answer
A and B

Explanation

The presence of dysuria, graft discomfort and tenderness are consistent with pyelonephritis. Despite the absence of overlying cellulitis, wound infection and underlying collection should still be considered in the differential diagnosis. Failure of sepsis resolution with appropriate antibiotic therapy would necessitate exclusion of a perinephric collection with an ultrasound, followed by a computerised tomography (CT) scan if required, or consideration of other foci of infection, including acute bacterial endocarditis. The ureteric stent and surgical sutures also serve as a nidus for infection (see Table 29.1). Furthermore, the presence of urinary stents allows for reflux of urine into the renal allograft. The chest X-ray finding of bibasal plate collapse is common post-operatively, and the absence of focal pulmonary symptoms and signs makes pneumonia an unlikely cause of infection in this case. Infection of a native fistula typically presents with pain, erythema and swelling. Clinical findings could include tracking cellulitis and a fluctuant mass, consistent with an abscess. None of these features was present in this case.

In the acute post-transplant period, infectious complications are similar to other standard surgical interventions involving non-immunosuppressed patients. Nosocomial bacterial and fungal infections of wounds, vascular access sites, urinary tracts and lungs are most common. In rare instances, the allograft is the source of infection. Examples include disseminated toxoplasmosis and bacterial infections, with the potential to seed to the vascular suture anastomosis and risking a mycotic aneurysm. As such, donor screening is imperative to exclude possible bacteraemia and fungaemia. The recipient is also assessed pre-operatively to exclude possible sepsis.

The risk of opportunistic and unconventional infections increases after the first month of transplantation. Particular opportunistic infectious agents within the first six months include CMV, Varicella-zoster virus (VZV), *Nocardia*, *Listeria*, *Pneumocystis* and *Mycobacterium*. Six months after transplantation, the majority of recipients share similar infectious complications as per the general population. Acute opportunistic infections are relatively uncommon unless significant exposure to a pathogen has occurred. In addition, roughly 10% of recipients have chronic infection with CMV, herpes simplex virus (HSV), VZV, EBV and possibly papillomavirus, leading to infection of the allograft, various other organs and increased risk of malignancy.

 Clinical pearls

- The risk of infections in solid organ transplant recipients is determined by the net state of immunosuppression and level of exposure to a pathogen.
- These patients are at risk for standard pathogens as well as opportunistic infections.
- Acutely post-transplant, infectious complications are similar to any other post-operative events such as wound infections, urinary tract infection (UTI) from an indwelling catheter and pneumonia.
- Prophylaxis is effective in reducing certain infectious complications post-transplantation. Examples include valganciclovir (for CMV), isoniazid (for *Mycobacterium*), trimethoprim-sulfamethoxazole (for *Pneumocystis carinii* pneumonia, toxoplasmosis, *Nocardia* and UTIs), and topical antifungal therapy (for *Candida albicans*).
- Possible drug interactions with immunosuppressive medications via the P450 cytochrome enzyme should be taken into consideration with prescription of antibiotic, antifungal and antimycobacterial therapy (e.g. macrolides, ketoconazole, rifampicin and isoniazid).

LEVEL B

Case history continued ...

Clinical diagnosis of this patient is allograft pyelonephritis complicated by severe sepsis. A midstream specimen of urine culture shows *E. coli* resistant to trimethoprim-sulfamethoxazole. The patient is treated with intravenous ceftriaxone and fluids, with resolution of sepsis and improvement in haemo-dynamics, and serum creatinine level returns to 150 µmol/L. He is discharged and completes a course of oral antibiotics. The ureteric stent is removed at week 3 following the transplant without any complications.

On routine follow-up at 3 weeks, creatinine has suddenly risen to 300 µmol/L compared with 150 µmol/L 2 days prior. Renal biopsy was performed. Histology is consistent with vascular rejection. He is treated with 10 days of OKT3 with conversion from cyclosporine to tacrolimus. CMV prophylaxis with valganciclovir is continued for a further 3 months. Creatinine improves to a new baseline of 180 µmol/L.

Four months following the episode of rejection, he presents with fever (39°C), epigastric discomfort, elevated cholestatic liver enzymes and leucopenia. An abdominal ultrasound shows neither gallstones nor liver abnormalities.

Laboratory data

	Results	Reference range
WCC	1.0×10^9/L	(4.0–11.0)
Neutrophils	0.5×10^9/L	(1.8–7.5)
Alkaline phosphate (ALP)	220 U/L	(30–110)
Gamma glutamyltransferase (GGT)	300 U/L	(0–60)
Lactate dehydrogenase (LDH)	450 U/L	(110–230)

Question 3

What are the likely causes of neutropenia in this case?
- **(a)** Mycophenolate mofetil
- **(b)** Infection
- **(c)** Previous OKT3
- **(d)** Valganciclovir

Answer

A, B and D

Explanation

Mycophenolate mofetil is a non-competitive inhibitor of inosine monophosphate dehydrogenase, blocking *de novo* purine synthesis in lymphocytes, resulting in inhibition of cellular proliferation to antigenic stimuli. Up to 2% of patients develop severe neutropenia with mycophenolate mofetil, with the highest rate on doses of 3 g/day. Management requires dose reduction and in some cases withdrawal of the drug. Infection is a well-recognised cause of neutropenia, more commonly associated with viral infections. Generally this is a short-lived event with low risk of bacterial superinfection. Mechanisms include redistribution, sequestration, aggregation and destruction by circulating antibodies. OKT3 is a monoclonal antilymphocyte antibody used for induction therapy and for treatment of vascular or steroid-resistant rejection. A well-recognised haematological side effect of this agent is transient lymphopenia but not neutropenia. Lymphopenia occurs at the time of treatment and not 4 months later. Valganciclovir can be associated with neutropenia, especially in combination with antimetabolite therapy. The incidence is less than 5%, and management includes dose reduction or cessation.

Case history continued ...

The constellation of fever, leucopenia and cholestatic liver enzymes post cessation of valganciclovir raises the suspicion of CMV infection. A subsequent diagnostic test is performed and CMV infection is confirmed.

Question 4

What are this patient's risk factors for CMV infection?
(a) Previous OKT3
(b) Daclizumab induction
(c) Donor-positive allograft/recipient seronegative status
(d) EBV IgG seropositive status

Answer
A and C

Explanation

CMV infection is a common cause of febrile events following solid organ transplants, and is associated with a significant increase in morbidity and mortality. CMV has direct and indirect pathogenic effects, via expression of various cytokines, chemokines and growth factors. Up to two-thirds of adults are seropositive at time of transplantation. Multiple organ involvement has been observed, including hepatitis, pneumonitis, cutaneous vasculitis and bone marrow suppression. Use of OKT3 is associated with a significantly increased risk of CMV infection, and prophylaxis against CMV is routinely used following lymphocyte-depleting antibody therapy.

Reasons for the increased risk of CMV infection in this setting include reduction of anti-CMV T-cell lymphocyte activity as well as TNF-α-stimulated CMV reactivation from its latent state. Daclizumab, a humanised IL-2 receptor antagonist, has been shown to reduce acute rejection rates compared to a placebo when used as induction therapy. Unlike OKT3, it is not associated with cytokine release or lymphocyte depletion, and does not increase the risk of subsequent CMV infection.

CMV seronegative recipients from CMV seropositive donors are at greatest risk of CMV infection. Without prophylaxis, 70 to 90% of seronegative recipients from a positive donor will develop infection, with 30 to 50% progressing to develop CMV disease. Of these, 30% will subsequently develop pneumonia with 15% progressing to death in the absence of prophylaxis or treatment. As such, prophylaxis for this donor/recipient combination is routine in many transplant units. Valganciclovir and ganciclovir have both been shown to decrease the risk of developing infection and disease during prophylaxis. Despite this, there is an increase rate of viraemia in patients once prophylaxis is ceased. EBV seropositive status is not known to be associated with an increased risk of CMV infection.

Question 5

Which of the following is/are a suitable diagnostic test/s in this situation?
(a) Viral culture
(b) pp65 antigenaemia
(c) CMV serology
(d) Polymerase chain reaction (PCR)

Answer
B and D

Explanation

Commonly used assays in the immunocompromised population examine for viraemia, antigenaemia, mRNA and DNA. For the purpose of diagnosis, molecular methods offer reliable and rapid results. In this case, the best diagnostic test would be quantitative CMV PCR. The use of CMV PCR provides a quantification of viral load, with several studies showing good correlation between high titres of viral DNA and clinical manifestations in various solid organ transplant recipients. CMV serology requires a fourfold increase in anti-CMV IgG titres or newly detected IgM antibodies. Serology is an unreliable tool in the immunocompromised patients and thus not used for the purpose of diagnosis. IgM anti-CMV antibodies may be present for up to 2 years post seroconversion, and therefore the timing of acute infection may be difficult to ascertain in the absence of a recent IgM serology assay. Host leucocytes serve as reservoirs for CMV. Antigenaemia assay for pp65, a late structural antigen, quantifies leucocytes positive for CMV and provides an indirect assessment of viral load. It is a sensitive tool providing rapid and reliable results, with 95% sensitivity and specificity. In the setting of neutropenia, however, its sensitivity is diminished. Nonetheless, this test could be performed pending a quantitative PCR result as results are available within several hours. CMV culture, which reflects viral cytopathic effect, could be obtained from urine, throat and buffy coat, or bronchoalveolar lavage specimens in cases of pneumonia. Using the rapid shell vial culture technique, a result can be obtained within 24 to 48 hours. It may be useful in cases of resistance but has been superseded by molecular techniques.

Question 6

What are the appropriate treatment options now?
(a) Cease mycophenolate mofetil
(b) Cease tacrolimus
(c) Commence IV ganciclovir
(d) CMV hyperimmune globulin

Answer

A and C

Explanation

It is standard practice to reduce or cease antimetabolite therapy with severe CMV disease or significant neutropenia. Neutropenia in CMV disease is usually a direct effect of the virus itself and is a marker of severe disease. There is evidence that mycophenolate increases the frequency of CMV infection, especially with doses above 3 g/day. The decision whether to cease calcineurin inhibitors is controversial. Calcineurin inhibitors (CNIs) do not activate CMV from latency, but enhance proliferation, persistence and spread of activated virus. Generally CNIs are continued while antimetabolite dose is reduced unless infection leads to life-threatening illness. Uncontrolled trials have shown benefit for intravenous ganciclovir in the treatment of organ involvement with CMV disease. Intravenous therapy over 2 to 3 weeks has shown significant improvement in histology and clearance of viraemia in various forms of solid organ transplants. Clearance of viraemia is ideal before cessation of intravenous therapy is possible. This is necessary to prevent relapse and limit resistance to ganciclovir. Commonly either oral valganciclovir or oral ganciclovir is continued for a few weeks to months post intravenous therapy. A product obtained from human sera, CMV hyperimmune globulin, contains high levels of anti-CMV antibodies. It has been shown to reduce the incidence of CMV disease, leucopenia, fungal and bacterial superinfection. However, CMV hyperimmune globulin has not been shown to decrease CMV seroconversion or infection, reflecting its capability to prevent disease development and not infection. CMV hyperimmune globulin can be used as add-on therapy with severe or antiviral refractory disease, but does not have a role as primary therapy.

Clinical pearls

- CMV infection typically occurs 1 to 3 months following transplantation or cessation of prophylaxis.
- Recipients at highest risk of CMV infection are CMV seronegative recipients from seropositive donors and those who receive lymphocyte depleting therapy.
- Antiviral prophylaxis is effective in reducing CMV infection and disease but viraemia is a common event once prophylaxis is ceased.

LEVEL C

Case history continued ...

The patient is treated with intravenous ganciclovir for 2 weeks. Symptoms resolve with normalisation of WCC and liver function tests. Valganciclovir is restarted and he completes a 3-month course. Mycophenolate mofetil is recommenced with gradual dose escalation to 1 g twice daily. WCC remains within normal limits.

Over the course of the next 6 months, renal function deteriorates to a serum creatinine of 220 µmol/L. A renal allograft biopsy shows marked interstitial fibrosis and a tubulointerstitial inflammatory infiltrate with tubulitis. The histopathologist observes what appears to be viral inclusions in some tubular cells, and raises the possibility of BK virus (BKV) infection.

Question 7

What histological features are more commonly associated with BK nephropathy?
- **(a)** Cytoplasmic inclusions
- **(b)** Nuclear inclusions
- **(c)** Perinuclear halo
- **(d)** Epithelial cell lysis

Answer
B and D

Explanation

Polyoma virus associated nephropathy (PVAN) affects up to 10% of renal allografts, with progressive graft dysfunction occurring in up to 60 to 80% of patients. The majority of cases occur within the first year following transplantation. The development of BK nephropathy reflects over immunosuppression, highlighting the difficult balance between prevention of rejection and infectious complications. Viruria, which reflects the host's immune status, can precede viraemia and PVAN by several months.

Histological features of BK nephropathy reflect typical viral cytopathic changes. BK virions are transported into the perinuclear cisterna, with subsequent replication within the cellular nucleus, and hence are more typically associated on light microscopy with enlarged nucleus and gelatinous basophilic intranuclear inclusions. Intracytoplasmic inclusions are more typical of CMV, while HSV can present with both. On light microscopy, a perinuclear halo can be seen with BK nephropathy. However, this is a more typical feature of CMV. Further differentiation is assisted by greater nuclear/cytoplasmic ratio in BK-infected cells. BKV exhibits tropism for uroepithelial cells, with prominent cytopathic effects of the renal tubular epithelium and the urothelium. Histological findings can be quite focal, and the absence of PVAN on biopsy specimen does not exclude disease. Suspicion needs to be maintained and a presumptive diagnosis should be made in the presence of sustained viraemia.

Question 8

Which of the following confirm(s) the diagnosis of BK nephropathy?

(a) Positive plasma BKV DNA PCR
(b) Positive urine BKV mRNA PCR
(c) Immunohistochemistry for Simian virus Large T-cell antigen (SV LT-ag)
(d) Decoy cells in the urine

Answer

C

Explanation

Plasma BKV DNA and urine mRNA PCR are both useful screening tests for the diagnosis of PVAN, with absence of viral replication having a negative predictive value close to 100%. The positive predictive value for PVAN using plasma and urine DNA PCR is 60 and 40% respectively. Persistent plasma BKV DNA viral loads of >10 000 copies/mL for ≥4 weeks or urine BKV VP-1 mRNA loads of >6.5 × 10^5 copies/ng of total RNA has been shown to have a >93% sensitivity and specificity for histologically confirmed PVAN. Simian virus 40 (SV40) is a polyoma virus which was initially isolated as a contaminant of rhesus monkey kidney cells used to prepare the Salk and Sabin vaccines. Large T-cell antigen (LT-ag) is an 'early' non-structural or enzymatic protein that is essential for viral replication, cell immortalisation and latency. Immunohistochemistry for SV-40 LT-ag detects all forms of polyoma virus on biopsy specimens due to cross-reactivity between SV40 and both BK and JC virus. It is currently considered the best confirmatory assay for the diagnosis of PVAN. Specific monoclonal antibody assays can be used to differentiate the various species of polyoma viruses on biopsy, with BKV the aetiological species in nearly all cases. Decoy cells are BKV-infected renal tubular and urothelial cells that are shed into the urine, though CMV and adenovirus can cause similar changes. Most decoy cells show an enlarged nucleus with basophilic inclusion surrounded by chromatin that confers a ground-glass or gelatinous appearance. The positive predictive value for decoy cells for the diagnosis of PVAN is only 20%, but its absence confers a negative predictive value of 100% and may be used as a screening test for PVAN.

Question 9

What are reasonable treatment options for BK nephropathy?

(a) Decrease immunosuppression
(b) High-dose steroids to clear interstitial nephritis
(c) Valganciclovir
(d) Cidofovir

Answer

A and D

Explanation

Reduction in the intensity of immunosuppression, with the aim of immune reconstitution, is presently the primary intervention in the management of PVAN, with some evidence showing clearance of viraemia in up to 80% of patients with BKV infection. At present, there are no randomised or well-designed trials to guide the treatment of this condition, and the advantage of reduction of immunosuppression has to be weighed against the risk of further rejection. In this case, an appropriate plan would be to reduce the dose of mycophenolate and tacrolimus or replace mycophenolate with azathioprine. Serial monitoring of plasma BK DNA PCR fortnightly is recommended to assess response to treatment. If inadequate response is obtained, then mycophenolate should be ceased. The exact role of steroids in PVAN is unclear with a possible association between increased prednisolone use for rejection therapy and risk of PVAN. However, steroid therapy is generally continued at the lowest possible dose.

Evidence for the role of antiviral therapy in the treatment of PVAN is scant. Cidofovir, a nucleotide analogue of cytosine, has activity against multiple DNA viruses. Small studies have shown efficacy for cidofovir in the treatment of PVAN with moderate in vitro activity against BKV. Its use is complicated by increased risk of renal failure and proteinuria. This can be minimised by fluid loading pre-treatment. In cases of PVAN refractory to reduction in immunosuppression, treatment with low-dose cidofovir could be used. More recently, leflunomide has shown some efficacy in the treatment of PVAN in small studies. Leflunomide exerts its immunosuppressive effect via its active metabolite A77 1726. Its mechanism of action includes inhibition of dihydro-orotate dehydrogenase, leading to decreased levels of rUMP (reverse uridine monophosphate) and lymphocyte arrest in the G1 phase. A77 1726 antiviral activity occurs via inhibition of viral envelope assembly, with moderate in vitro activity against BKV. However, BKV lacks a nuclear envelope. Treatment with leflunomide, with drug levels of 40 µg/mL, has been shown to reduce or clear viral load. In a few patients with subtherapeutic drug levels (under 40 µg/mL), combination therapy with cidofovir has been beneficial. However, most patients had reduction of immunosuppression prior to treatment with leflunomide, which could potentially introduce bias to the primary outcome measure. There has been no published study assessing the role of valganciclovir in the treatment of BK nephropathy. Ciprofloxacin, a quinolone antibiotic, with some in vitro activity against SV helicase, has demonstrated efficacy against BK nephropathy in limited case studies.

 Clinical pearls

- PVAN affects up to 10% of renal allografts, with progressive graft dysfunction occurring in 60 to 80% of patients.
- The majority of cases occur within the first year following transplantation.
- PVAN can be difficult to differentiate from acute cellular rejection. Typical changes of acute rejection in areas lacking polyoma virus replication may assist in the differentiation of the two conditions.
- Reduction in immunosuppression is essential in suspected or established PVAN to prevent progressive graft dysfunction.

Bibliography

Level A

1. Fishman, J.A. & Rubin, R.H. (1998) Infection in organ transplant recipients. N Engl J Med. 338(24), 1741–51.
2. Bernabeu-Wittel, M., Naranjo, M., Cisneros, J.M., Naranjo, M., Cisneros, J.M., Cañas, E., Gentil, M.A., Algarra, G., Pereira, P., González-Roncero, F.J., de Alarcón, A. & Pachón, J. (2002) Infections in renal transplant recipients receiving mycophenolate versus azathioprine-based immunosuppression. Eur J Clin Microbiol Infect Dis. 21, 173–80.

Level B

3. Snydman, D.R., Werner, B.G., Heinze-Lacey, B., Berardi, V.P., Tilney, N.L., Kirkman, R.L., Milford, E.L., Cho, S.I., Bush, H.L. Jr., Levey, A.S., et al. (1987) Use of cytomegalovirus immune globulin to prevent cytomegalovirus disease in renal-transplant recipients. N Engl J Med. 22 Oct., 317(17), 1049–54.

4. Snydman, D.R. (1988) Ganciclovir therapy for cytomegalovirus disease associated with renal transplants. Rev Infect Dis. Jul–Aug., 10 (Supp. 3), S554–62.

5. Gandhi, M.K. & Khanna, R. (2004) Human cytomegalovirus: clinical aspects, immune regulation, and emerging treatments. Lancet Infect Diseases. Dec. 4, 725–38.

Level C

6. Hirsch, H.H. & Suthanthiran, M. (2005) Polyomavirus-associated nephropathy in renal transplantation: interdisciplinary analyses and recommendations. Transplantation. May, 79(10), 1277–86.

7. Hirsch, H.H. (2005) BK virus: opportunity makes a pathogen. Clin Infec Dis. 41, 354–60.

8. Drachenberg, C.B., Hirsch, H.H., Ramos, E. & Papadimitriou, J.C. (2005) Polyomavirus disease in renal transplantation. Review of pathological findings and diagnostic methods. Hum Pathol. 36, 1245–55.

9. Hariharan, S. (2006) BK virus nephritis after renal transplantation. Kidney Int. 69, 655–62.

Case 30
Post-transplant malignancy

KARUMATHIL MURALI AND ANGELA WEBSTER

LEVEL A

Case study

The patient is diagnosed with systemic lupus erythematosus (SLE) after present-ing with arthralgia and weight loss at 26 years of age. He is initially treated with steroids, but following the development of renal involvement (class IV lupus nephritis), he receives high-dose steroids and intravenous cyclophosphamide (for 6 months) and two courses of oral chlorambucil (for 9 months) followed by prolonged therapy with azathioprine. Unfortunately, despite all this therapy his renal disease progresses. At 36 years of age he undergoes left hip replacement for steroid-induced avascular necrosis of the femoral head, and 5 years later he commences dialysis. At 47 years of age he receives a cadaveric kidney transplant. Immunosuppression consists of tacrolimus, mycophenolate mofetil (MMF) and prednisolone. Over the next 4 years his graft function remains stable with a creatinine of 150 to 200 μmol/L. He requires femoro-popliteal bypass surgery for symptomatic peripheral vascular disease. He develops actinic keratosis of his right hand and viral warts involving face, hands and feet in the third post-transplant year.

Question 1

Which of the following statements is true about skin cancers in context of this patient's clinical course?
- **(a)** Basal cell cancer (BCC) is the most common skin cancer after transplantation.
- **(b)** Risk of skin cancer is highest in the first five years after transplantation when immunosuppression is most intense.
- **(c)** Viral warts are premalignant lesions and require intervention.
- **(d)** Risk of skin cancer in this patient is higher than average since his primary renal disease was due to SLE.

Answer
C

Explanation

Following kidney transplantation patients are maintained on immunosuppressive medications to prevent rejection of the 'foreign' organ. However, the immune system also has an important role in fighting infections and preventing cancers. There is an active 'immune surveillance' against cancer, which is blunted by immunosuppressants. The incidence of certain malignancies such as non-melanomatous skin cancers (NMSC), Kaposi's sarcoma and non-Hodgkin's lymphoma (NHL) is increased twentyfold in renal transplant recipients compared to the general population. Incidence of cancer rates at twenty-five body sites have been demonstrated to be increased in transplant patients. Melanoma, renal cell cancer, leukaemia, hepatobiliary cancers, uterine, cervical, vulvo-vaginal cancer and so on were shown to be up to 3 to 5 times more common than in the general population. Interestingly, the incidence of breast and prostate cancer were not significantly increased in transplant recipients. There is marked geographical variation in the commonest type of cancers observed in transplant recipients around the world (e.g. NMSC and lymphoma in Australia, lymphoma and renal cell cancer in the United Kingdom, liver and stomach cancer in Japan, Kaposi's sarcoma and lymphoma in Saudi Arabia).

Risk of NMSC increases with duration of immunosuppression rather than its intensity and at least one NMSC lesion occurs in up to 15% of transplant recipients by 5 years, rising to 70% by 20 years after transplantation. In the general population, BCC is three times more common than squamous cell cancer (SCC), whereas in the transplant population SCC is more common (2:1) than BCC.

SCC develops frequently at the site of warts or actinic keratosis. Human papilloma virus (HPV) has been implicated in most warts in transplant recipients. Risk of recurrence of warts is very high in this population. HPV is associated with a number of benign and premalignant skin lesions in transplant patients in whom Bowen's disease, premalignant keratoses and keratoacanthomas are common. Transplant recipients with premalignant lesions should be referred early to a dermatologist for active treatment and surveillance. The major risk factors for development of SCC in this population include white race, male gender, smoking, childhood sunburn and residence in hot climate. Primary prevention strategies include encouraging self-awareness, minimisation of sun exposure, use of protective clothing and use of an effective sunscreen (protection factor ≥ 30) for unclothed part of body parts (head, neck, hands and arm).

Underlying kidney diseases such as autosomal dominant polycystic kidney disease (ADPKD) are associated with greater risks of skin cancer, but SLE per se is not associated with any such risk. Moreover, prolonged immunosuppressive therapy administered for SLE, especially azathioprine, might have increased his risk of developing SCC in the future.

Case history continued ...

At 51 years of age he presents with lower abdominal pain and abdominal distension. An abdominal X-ray shows multiple air fluid levels suggestive of small bowel obstruction. A computerised tomography (CT) scan of the abdomen shows thickening of the wall of the small bowel. The intestinal obstruction responds to conservative management. Upper and lower gastro-intestinal endoscopies reveal no abnormalities. A laparoscopic exploration shows marked jejunal thickening and a resection anastomosis is performed. The histology is shown in Figure 30.1. The patient was known to have Epstein-Barr virus (EBV) and Cytomegalovirus (CMV) IgG antibodies at the time of transplantation. The donor was similarly positive for these antibodies. A pathological diagnosis of post-transplant lymphoproliferative disease is made and cell surface markers characterise it as a B-cell lymphoma.

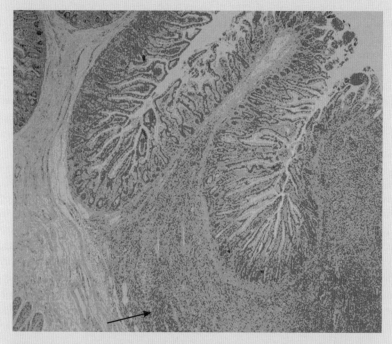

Figure 30.1 Dense lymphomatous infiltrates in the centre (shown by arrow) compared to normal architecture of the bowel wall elsewhere

Question 2

Regarding this presentation, which of the following statements is/are true?

(a) Non-Hodgkin's lymphoma is more common than Hodgkin lymphoma in transplant recipients.

(b) The small intestine is a common site of involvement for lymphoma in transplant recipients.

(c) Lymphoma could have been transmitted from the donor of the kidney.

(d) The term post-transplant lymphoproliferative disease refers to either Hodgkin lymphoma or NHL in a transplant recipient.

Answer

A and B

Explanation

Excluding NMSC, post-transplant lymphoproliferative disorder (PTLD) is the most common malignancy seen in transplant recipients. According to the World Health Organization reclassification of malignant lymphomas in 2001, PTLD encompasses a continuous spectrum of both hyperplastic and neoplastic entities, mostly but not exclusively EBV-associated lymphoid proliferation, including post-transplant infectious mononucleosis syndrome, EBV-positive plasma cell hyperplasia, polymorphic PTLD, monomorphic PTLD (including myeloma) and Hodgkin lymphoma. Non-Hodgkin's lymphoma accounts for 65% of lymphomas in the general population whereas it constitutes almost 93% of lymphomas (monomorphic PTLD) in transplant recipients. Most of these are B-cell lymphomas. Extranodal disease is common in up to 30 to 70% of patients and more than 50% present with extranodal masses. The small intestine has abundant lymphoid tissue in the form of Peyer's patches and the gastrointestinal tract is the predominant site of extranodal disease in non-Hodgkin's lymphoma.

EBV has been causally associated with Burkitt's lymphoma (a type of aggressive childhood non-Hodgkin's lymphoma common in equatorial Africa), nasopharyngeal carcinoma and some cases of Hodgkin lymphoma. Unlike other members of the herpesvirus family, EBV has the ability to transform human B cells and initiate a cycle of proliferation, which is initially polyclonal but in the immunocompromised host can evolve into monoclonal proliferation culminating in PTLD.

Lymphomas, like any other cancers, can be transmitted through transplanted organ, even though kidneys are devoid of large amounts of lymphoid tissue. For this reason, cadaveric donors with cancers (except the most localised brain tumours) are not generally accepted for organ donation. However, most transplanted cancers will declare themselves in the first few months following transplantation. Cancer occurring 5 years post-transplant, as in this case, would be very unlikely to be of donor origin.

Clinical pearls

- The incidence of non-melanomatous skin cancers (NMSC), Kaposi's sarcoma and non-Hodgkin's lymphoma is increased twentyfold in transplant recipients.
- SCC is more common than BCC post-transplant.
- Cancers transmitted through the transplanted organ usually declare themselves within the first few post-transplant months.
- Post-transplant lymphoproliferative disorder (PTLD) includes both hyperplastic and neoplastic diseases, frequently associated with EBV.
- NMSC and PTLD are the most common post-transplant malignancies.

Question 3

Which of the following statements is/are true regarding evidence of EBV infection and the development of PTLD in the case presented?

(a) Most patients who have positive anti-EBV IgG antibodies give a past history of infectious mononucleosis.

(b) Positive anti-EBV IgG at the time of transplantation suggests that the patient is at high risk of developing EBV reactivation and EBV-related PTLD after transplantation.

(c) Serial measurement of anti-EBV IgG and IgM titres would be the best way to determine whether or not the PTLD is due to progressive EBV infection.

(d) Negative EBV polymerase chain reaction (PCR) will exclude progressive EBV infection as a cause of PTLD.

Answer

D

Explanation

Most EBV infections are subclinical and unapparent. Approximately 90 to 95% of adults become anti-EBV IgG positive by 40 years, yet very few had symptomatic infectious mononucleosis, which is the classic clinical syndrome of acute EBV infection.

In order to identify patients at high risk of developing opportunistic viral infections after transplantation, IgG antibodies against EBV and CMV are routinely tested prior to transplantation. The presence of anti-EBV IgG antibodies indicates past infection with the virus. An anti-EBV IgM antibody indicates acute EBV infection; it peaks early in the course of illness and wanes about 3 months after infection. Subsequently, anti-EBV IgG antibodies appear about 6 to 12 weeks after infection and persist for life. Classically, EBV infection does not lead to complete viral elimination or destruction of the infected cells and therefore the virus can remain dormant inside infected cells for several years. For most viral infections, IgG antibodies are protective and their level in sufficient titres implies immunity against re-infection or severe infection. Patients who are positive for anti-EBV IgG antibody at the time of transplantation have some immunity against EBV and are therefore at lower risk of developing PTLD. At the same time this protection may be offset by aggressive immunosuppression (allowing reactivation of the dormant virus and leading to the development of PTLD).

The most clearly defined risk factor for development for PTLD after transplantation, however, is primary infection occurring after transplant in a person not previously exposed to EBV. Such subjects are anti-EBV IgG negative at time of transplant and receive an organ from an EBV-positive donor. In this setting, the EBV infection is transmitted from the donor to the recipient, who has no protective antibodies; fuelled by heavy immunosuppression, viral replication proceeds unabated, predisposing the patient to PTLD. Pre-transplant EBV seronegativity increases the risk of PTLD 10- to 70-fold compared to EBV seropositive recipients, when they receive organs from EBV seropositive donors. The cells of the allograft which carry the dormant virus are the actual source of primary infection. For this reason, risk of PTLD is higher with liver (2 to 4%) and lung (up to 30%) transplants than with kidney (1 to 2%) transplants, because these organs are heavier, have more lymphoid cells and therefore have higher viral load.

Although the presence of anti-EBV IgM antibodies or a rising anti-EBV IgG titre may indicate recent infection or reactivation, it is impractical to use this sort of information obtained by serial testing in making a diagnosis in this patient's setting. Given anti-EBV IgG antibodies were present in our subject pre-transplant, we know he has previously been exposed to the virus. Anti-EBV IgG antibodies would still be detectable and looking for a change in the titre is not a reliable or quick way of analysing the situation. Because of concurrent immunosuppression, he may not mount an appropriate anti-EBV IgM antibody response even if he has reactivation of EBV. Thus these serological tests are less helpful in detecting progressive EBV infection.

Serum EBV PCR is a very sensitive assay which detects active infection. A negative EBV PCR in a patient with post-transplant lymphoma has good negative predictive value for excluding progressive EBV infection as a cause of PTLD, but the specificity of higher EBV titres is poor, as many transplant recipients have at least transient circulating EBV without evidence of PTLD.

 Clinical pearls

- The gold standard investigation to determine the role of EBV infection in a patient's PTLD is histological demonstration of the viral genome in tumour tissue.

- Pre-transplant EBV seronegativity (versus seropositivity) increases the risk of PTLD 10- to 70-fold in recipients of EBV seropositive donors.
- Viral load is a determinant of risk of PTLD.

LEVEL B

Question 4

Regarding skin cancers in transplant recipients, which of the following statements is/are true?

(a) Clinical outcome of SCC in transplant recipients is similar to that in the general population.

(b) Incidence of rarer neuroendocrine cancers of skin such as Merkel cell carcinoma is increased after transplantation.

(c) Topical retinoid creams can control actinic keratosis and prevent recurrence of SCC in transplant recipients.

(d) Development of a BCC does not increase the likelihood of a future SCC in a transplant recipient.

(e) Among immunosuppressants, calcineurin inhibitors predispose most to NMSC.

Answer

B and C

Explanation

Squamous cell cancer occurs about 10 to 15 years earlier in transplant recipients than in the general population. There is a higher incidence of multiple lesions, local recurrence, metastatic disease and risk of mortality. Surprisingly, BCC does not follow a more aggressive course in transplant recipients. However, in both the general population and transplant recipients a prior BCC increases risk of a subsequent SCC as well as melanoma.

Rarer skin cancers such as Merkel cell carcinoma, malignant fibrous histiocytoma, Kaposi's sarcoma and cutaneous lymphoma occur with increased frequency in transplant recipients. Merkel cell carcinoma is more prevalent in men, develops at an earlier age than in general population and presents typically as an asymptomatic nodule on the head and neck or arms.

Topical retinoids such as isotretinoin and tretinoin do reduce actinic keratosis and therefore recurrence risk of SCC. Imiquimod cream, a topical immune response modifier used to treat anogenital warts, has also been shown to reduce actinic keratosis. The principal advantage of topical retinoids is the avoidance of systemic toxicity.

There is no convincing evidence that any specific component of maintenance immunosuppression is solely responsible for increased NMSC risk. Azathioprine may increase risk of SCC by a mechanism thought to be mediated by inhibition of repair splicing and induction of codon misreads in DNA. Calcineurin inhibitors may promote cancer progression principally via production of transforming growth factor β (TGF-β) but this effect is not specific for skin cancers. Sirolimus suppresses growth of many tumours in animal models by its anti-proliferative effect.

Question 5

Which of the following statements is/are true regarding the approach to PTLD in this patient?
(a) Disease onset 5 years after transplantation is very unusual for PTLD.
(b) The majority of PTLD occurring within 1 year of transplantation are EBV-related.
(c) Central nervous system involvement is common in post-transplant lymphoma and a CT brain scan is an essential part of investigations.
(d) A positron emission tomography (PET) scan is useful in the initial diagnosis of PTLD but not useful in evaluating response to treatment.

Answer
B and C

Explanation

PTLD occurs in a bimodal distribution with time following transplantation, the first peak occurring within the first 2 years and a second peak after 5 years. More than half occur within the first 2 years and these are more likely to be associated with EBV than those developing after 5 years. Late-onset PTLD appears to occur more frequently in patients older than 49 years of age than in those younger than 20 years. The reason for early-onset PTLD being more common in paediatric transplant recipients could be that many of them are EBV-negative and chances of primary infection following transplant from EBV-positive donors are high.

The pattern of organ involvement in post-transplant lymphoma differs from that of NHL in the general population. Central nervous system involvement is rare in NHL in the general population, whereas up to 25% of transplant patients have neurological disease. Demonstration of gadolinium-enhancing lesions on CT scan of the brain, positive analysis of spinal fluid for EBV by PCR and positive cytology with cell markers by flow cytometry will help to establish a diagnosis of CNS lymphoma. While it is therefore essential to perform a CT scan of the brain in PTLD, false negative scans can occur in up to 10% of cases.

Approximately 25% of PTLD infiltrates the allograft and can contribute to organ failure. The Collaborative Transplant Study demonstrated that renal lymphoma developed in 14.2% of renal transplant recipients versus 0.7% of heart transplant recipients. Allograft involvement occurs in a vast majority (>80%) of lung and intestinal transplant recipients. When PTLD occurs in the transplanted organ, the disease is more likely to be EBV-associated, it more often arises in cells of donor origin and it manifests early after transplantation. Response to reduction of immunosuppression in this situation is likely to be good and associated with better prognosis.

Positron emission tomography using 18F-fluorodeoxyglucose is very useful in detecting nodal and extra nodal involvement in aggressive forms of NHL as well as Hodgkin's lymphoma, and is superior to gallium and CT scan. Its role in indolent lymphomas and less-aggressive forms of NHL is less well defined. The most important role of PET scan is in monitoring patients after chemotherapy for lymphoma. Following completion of treatment, some patients with NHL may have residual masses on CT scans containing only fibrotic tissue or non-viable tumour and patients may be erroneously considered as not having attained complete remission. Functional imaging of these sites using PET scanning or combined PET/CT scanning will clarify the issue in most cases. Furthermore, PET scan can detect tumour activity well before macroscopic recurrence and is useful for evaluation of patients with suspected recurrence, but it has no role in routine follow-up of patients in remission.

Question 6

Which of the following therapeutic measures would be appropriate for this patient at this stage of disease?
(a) Complete withdrawal of immunosuppression
(b) Cytotoxic chemotherapy for the lymphoma
(c) Intravenous acyclovir followed by oral acyclovir
(d) Ganciclovir

Answer
B

Explanation

Whether the lymphoma is related to EBV or not, it would a logical step in the setting of a cancer to cut down the immunosuppression with the hope that this will give a chance for the body to fight the cancer by reconstitution of T-cell function. There is a risk of rejection with such approach, which has to be balanced against risk of progression of malignancy. However, complete withdrawal of immunosuppression is rarely practised, which would in most instances result in rejection and graft loss leading to severe patient morbidity.

The first step in many cancers occurring in a post-transplant patient would be reduction of immunosuppression. Whether a given cancer would respond to scaling down of immunosuppression depends on a number of factors: the type and stage of cancer, timing of its occurrence in relation to transplant, whether infection might be playing a role in the genesis of cancer and so on. Although the response is best with infection-related cancers like EBV-related PTLD, some patients respond dramatically even if the cancer is not related to an infection. Less aggressive anti-B-cell therapy with rituximab may be appropriate at this stage and more aggressive cytotoxic therapy should always be offered for patients who fail to respond to reduction of immunosuppression.

Anecdotal use of antiviral agents in PTLD has been reported. Acyclovir is a nucleoside analogue which inhibits EBV-DNA polymerase and inhibits lytic infection, but has no effect on latent infection. In the majority of EBV-associated malignancies in which the life cycle of the virus has been characterised, there is little evidence for lytic infection, which makes therapy with acyclovir in PTLD a futile exercise. Ganciclovir does not offer any advantages over acyclovir unlike with CMV, and is not useful in treatment. However, there are reports of the use of ganciclovir for prophylaxis against PTLD in high-risk patients (donor positive, recipient negative for EBV). There is one report of successful treatment with foscarnet of PTLD in a heart transplant recipient, without any reduction of immunosuppression.

Question 7

Which of the other following cancers occurring in solid organ transplant patients could be linked to persistent viral infections?
(a) Kaposi's sarcoma
(b) Cancer of uterine cervix
(c) Gastric cancer
(d) Hepatocellular cancer
(e) Nasopharyngeal cancer

Answer
A, B, D and E

Explanation

Viruses in addition to EBV have been linked to various cancers in transplant recipients. For example, Kaposi's sarcoma occurs after solid organ transplantation and is thought to be transmitted by donor progenitor cells infected with human herpesvirus 8 (HHV-8). Transmission of HHV-8 virus infection from renal transplant donor to recipient has been documented with seroconversion occurring in up to 25% of patients. Tumorigenesis may occur via HHV-8 production of virally encoded anti-apoptotic proteins. HHV-8 infection is necessary but not sufficient for development of Kaposi's sarcoma. A modulatory effect of other concomitant viral infections, such as HHV-6, and immune dysfunction associated with anti-rejection therapy could play a role in its development. HHV-8 has also been implicated in multiple myeloma, primary effusion lymphoma and multi-centric Castleman's disease.

Cancer of the uterine cervix has been linked to human papilloma virus, which has also been implicated in anal, penile and oropharyngeal cancer. Serotypes HPV-16 (50%) and HPV-18 (20%) account for the majority of cancers. The E6 and E7 proteins of many HPV strains interact with p53 and Rb protein of cells, which have a regulatory role in cell growth and apoptosis leading to immortalisation of human cells progressing to malignancy in the context of immunosuppression.

Hepatocellular cancer has been shown to be caused by hepatitis B and C, both in the general population and in transplant recipients. Nasopharyngeal cancer is relatively rare in most populations but is the most common cause in Southern China. A large body of highly consistent evidence supports the role of EBV as the primary aetiological agent in the pathogenesis of nasopharyngeal carcinoma. EBV is present in clonal form in pre-malignant nasopharyngeal dysplasia and in every anaplastic nasopharyngeal carcinoma cell. Gastric cancer has been linked in the general population to *Helicobacter pylori*, a bacterium.

Genetic factors which play an important role in the development of cancers in the general population are important in transplant recipients as well. This is evidenced by the observation that patients who had an invasive carcinoma before transplantation have a much higher risk (relative risk 2.38) of developing a second invasive carcinoma *de novo* after transplantation. However, a significant contribution to the increased risk of cancers in transplant recipients appears to have arisen from the increased predisposition to opportunistic viral infections.

Clinical pearls

- PTLD has a bimodal distribution with time post-transplantation.
- Twenty-five per cent of PTLD infiltrate the allograft.
- Kaposi's sarcoma, cervical cancer, nasopharyngeal cancer and hepatoma may be caused by viruses.

LEVEL C

Question 8

Which of the following is true regarding skin cancers in transplant recipients?

(a) Oral acitretin is well tolerated and generally free from any serious side effects.

(b) Female patients receiving systemic retinoids need counselling in terms of pregnancy due to potential teratogenic effects.

(c) The benefit of acitretin therapy persists long after the treatment is ceased.

(d) Retinoids are capable of preventing skin cancer by virtue of their anti-proliferative effect.

Answer
B

Explanation

Retinoids act by inducing growth arrest, promoting apoptosis of tumour cells, modulating the immune response or a combination of these events. Topical retinoids are less effective than systemic retinoids in their ability to prevent actinic keratosis and skin cancers. However, up to 20% of patients initiated on systemic retinoids withdraw treatment due to adverse drug events, which include rash, skin peeling, dyslipidaemia and hepatotoxicity. They may have some adverse impact on renal allograft function as well.

Both commonly used systemic retinoids, acitretin and isotretinoin, are proven teratogens and contraindicated during pregnancy and unsafe during lactation. The teratogenic effect of acitretin may last up to 3 years, while that of isotretinoin up to 1 month after the drug is ceased, and pregnancy should be avoided during this period.

Many studies have documented a rebound effect on recurrence of both keratosis and SCC after systemic retinoids are discontinued.

Question 9

Which of the following conditions are associated with increasing risk of PTLD in renal transplant recipients?
(a) Degree of HLA match
(b) CMV serostatus and mismatch (donor positive, recipient negative for anti-CMV IgG antibody)
(c) Hepatitis C infection prior to transplantation
(d) Use of interleukin-2 (IL-2) receptor blockers to prevent rejection
(e) Monoclonal gammopathy after transplantation

Answer
B, C and E

Explanation

In bone marrow transplantation, the relative risk of PTLD is increased four times for recipients of an unrelated or HLA-mismatched related donor, but in solid organ transplantation HLA mismatching per se does not appear to influence the risk of PTLD. However, perfectly matched transplants may be associated with fewer rejection episodes and less-intensive immunosuppression which indirectly reduces the risk of PTLD.

CMV has no proven causal role in PTLD, but CMV seromismatch (donor positive, recipient negative) and post-transplant CMV disease are associated with a 2- to 7-fold increased risk of PTLD. CMV disease may just be a marker of over-immunosuppression or it might be a confounding factor; CMV seroprevalence being related to age, young recipients being more often negative for both CMV and EBV, putting them at higher risk of EBV-related PTLD. Similarly, hepatitis C infection, though it is difficult to establish a causal role, has been implicated as a risk factor for PTLD.

Intensity of overall immunosuppression is the major modifiable determinant of post-transplant malignancy. The effect of anti-lymphocyte products, including monoclonal OKT3 and polyclonal anti-thymocyte globulin (ATG) are associated with a higher relative risk of PTLD. The same risk has not been shown for monoclonal interleukin-2 (IL-2) receptor blockers such as basiliximab and dacluzimab according to current data. It is unclear whether IL-2 receptor blockers have a quantitatively similar net immunosuppressive capacity as OKT3 or ATG, but it seems likely they offer the best risk to benefit ratio for transplant recipients in terms of graft survival and risk of PTLD. According to current data, drugs such as MMF and sirolimus have not been associated with increased incidence of PTLD. Sirolimus because of its anti-proliferative, anti-angiogenesis activity could have beneficial effects in some tumours and it is commonly used in patients with Kaposi's sarcoma following transplantation.

The increased incidence of monoclonal gammopathies after transplantation is well known. In the general population monoclonal gammopathy is associated with subsequent development of myeloma, amyloidosis, macroglobulinaemia and lymphoma. In liver transplant recipients, development of an abnormal immunoglobulin has been described to be associated with up to sixty-five times increased risk of developing EBV-associated PTLD.

Question 10

Which of the following management strategies is/are appropriate at this stage of disease?

(a) Withdraw prednisolone and mycophenolate while continuing tacrolimus as withdrawal of this agent would carry the highest risk of rejection.

(b) Discontinue tacrolimus and reduce other immunosuppressive agents as he is more likely to die from PTLD than from rejection.

(c) Allograft nephrectomy followed by complete withdrawal of immunosuppression.

(d) Anti-B-cell agents like anti-CD20 antibody (rituximab).

Answer

B and D

Explanation

Though most nephrologists would scale down the immunosuppression when a post-transplant malignancy is identified as in this setting, there is no standardised approach to immunosuppressant management, and treatment is often combined with other therapeutic interventions. There are no randomised controlled trials in this area and the extent to which immunosuppression should be curtailed, and the duration of the reduction, is pragmatic. Most observational data have suggested cessation of azathioprine or MMF with reduction of calcineurin inhibitor by at least 50%, and current international guidelines are based on this approach. For recipients where transplant loss is not immediately life threatening, as with kidney or pancreas grafts, the option of stopping all immunosuppressive agents exists. However, this is rarely practised. There is no evidence that reduction of immunosuppression alters outcome.

Occasionally allograft may be the only site of involvement of PTLD and in many of these cases the tumour originates from donor cells and most of them are EBV-related. Overall survival was 69% for allograft involvement alone versus 36% for other organ involvement plus allograft, according to data from the Israel Penn (Cincinnati) transplant tumour registry. In patients with allograft involvement, survival was about 80% when treated with allograft nephrectomy alone versus 53% when treated without allograft removal. Except in this rare scenario, allograft nephrectomy is rarely performed in the treatment course of PTLD. Complete withdrawal of immunosuppression does not guarantee a cure from PTLD but almost always guarantees return to dialysis.

The role of full-scale aggressive cytotoxic chemotherapy is debatable as the first-line approach to a patient with PTLD. Rituximab becomes a logical choice in this setting. Rituximab or anti-CD20 human/mouse chimeric monoclonal antibody kills B cells predominantly through antibody-mediated cytotoxicity; complement dependent cytotoxicity (CDC) and apoptosis also play a role in its anti-B-cell activity. The drug is detectable in serum 3 to 6 months after treatment and B-cell recovery is delayed by up to 6 to 12 months. Current guidelines suggest that rituximab be used for all CD20-positive lymphomas. CD20 is a hydrophobic transmembrane phosphoprotein with a molecular mass of approximately 35 kDa present on pre-B- and mature B-lymphocytes. It is not expressed on haematopoietic stem cells or other normal tissues. CD20 regulates cell cycle initiation and may function as a calcium channel.

There is evidence from phase two trials (but not randomised trials) that response to treatment with rituximab is of the order of 40 to 50% at 3 months, and patients treated with rituximab and chemotherapy have a low relapse rate when compared to those receiving chemotherapy alone. It has been suggested that efficacy may improve if rituximab is used as a first-line agent and duration of therapy is extended beyond 30 days. Factors that may predict a favourable response to rituximab include a short duration between organ transplantation and onset of PTLD, localised disease and absence of CNS involvement.

There are anecdotal reports of the successful use of intravenous immunoglobulin, usually in conjunction with other treatment modalities, to treat (and prevent) PTLD.

 Clinical pearl

- Rituximab is a unique drug that can be used as an anti-rejection agent as well as anti-cancer (B-cell lymphoma) therapy.

Case history continued . . .

The patient's tacrolimus is discontinued, mycophenolate is converted to azathioprine and prednisolone is continued. He is given rituximab every week for 4 weeks. No anti-viral therapy is administered. He receives no further specific cytotoxic chemotherapy for lymphoma at this stage but remains on follow-up. PET scan done 6 weeks after initial treatment shows no evidence of residual disease. CT scan of chest and brain shows no lesions. Bone marrow shows no

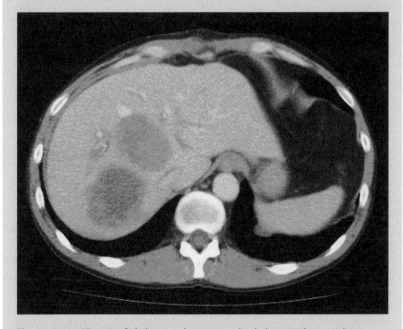

Figure 30.2 CT scan of abdomen showing multiple hepatic lesions due to recurrence of NHL

lymphomatous deposits. His renal function remains stable with a creatinine of approximately 200 μmol/L.

Unfortunately, after six months, he returns with high-grade fever, acute right upper quadrant abdominal pain and vomiting. He has also experienced night sweats and weight loss over several weeks. On examination he is febrile, with tender hepatomegaly. Total white cell count is normal, cultures of blood and urine are negative, his renal function is unchanged and liver functions are deranged (elevated transaminase levels). A CT scan of his abdomen shows the above appearance in the liver in addition to two significant mesenteric lymph nodes (see Fig. 30.2). There are no supraclavicular or other clinically palpable lymph nodes. Excision biopsy of lymph node and liver lesion shows recurrence of B-cell lymphoma.

Question 11

Which of the following management considerations for this patient at this stage is/are true or appropriate?

(a) Further reduction of immunosuppression

(b) Aggressive chemotherapy using CHOP/ABVD regimens

(c) A second course of rituximab

(d) If his renal allograft fails in response to downscaling immunosuppression, he is not a candidate for re-transplantation

Answer
A, B and C

Explanation

Further reduction in immunosuppression would be a reasonable step in view of the recurrence of lymphoma, though there is no evidence that such a strategy leads to improved outcomes. The fear of rejection would be unreasonable as his life span is going to be cut short by his recurrent cancer. Furthermore, cytotoxic chemotherapy for lymphoma would have an immunosuppressive effect of its own. For organs where consequences of graft failure are grave, such as the lung and heart, extreme caution should be exercised in scaling down immunosuppression.

Given recurrence in such a short time, there is a strong case for aggressive cytotoxic chemotherapy considering his young age. Mortality with monoclonal PTLD can be as high as 80%. For patients with localised disease and those with central nervous system involvement, involved field radiation therapy may be beneficial. In view of previous good response to rituximab, it may be worth considering its use again, especially so if the tumour is CD20-positive. Despite all these measures his prognosis remains guarded.

There is no contraindication to re-transplantation if chances of PTLD recurrence are low. A retrospective study of six renal transplant patients who were re-transplanted 50 to 128 months after successful treatment of PTLD showed good patient and graft survival. Five out of six patients had PTLD confined to their graft and had undergone allograft nephrectomy in addition to other treatments for their PTLD. A large cohort study based on the United Network of Organ Sharing (UNOS) database reported sixty-nine patients who were successfully treated for PTLD and who underwent re-transplantation with overall patient and graft survival of 86 and 74% respectively.

Case history continued ...

His azathioprine is ceased, and chemotherapy with R-CHOP (rituximab, cyclo-phosphamide, doxorubicin, vincristine, prednisolone) is administered. He suffers two episodes of febrile neutropenia which are successfully treated. He remains in follow-up, with his serum creatinine remaining at baseline around 200 μmol/L. He has been given a very guarded prognosis in view of prompt recurrence of B-cell lymphoma in such a short interval.

Question 12

Which of the following statements is/are true regarding screening for cancers in transplant recipients?

(a) Cancer screening in transplant recipients is not indicated since screening programs have been validated for cost-effectiveness only in the general population.

(b) Annual screening for breast cancer should begin at 40 years of age in standard-risk transplant recipients, about 10 years earlier than in the general population.

(c) Patients with polycystic kidney disease who undergo transplantation should undergo annual ultrasound scan of abdomen and urine cytology as they are at high risk of renal cell cancer.

(d) Lung cancer screening is not indicated in renal transplant recipients who are smokers.

Answer

D

Explanation

The objective of cancer screening in high-risk populations is to facilitate early detection, which would enhance the chances of curative treatment and improve outcomes. Though cost-effectiveness of screening programs has been validated for the general population, transplant recipients are at markedly increased risk for many different type of cancers and it is illogical to deny them the benefits of cancer screening. Various recommendations for screening of transplant recipients for cancer are in place, though these are not based on randomised controlled trial data, but rather based on observational data and expert opinion.

Breast cancer risk is not particularly increased in the transplant population and therefore should follow the same guidelines as in the general population. Skin cancer, which is the most common post-transplant malignancy, is best screened by monthly self-examination and annual physical examination. All women over 18 years of age and those under 18 years who are sexually active should ideally undergo annual pelvic examination and PAP smear.

Screening for urinary tract cancer is indicated only in patients with analgesic nephropathy due to the high incidence of urothelial cancers in this population. Patients who had been exposed to prolonged therapy with cyclophosphamide and those with nephropathy due to Chinese herbs are also at high risk. Patients with polycystic kidney disease are not at any higher risk of renal cell cancer than the general population, unlike patients with acquired cystic disease. They do not require any screening procedures to detect early renal cell cancers. Patients with von Hippel-Lindau disease are at very high risk of multiple cancers and should be screened by detailed annual clinical assessment and radiological tests if necessary.

Benefits of screening for lung cancer are unclear even in the general population. Many randomised controlled trials have failed to show any benefit in terms of mortality from lung cancer, despite improvement in detection of early lesions. In this setting, screening in transplant recipients would not be justified.

Bibliography

Level A

1. Morath, C., Mueller, M., Goldschmidt, H., Schwenger, V., Opelz, G. & Zeier, M. (2004) Malignancy in Renal Transplantation. J Am Soc Nephrol. 15, 1582–8.
2. Kotton, C.N. & Fishman, J.A. (2005) Viral infection in the renal transplant recipient. J Am Soc Nephrol. 16, 1758–74.
3. Jaffe, E.S., Harris, N.L., Stein H. & Vardiman, J.W.; World Health Organization Classification of Tumours. (2001) *Pathology and Genetics: Haematopoietic and Lymphoid Tissues*. Lyon: IARC Press.

Level B

4. Vajdic, C.M., McDonald, S.P., McCredie, M.R., van Leeuwen, M.T., Stewart, J.H., Law, M., Chapman, J.R., Webster, A.C., Kaldor, J.M. & Grulich, A.E. (2006) Cancer incidence before and after kidney transplantation. JAMA. 296, 2823–31.
5. Euvard, S., Kanitakis, J. & Claudy, A. (2003) Skin cancers after organ transplantation. N Eng J Med. 348, 1681–91.
6. Moloney, F.J., Keane, S., O'Kelly, P., Conlon, P.J. & Murphy, G.M. (2005) The impact of skin disease following renal transplantation on quality of life. British Journal of Dermatology. 153, 574–8.

7. Lim, W.H., Russ, G.R. & Coates, P.T. (2006) Review of Epstein-Barr virus and post-transplant lymphoproliferative disorder post-solid organ transplantation. Nephrology. 11, 355–66.

Level C

8. Chen, K., Craig, J.C. & Shumack, S. (2005) Oral retinoids for the prevention of skin cancers in solid organ transplant recipients: a systematic review of randomized controlled trials. British Journal of Dermatology. 152, 518–23.

9. Webster, A.C., Playford, E.G., Higgins, G., Chapman, J.R. & Craig, J.C. (2004) Interleukin 2 receptor antagonists for renal transplant recipients: a meta-analysis of randomized trials. Transplantation. 77, 166–76.

10. Svoboda, J., Kotloff, R. & Tsai, D.E. (2006) Management of patients with post-transplant lymphoproliferative disorder: the role of rituximab. Transpl Int. 19, 259–69.

11. Trofe, J., Buell, J.F., Beebe, T.M., Hanaway, M.J., First, M.R., Alloway, R.R., Gross, T.G., Succop, P. & Woodle, E.S. (2005) Analysis of factors that influence survival with post-transplant lymphoproliferative disorder in renal transplant recipients: the Israel Penn International Transplant Tumor Registry experience. Am J Transplant. 5, 775–80.

12. Kasiske, B.L., Vazques, M.A., Harmon, W.E., Brown, R.S., Danovitch, G.M., Gaston, R.S., Roth, D., Scandling, J.D. & Singer, G.G. (2000) Recommendations for the outpatient surveillance of renal transplant recipients. American Society of Transplantation guidelines. J Am Soc Nephrol. 15, S1–86.

13. Webster, A.C., Craig, J.C., Simpson, J.M., Jones, M.P. & Chapman J.R. (2007) Identifying high risk groups and quantifying absolute risk of cancer after kidney transplantation: A Cohort Study of 15183 Recipients. Am J Transpl. 9, 2140–51.

Case 31
Other complications of immunosuppression

JOHN KANELLIS

LEVEL A

Case history

The patient is a 70 kg, 46-year-old man with hypertension and previous end-stage renal failure secondary to reflux nephropathy. A kidney transplant performed 14 years ago (live donation from his mother, 3/6 human leukocyte antigen, HLA, match) worked well until 2 years ago. This was despite some early rejection in the first year which was treated successfully with two separate courses of pulse steroids (daily intravenous injections for 3 days on both occasions).

Unfortunately, over the last 2 years his renal function has gradually deteriorated with his most recent tests showing the following.

Laboratory data

	Results	Reference range
Urea	20.5 mmol/L	(2.5–9.6)
Creatinine	350 µmol/L	(40–120)
Haemoglobin	81 g/L	(130–180)
Mean red cell volume	67 fL	(78–98)
Total white cell count	4.1×10^9/L	$(4–12 \times 10^9$/L)
Platelets	175×10^9/L	$(150–400 \times 10^9$/L)

A renal biopsy performed 18 months ago (creatinine 260 µmol/L) revealed typical features of chronic allograft nephropathy (CAN) with moderate tubulointerstitial fibrosis, tubular atrophy and some glomerular damage. His haemoglobin and mean red cell volume were normal at that time and no adjustments were made to his immunosuppressive regimen. This has consisted of azathioprine 75 mg daily and prednisolone 5 mg daily for the last 5 years. He has never taken calcineurin inhibitors (CNIs) such as cyclosporin or tacrolimus. Recent oedema has been treated with some diuretics and with salt and fluid restriction.

Question 1

In considering the following list of his known problems, which two of these are *most likely* to have arisen largely because of his immunosuppression?

(a) Hyperparathyroidism
(b) Unilateral hip pain
(c) Microcytic anaemia
(d) Cataracts
(e) Hypertension

Answer

B and D

Explanation

The patient has significant renal impairment and may have poor control of his serum calcium and phosphate levels. This will provide a major stimulus for the development of secondary hyperparathyroidism and renal bone disease, although these conditions are not related to his immunosuppression (answer A incorrect). However, complicating his bone disease may be problems induced by long-term steroid therapy including osteopenia and osteonecrosis (avascular necrosis). Osteonecrosis commonly affects the femoral head, lower femur and tibia. In this case, the hip pain may be a manifestation of avascular necrosis of the femoral head (answer B correct). Prior to the routine use of cyclosporin, this occurred in up to 10 to 15% of transplanted patients. Hip replacement surgery was often necessary.

Steroid use is also associated with the development of ophthalmologic problems including cataracts and glaucoma (answer D correct). Other steroid-related problems include glucose intolerance, weight gain and mood disorder.

While azathioprine can cause myelosuppression leading to leucopenia, thrombocytopenia and anaemia, the anaemia is generally macrocytic (answer C incorrect). Macrocytosis can also occur in the absence of anaemia and is due to direct toxic effects of azathioprine on the bone marrow. In this gentleman, a new microcytic anaemia suggests he has iron deficiency. This is most commonly due to chronic blood loss (e.g. gastrointestinal bleeding) and is unlikely to be directly related to his immunosuppressive drugs. Low dose, long-term steroids are not likely to cause peptic ulceration. The degree of anaemia also appears to be more severe than would be expected for his level of renal failure. Anaemia due to chronic renal failure is typically normochromic and normocytic.

Hypertension is common in renal transplant recipients and is usually multifactorial. While steroid use can promote sodium and water retention with resultant elevation in blood pressure, it is not likely to be the main factor causing hypertension in this patient who also has poor transplant function and reflux nephropathy as underlying problems (answer E incorrect).

Clinical pearls

- Patients at high risk for steroid-related bone problems post-transplant include post-menopausal females, the elderly and patients previously on steroids (e.g. previous lupus or vasculitis).
- Azathioprine use commonly leads to macrocytosis of red cells and to mild anaemia and thrombocytopenia. Lymphopenia is also common. Megaloblastic changes and myelodysplasia may be seen on bone marrow examination.

Case history continued ...

Gout has also become a major problem for the patient. He has had three episodes of joint pain and inflammation in the last 6 months affecting his hands, feet and right knee (aspiration excluded infection and showed uric acid crystals). The first episode was treated briefly but incompletely with colchicine (diarrhoea developed as a side effect). The next two episodes responded well to a short-term increase in his steroid dose (to 20 mg/day for 3 days).

Question 2

In considering the use of allopurinol to manage his gout, which of the following statements is/are true?

(a) Allopurinol can be safely started once an acute attack settles.

(b) Allopurinol and azathioprine are both metabolised by the cytochrome P-450 pathway.

(c) If azathioprine is continued, a major adjustment in the azathioprine dose will be required once allopurinol is commenced.

(d) Using a non steroidal anti-inflammatory drug and ceasing the diuretic are better alternatives to using allopurinol in this patient.

(e) Mycophenolate mofetil (MMF) or mycophenolic acid (MPA) without dose adjustment could be used in place of azathioprine once allopurinol is commenced.

Answer

C and E

Explanation

Gout is a common disorder which can be exacerbated in transplant patients by CNIs and diuretic treatment. Azathioprine and steroids are not associated with an increased incidence of gout.

Allopurinol is a xanthine oxidase inhibitor which blocks the metabolism of purines and decreases uric acid production. In managing gout in transplant patients, it should be remembered that allopurinol interferes with the metabolism of azathioprine (answer A incorrect). Azathioprine is converted to 6-mercaptopurine (an active immunosuppressant and bone marrow toxin) which is then metabolised by xanthine oxidase to the inactive metabolite thiouric acid. The concomitant use of azathioprine and allopurinol should therefore be avoided or the dose of azathioprine should be significantly reduced by 50 to 75% (answer C correct), followed by close monitoring of the full blood count, to avoid severe bone marrow toxicity due to markedly increased circulating concentrations of 6-mercaptopurine. The cytochrome P-450 pathway is of no relevance to the metabolism of azathioprine or allopurinol (answer B incorrect).

Non-steroidal anti-inflammatory drugs are very effective for treating acute gout but in this patient with significant renal impairment, they should be avoided as they may further worsen renal function and exacerbate oedema (answer D incorrect). Ceasing the diuretic may help reduce the tendency for gout in this patient but he will still need his oedema managed somehow.

 Clinical pearls

- Azathioprine is rapidly converted to 6-mercaptoprine (6MP), a purine analogue which is largely responsible for the immunosuppressive action of azathioprine. 6MP interrupts the synthesis (S) phase of the lymphocyte cell cycle by disrupting nucleotide synthesis.
- As 6MP is metabolised by xanthine oxidase, continued use of azathioprine with allopurinol (a xanthine oxidase inhibitor) will lead to marked bone marrow suppression unless the dose of azathioprine is reduced by up to 75%.
- MMF (and the active metabolite MPA) is not metabolised by xanthine oxidase. It is therefore an easier drug than azathioprine to manage with concurrent allopurinol administration.
- CNIs are associated with hyperuricaemia and increase the likelihood of gout. This is due to decreased renal uric acid clearance, through both glomerular haemodynamic and renal tubular effects of the CNIs.
- MMF/MPA has largely replaced azathioprine in modern immunosuppressive regimens. It is not metabolised by xanthine oxidase and does not interact with allopurinol. Allopurinol and MMF/MPA can be used together without the need for dose adjustment (answer E correct).

Question 3

Azathioprine is ceased and the patient is commenced on MMF in order to put him on allopurinol. Common side effects of MMF/MPA that the patient should be made aware of include:

(a) diarrhoea, bloating, gastrointestinal upset
(b) hair loss
(c) neurotoxicity
(d) leucopenia
(e) nephrotoxicity.

Answer

A and D

Explanation

The predominant side effects of MMF/MPA are those affecting the gastrointestinal and haematopoietic systems (answers A and D correct). Both of these are dose-related.

Abdominal discomfort, nausea and diarrhoea are relatively common side effects of MMF/MPA that can be improved by dose reduction, dosing with food or by dividing up the daily dose into more frequent, smaller amounts (e.g. twice-a-day regimen changed to three-times-a-day regimen, with no change in total daily dose).

Leucopenia predominantly occurs due to the inhibition of inosine monophosphate dehydrogenase in lymphocytes. This enzyme synthesises guanosine monophosphate (GMP) from inosine monophosphate (IMP). GMP and its derivatives (e.g. GTP) are required for nucleotide synthesis. While there are 'salvage' pathways for the production of these molecules directly from guanine in other cells, lymphocytes lack these alternative pathways and are more susceptible to the effects of MMF/MPA.

More widespread effects of MMF/MPA on the bone marrow (manifest as anaemia, neutropenia and thrombocytopenia) can occur but are less common. Dose reduction usually improves these complications.

Neurotoxicity and nephrotoxicity are side effects of the CNIs (answers C and E incorrect). Tacrolimus causes hair loss (alopecia) while cyclosporin is associated with hirsutism. The use of MMF/MPA is not associated with any of these problems (answer B incorrect).

Clinical pearls

- Diarrhoea in transplant patients may be related to immunosuppression, but may also be due to infective causes such as cytomegalovirus (CMV). Other medications can also cause diarrhoea (e.g. valganciclovir, which is commonly used for CMV prophylaxis).

- Leucopenia in transplant patients can arise due to multiple factors including immunosuppressive drugs (MMF/MPA) and active viral infection (e.g. CMV). Other medications are also commonly implicated and include valganciclovir and cotrimoxazole (commonly used for pneumocystis prophylaxis).

Case history continued ...

After further deterioration in renal function and a short period of time on maintenance dialysis, a second live donor kidney transplant is performed (70-year-old father as donor, glomerular filtration rate, GFR, of 100 mL/min, 3/6 HLA match). The immunosuppressive regimen for the new transplant consists of tacrolimus, MMF and prednisolone.

Question 4

Possible complications related to tacrolimus use may include:
(a) electrolyte abnormalities
(b) lipid abnormalities
(c) gingival hyperplasia (gum hypertrophy)
(d) hypertension
(e) diabetes.

Answer
A, B, D and E

Explanation

In general, the side effects of tacrolimus are similar to those of cyclosporin (both are CNIs). One difference involves cosmetic effects such as gum side effects and hypertrichosis/hirsutism. These are generally seen with cyclosporin but not with tacrolimus (answer C incorrect).

Both cyclosporin and tacrolimus have been implicated in post-transplant diabetes mellitus (PTDM); however, tacrolimus is more diabetogenic than cyclosporin (answer E correct). The co-administration of steroids also contributes to the development of this problem. Glucose intolerance is generally at its worst in the early post-transplant period when doses of CNI drugs and steroids are both high.

The CNIs commonly worsen blood pressure control in patients following transplantation, an effect which is dose-related (answer D correct). Sodium retention and volume expansion occur and there is evidence for increased sympathetic activity. Intrarenal vasoconstriction, particularly affecting the afferent arteriole, is also implicated.

Lipid abnormalities following transplantation are common and are usually due to multiple factors. CNIs have been found to promote an increase in total as well as low-density lipoprotein (LDL) cholesterol (answer B correct). Other factors potentially affecting lipid levels following transplantation include steroid therapy, antihypertensives (e.g. beta-blockers, thiazides) and the presence of proteinuria or renal impairment. Dietary habits often change significantly following transplantation and this also needs to be considered and targeted in treating hyperlipidaemia.

CNIs are commonly associated with a variety of electrolyte abnormalities including hyperkalaemia, hypophosphataemia, hypomagnesaemia and hyperchloraemic acidosis (answer A correct). These alterations are all dose-related and are usually manageable with gradual dose adjustment and with supplementation where necessary (e.g. magnesium).

 ### Clinical pearls

- Cardiovascular disease remains one of the major causes of premature death in renal transplant recipients. Multiple factors contribute to this risk including side effects associated with immunosuppressive medications (e.g. diabetes and glucose intolerance, hypertension and lipid abnormalities).
- Major differences between tacrolimus and cyclosporin include cosmetic side effects (cyclosporin worse) and relative diabetogenicity (tacrolimus worse). As immunosuppressants, tacrolimus is more powerful and therefore the risk of rejection is lower with this agent. However, the risk of opportunistic infection is also increased with tacrolimus (e.g. polyoma virus nephropathy, CMV).

LEVEL B

Case history continued ...

It is now 3 weeks following the second transplant operation. Despite a slow but steady fall in the creatinine over the first 2 weeks (reaching 190 to 200 μmol/L) there has been no further improvement during the third week. The patient is well and a transplant ultrasound shows no evidence of obstruction. It is expected that the creatinine be better and a biopsy is considered. An initial biopsy was performed at implantation, following reperfusion.

Current results are as follows:

Urea	16.5 mmol/L	(2.5–9.6)
Creatinine	194 µmol/L	(40–120)
Tacrolimus (trough level)	10.7 µg/L	(target 10–15)
Haemoglobin	91 g/L	(130–180)
Mean red cell volume	89 fL	(78–98)
Total white cell count	10.8×10^9/L	$(4–12 \times 10^9$/L)
Platelets	165×10^9/L	$(150–400 \times 10^9$/L)
Blood film	No fragments, mild left shift of neutrophils	

Question 5

From the following list of possibilities, *which one is least likely* to be contributing to the suboptimal kidney function?

(a) Donor-related factors
(b) CNI-related factors
(c) Acute tubular necrosis
(d) Polyoma virus nephropathy
(e) Immunological factors

Answer

D

Explanation

Renal transplant dysfunction due to CNI is commonly encountered in the early post-transplant period (answer B incorrect). A biopsy will usually be necessary to separate this from acute rejection. The impact of nephrotoxicity will be heightened in the presence of other factors such as acute tubular necrosis or donor-related pathological changes. Haemolytic uraemic syndrome (HUS) can also occur as a complication of CNI use. The blood film (no fragments) and platelet count does not support this diagnosis but these are not always abnormal. (The left shift in neutrophils is most likely due to the steroids.)

Reversible graft dysfunction due to CNI in the early period after transplantation is caused by increased renal vascular resistance. This occurs predominantly at the afferent arteriole and results in a reduction in the glomerular filtration rate. Renal function usually improves with a decrease in the CNI dose. Therapeutic drug monitoring may help guide dose adjustments although nephrotoxicity can still occur even when CNI levels appear low.

The donor on this occasion was the 70-year-old father. While he may have been deemed suitable and had good renal function, there are likely to be pathological changes related to ageing which can impact on renal function (answer A incorrect). These include glomerulosclerosis (probably <20% of glomeruli as his GFR had been good enough to allow him to donate a kidney), vascular changes (mild hyalinosis and atheroma), mild interstitial fibrosis and tubular atrophy. A minor degree of these changes was present on the initial, implantation biopsy.

Acute tubular necrosis is commonly encountered in the first few days or weeks following transplantation and may be severe, leading to delayed graft function (DGF), which is defined as the need for ongoing dialysis post-transplantation. DGF is more common when the donor is cadaveric or when there have been haemodynamic problems requiring the use of ionotropes, hypovolaemia or prolonged ischaemia time. While this is not likely to be severe in the present case (good initial renal function and live donation) there may still be a degree of tubular injury contributing to the graft dysfunction (answer C incorrect).

Polyoma virus (or BK) nephropathy tends to present after the first month (answer D is therefore correct: it is least likely to be contributing). In a prospective study looking for active polyoma virus infection post-transplant, Gardner et al. (1984) found no positive cases prior to 4 weeks post transplant. In another study, Vasudev et al. (2005) found the median time to presentation was 318 days (range 48 to 1356 days).

Rejection could be underlying the suboptimal graft function and may be more likely in view of the history suggesting sensitisation (previous transplant). Both humoral and cellular rejection are possibilities and the only way to definitely exclude them is through a biopsy of the transplant (answer E incorrect).

Clinical pearls

- Histological features of acute CNI nephrotoxicity vary but include isometric tubular vacuolation, loss of tubular brush borders, vascular smooth muscle cell apoptosis, degeneration or hyalinosis. Where the biopsy is normal, 'functional toxicity' may be diagnosed and the CNI dose decreased, often with good effect.
- HUS is another possible manifestation of CNI 'toxicity'. There is often (not always) evidence of thrombotic microangiopathy on blood film, a falling platelet count and features of haemolysis (decreased haptoglobin, anaemia, elevated LDH). A renal biopsy usually shows arteriolopathy and glomerular microthrombi.
- If HUS occurs, alternatives to CNI may be required. Plasma exchange is often used. Differentiating HUS from severe antibody-mediated rejection is often difficult as some of the pathological features can look strikingly similar.

Case history continued ...

A renal biopsy performed a few days later, when the creatinine is suddenly 230 µmol/L, does show evidence of HUS. Tacrolimus is ceased and sirolimus (rapamycin) is commenced. The side effects of this drug (e.g. mouth ulcers, hyperlipidaemia, diarrhoea, myelosuppression, skin lesions, pneumonitis, lymphocoeles) are discussed with the patient.

Question 6

Other well-described complications associated with the use of sirolimus include:
(a) HUS
(b) oedema
(c) joint aches
(d) proteinuria
(e) hyperkalaemia.

Answer

A, B, C and D

Explanation

The mammalian target of rapamycin (mTOR) inhibitors, sirolimus and everolimus, are associated with a different toxicity profile to the CNI and antiproliferative drugs (MMF/MPA and azathioprine). Clinical experience with these drugs has rapidly increased over recent years and some of the complications seen in early studies are now less often encountered, possibly due to better patient selection (e.g. pneumonitis). As indicated, oedema, joint aches, skin reactions, mouth ulcers, lipid abnormalities and so on are all well-described complications (answers B and C correct).

Interestingly, HUS was a significant problem with sirolimus when it was first used because this was done in combination with CNI (answer A correct, with a caveat!). It is now known that mTOR inhibitors interact and enhance the toxicity of CNI drugs and great care is required if the drugs are to be used together. Many now advocate the use of mTOR inhibitors only in CNI-free regimens (particularly sirolimus) or with very significant CNI minimisation (particularly everolimus). The HUS previously described with sirolimus is generally not seen when it is used in CNI-free regimens. HUS is now a major indication for switching to mTOR inhibitors and ceasing CNI and this is generally considered to be a very effective strategy for managing this CNI-related complication.

Proteinuria (which may be nephrotic range) has been reported in studies where patients were switched from a CNI to mTOR inhibitors (answer D correct). In many cases this proteinuria reflected underlying renal pathology which was present prior to the switch. Despite their nephrotoxicity, CNI are also able to decrease proteinuria through their effects on glomerular haemodynamics, and their cessation would also be a factor underlying these cases of proteinuria. The incidence, pathophysiology and true significance of proteinuria which develops while taking mTOR inhibitors is still being examined and remains unclear. However, significant proteinuria (>800 mg in one study) is now seen as a contraindication for switching to mTOR inhibitors as it predicts a poor response to the switch.

Electrolyte abnormalities, thought to be due to tubular toxicity, are well described with mTOR inhibitors. These include hypophosphataemia and hypokalaemia (rather than hyperkalaemia; answer E is therefore incorrect).

 Clinical pearls

- mTOR inhibitors block the proliferation of cells in response to various molecular signals. The 'target of rapamycin' (TOR) is a key regulatory kinase-controlling cytokine-dependent cell division. Inhibition of TOR stops haematopoietic cells (and non-haematopoietic cells) from dividing and this accounts for its immunosuppressive actions.
- The antiproliferative effects of mTOR inhibitors also account for some of the side effects (wound-healing problems, prolongation of acute tubular necrosis) and potential benefits of these drugs (lower risk of malignancy, beneficial effects on smooth muscle cell proliferation).

LEVEL C

Question 7

Which of the following drug regimen alterations are known to require special consideration, potentially requiring a *decrease* in the dose of immunosuppressant?

(a) Sirolimus, after commencing diltiazem
(b) Tacrolimus, after commencing carbamazepine
(c) Tacrolimus, after commencing rifampicin
(d) MMF, after ceasing cyclosporin and commencing tacrolimus
(e) MMF, after ceasing cyclosporin and commencing sirolimus

Answer
A, D and E

Explanation

When prescribing CNIs as well as mTOR inhibitors, one must always consider the cytochrome P-450 IIIA (CYP3A) system and potential for drug interactions related to this metabolic pathway. CYP3A is found predominantly in the liver but it also resides in the intestinal tract. CYP3A in both sites contributes significantly to the metabolism of many drugs including CNI and mTOR inhibitors.

Carbamazepine and rifampicin are inducers of this pathway and will lead to increased metabolism of CNIs and mTOR inhibitors. This would require an increase in the respective immunosuppressive doses to maintain stable circulating concentrations (answers B and C incorrect). Other cytochrome P-450 inducers include barbiturates and phenytoin.

Inhibitors of CYP3A (or in some cases 'competitive' inhibitors) will decrease the metabolism of CNIs and mTOR inhibitors, requiring a decrease in the dose of immunosuppressant. These include calcium channel blockers (diltiazem, verapamil and, to a lesser extent, amlodipine), antifungals (ketoconazole, fluconazole, itraconazole), erythromycin and the antiretroviral drug ritonavir (answer A correct).

The immunosuppressive agent that is used along with MMF (e.g. cyclosporin, tacrolimus or sirolimus) needs to be considered carefully with regards to how this may affect the dose of MMF. Cyclosporin lowers mycophenolic acid (MPA) serum levels by decreasing its enterohepatic circulation (MPA absorption in the terminal ileum is blocked). For this reason, the dose of MMF or MPA to use in combination with cyclosporin is usually higher (e.g. 1 g twice daily initially) than that recommended for co-administration with tacrolimus or sirolimus (e.g. 500 to 750 mg twice daily). If cyclosporin is ceased in order to commence tacrolimus or sirolimus, the interaction involving the enterohepatic circulation is lost, and MPA levels will rise. The MMF/MPA dose should be lowered (by 25 to 50%) with this sort of switch (answers D and E correct).

It must also be remembered that MMF/MPA and mTOR inhibitors both have myelosuppressive effects. The combined use of these drugs has been shown to increase the incidence of clinically relevant anaemia, leucopenia and thrombocytopenia.

 Clinical pearls

- CNIs and mTOR inhibitors are prone to interact through the CYP3A system (inducers decrease immunosuppressant levels, inhibitors increase immunosuppressant levels).
- Cyclosporin also interacts by virtue of its effect on the enterohepatic circulation of MPA (lowering MPA levels). When ceasing cyclosporin in order to commence tacrolimus, sirolimus or everolimus, the dose of MMF/MPA may need to be lowered.

Case history continued ...

The initial response to switching the patient to sirolimus and ceasing tacrolimus because of HUS is excellent. The creatinine gradually falls to 142 μmol/L 14 days after the switch. However, despite therapeutic sirolimus concentrations, the creatinine gradually rises to 195 μmol/L over the following week and does not improve with daily steroid pulses over 3 days. A third renal biopsy (at 8 weeks post-transplant) now shows severe cellular and mild vascular rejection. There are no histological features of humoral rejection and no donor-specific HLA antibodies detectable in the patient's serum. A decision is made to use OKT3 (a mouse monoclonal anti-CD3 antibody) while temporarily ceasing the sirolimus, in order to treat the rejection.

Question 8

Which of the following is/are recognised side effects of OKT3 treatment?
(a) Thrombocytopenia
(b) Headache
(c) Pulmonary oedema
(d) Diarrhoea
(e) Serum sickness syndrome (arthralgia, urticaria, abdominal pain)

Answer

B, C and D

Explanation

The monoclonal anti-CD3 antibody OKT3 acts on mature T-cells as they possess the CD3 antigen. CD3 is required for T-cell activation and is closely linked to the T-cell receptor antigen recognition site.

Most patients experience fever and chills following the first dose (usually about 45 minutes to some hours after the dose). This usually subsides with subsequent doses. Diarrhoea can sometimes accompany this and persist for several days (answer D correct). The T-cell lysis that occurs following OKT3 therapy results in massive release of cytokines (e.g. interferon gamma, tumour necrosis factor) and activation of complement factors. This coincides with the acute flu-like syndrome seen after the initial dose. Corticosteroids, antipyretics and antihistamines can limit the severity of this initial reaction.

Non-cardiogenic pulmonary oedema following OKT3 administration is well described. Careful consideration of the patient's volume *prior* to administration of the OKT3 is therefore warranted, as this complication is more common in patients who are fluid overloaded. A chest X-ray and thorough examination are essential components of this assessment (answer C correct).

A range of neurological complications have been described including mild headache, aseptic meningitis and severe encephalopathy (answer B correct). These are usually self limiting. A lumbar puncture may be necessary to exclude infection and often this will show a mild CSF leucocytosis.

Thrombocytopenia and leucopenia are complications associated with polyclonal antilymphocyte preparations (polyclonal antibodies raised against T cells. e.g. antithymocyte globulin or ATG) and not with the use of the monoclonal antibody, OKT3 (answer A incorrect). Similarly, serum sickness is a recognised (though uncommon) complication of polyclonal antilymphocyte preparations (answer E incorrect). This is due to immune complex formation resulting from the large amount of foreign proteins in the polyclonal preparations (as opposed to the relative purity of the monoclonal OKT3 preparation).

Clinical pearls

- Human anti-mouse antibodies (HAMA) develop following OKT3 therapy (detectable about a week after completion). Subsequent courses of OKT3 (potentially required if rejection returns) may result in an anaphylactic reaction or be ineffective. HAMA titres should be assessed if a repeat course of OKT3 is contemplated and OKT3 reuse should be avoided if HAMA titres are very high.
- CD3 counts can be monitored (by flow cytometry) during OKT3 therapy. Usually CD3 cells are absent by day 3 to 5 of treatment. If CD3 positive cells persist or return during therapy, the OKT3 dose may need to be increased.

Bibliography

Level A

1. Danovitch, G.M. (2005) Immunosuppressive medications and protocols for kidney transplantation. *Handbook of Kidney Transplantation*, 4th edn, Danovich, G.M. (ed.). Philadelphia: Lippincott Williams and Wilkins. 72–134.
2. Mathew, T.H. (2001) Mycophenolate mofetil. *Kidney Transplantation: Principles and Practice*, 5th edn, Morris, P.J. (ed.). Philadelphia: WB Saunders Co.. 263–78.
3. Morris, P.J. (2001) Azathioprine and steroids. *Kidney Transplantation: Principles and Practice*, 5th edn, Morris, P.J. (ed.). Philadelphia: WB Saunders Co. 217–26.

Level B

4. Gardner, S.D., Mackenzie, E.F., Smith, C. & Porter, A.A. (1984) Prospective study of human polyomavirus BK and JC and cytomegalovirus in renal transplant recipients. J Clin Pathol. 37, 578–86.
5. Kulkarni, S., Kopelan, A. & Woodle, E.S. (2001) Tacrolimus therapy in renal transplantation. *Kidney Transplantation: Principles and Practice*, 5th edn, Morris, P.J. (ed.). Philadelphia: WB Saunders Co. 251–62.

6. Lee, V.W. & Chapman, J.R. (2005) Sirolimus: its role in nephrology. Nephrology (Carlton). 10(6), 606–14.
7. Vasudev, B., Hariharan, S., Hussain, S.A., Zhu, Y.R., Bresnahan, B.A. & Cohen, E.P. (2005) BK virus nephritis: risk factors, timing, and outcome in renal transplant recipients. Kidney Int. 68(4), 1834–9.

Level C
8. Abrahamian, G.A. & Cosimi, A.B. (2001) Antilymphocyte globulin and monoclonal antibodies. *Kidney Transplantation: Principles and Practice*, 5th edn, Morris, P.J. (ed.). Philadelphia: WB Saunders Co. 289–309.

Case 32
Chronic allograft dysfunction

STEVE CHADBAN

LEVEL A

Case history

The patient first presents at 18 years of age following an episode of macroscopic haematuria, which occurs during the course of a typical viral upper respiratory tract infection. Proteinuria is also detected, a kidney biopsy performed and IgA nephropathy confirmed.

At 35 years of age, the patient reaches end-stage kidney failure and is commenced on haemodialysis. Two years later he receives a deceased donor kidney transplant. The donor is male, aged 32 and died as a result of a closed head injury. The transplant procedure is uncomplicated, the graft works immediately and the patient receives cyclosporin, azathioprine and prednisone for immunosuppression.

Question 1

Which of the patient's immunosuppressive medications could damage his kidney transplant in the long term?
(a) Prednisone
(b) Cyclosporin
(c) Azathioprine

Answer

B

Explanation

Prednisone and azathioprine are not directly nephrotoxic (answers A and C incorrect). In contrast, cyclosporin and the other commonly used calcineurin inhibitor tacrolimus exert both acute and chronic nephrotoxicity (answer B correct). Acute toxicity causes a rise in serum creatinine but little structural damage to the kidney and is therefore largely reversible by decreasing drug exposure. Chronic toxicity causes characteristic arteriolar hyalinosis, tubular vacuolation and interstitial fibrosis and is generally not completely reversible.

Evidence of chronic toxicity is almost universal by 1 year after transplant if moderately high drug exposure is maintained (Nankivell 2003).

Clinical pearl

- The calcineurin inhibitors, cyclosporin and tacrolimus, are the most effective agents for the prevention of acute rejection and are therefore the cornerstone of current anti-rejection strategies for kidney transplant recipients. They are best used at high exposure early after transplantation when the risk of acute rejection is greatest, then tapered significantly (or even withdrawn) over the longer term to minimise the risk of chronic nephrotoxicity. The dose should be determined by measuring the drug concentration in blood (pharmacokinetic monitoring).

Case history continued ...

Two weeks after transplantation, a transplant biopsy is performed because of a rise in serum creatinine, and this reveals changes consistent with mild, tubulointerstitial acute rejection (Banff 1a), featuring a leucocytic infiltrate occupying 25% of the interstitium and moderate tubulitis. He is treated with three daily pulses of methylprednisolone and the serum creatinine returns to its baseline value of 100 µmol/L.

Over the following 12 months, the serum creatinine remains between 90 and 110 µmol/L and the doses of immunosuppressive drugs are decreased to cyclosporin 125 mg twice daily, azathioprine 100 mg/day and prednisone 10 mg/day. There are no other complications. The patient enjoys good health and returns to work.

Question 2

Which of the following statements is/are true? Greater than 90% of kidney transplant recipients:

(a) survive the first year post-transplant
(b) have a functioning kidney transplant (i.e. do not require dialysis) for at least 1 year after transplant
(c) experience acute rejection during the first year post-transplant.

Answer
A and B

Explanation

Current 1-year patient survival in Australia is approximately 98% (Briganti et al. 2002) (answer A correct). Approximately 95% of kidney transplant recipients in Australia have a functioning kidney transplant (i.e. do not require dialysis) for at least 1 year after transplant (Briganti et al. 2002) (answer B correct). Approximately 25% of kidney transplant recipients are diagnosed with acute rejection, and this can be effectively treated in over 90% of cases (answer C incorrect).

Clinical pearl

- Approximately 95% of kidney transplant recipients in Australia survive the first post-transplant year with a functioning graft; however, 4 to 5% either die or lose graft function per annum thereafter (Briganti et al. 2002).

Case history continued ...

Over the next 6 years, the patient continues to enjoy good heath, serum creatinine remains within the range of 90 to 110 µmol/L and no further changes are made to his immunosuppression. Blood pressure (BP) is checked regularly and averages 120/75 mmHg.

Creatinine is 118 µmol/L at the patient's next visit and his BP is 135/85 mmHg, with no other change in clinical condition and no intercurrent illnesses. Two months later the creatinine is 129 µmol/L, BP has risen further to 140/90 mmHg and general examination is unremarkable.

Question 3

Which of the following statements is/are true?
(a) It is normal for serum creatinine to increase over time.
(b) The glomerular filtration rate (GFR) would be normal.
(c) It is normal for BP to rise over time.
(d) BP of 140/90 mmHg is abnormal and requires management.

Answer
D

Explanation

Serum creatinine should remain stable and a significant rise, which this is, indicates graft dysfunction and a cause should be identified (answer A incorrect). If measured, or estimated, the GFR would be subnormal. Indeed, the

MDRD estimate of GFR in this case (Cr 129, male aged 44) is 49 mL/min/ 1.73 m^2 (answer B incorrect).

The prevalence of hypertension does increase with age; however, hypertension is pathological at any age. In this setting, graft pathology causing a decrease in GFR and hypertension must be considered (answer C incorrect). Most guidelines recommend keeping BP <130/80 mmHg in a kidney transplant recipient (answer D correct).

Clinical pearls

- eGFR is a more sensitive measure of kidney function than serum creatinine.
- Aim to keep BP <130/80 mmHg in kidney transplant recipients.

Case history continued ...

Some tests are performed. A cyclosporin C2 concentration is 900 ng/mL, midstream urine shows 10 to 100 × 10⁶/L red blood count, spot urine albumin/creatinine ratio (ACR) is 60 mg/mmol (normal <3, microalbuminuria 3 to 30, albuminuria >30), and an ultrasound shows a transplant kidney of 10 cm in length with normal flows in the renal artery, resistive index in cortex of 0.75 (normal) and no evidence of hydronephrosis.

Question 4

Likely diagnoses include which of the following?
(a) CSA toxicity
(b) Acute rejection
(c) Chronic allograft nephropathy (CAN)
(d) Recurrent IgA nephropathy
(e) Obstruction
(f) BK nephropathy

Answer
A, C and D

Explanation

The cyclosporin concentration (C2 value of 900 ng/mL) is on the high side for a patient over 6 years post transplant and may have caused toxicity (answer A correct). Acute rejection does not cause albuminuria or haematuria (answer B incorrect). CAN typically causes proteinuria, hypertension and decreasing GFR, though haematuria is not typical and is more suggestive of glomerulonephritis (answer C correct). Recurrence of IgA nephropathy is common and classically presents with declining GFR, hypertension, proteinuria and haematuria (answer D correct). Obstruction is uncommon in a young man and is effectively excluded by a normal ultrasound (answer E incorrect). BK nephropathy does not typically cause albuminuria (answer F incorrect).

Question 5

The next step in managing the patient should be:
(a) pulse steroids
(b) reduction in cyclosporin dose
(c) kidney biopsy
(d) transplant renal angiogram.

Answer
B and C

Explanation

Pulse steroids are used to treat acute rejection, which is an unlikely diagnosis in this case. This treatment is not useful for the management of chronic allograft nephropathy or recurrent IgA nephropathy (answer A incorrect). Although cyclosporin toxicity does not explain all features of this presentation, it is likely to be contributing to graft dysfunction and therefore a reduction in dose is appropriate (answer B correct). A biopsy of the transplant kidney is a low-risk procedure and will provide useful information regarding the diagnosis and prognosis in this case (answer C correct).

As transplant renal artery stenosis is not a likely diagnosis in this case, angiography is not indicated (answer D incorrect). Any procedure that involves the use of nephrotoxic agents, such as radio-contrast, should be avoided if possible as it will further compromise transplant function.

Case history continued ...

A kidney biopsy is performed and two diagnoses are made: recurrent IgA nephropathy plus cyclosporin toxicity.

Question 6

Which of the following may be beneficial in managing the patient?
(a) Stop the cyclosporin
(b) Add an angiotensin-converting enzyme inhibitor (ACEi)

Answer
Both are correct

Explanation

Minimising or ceasing the cyclosporin will retard further CSA nephrotoxicity (answer A correct). CSA is not known to be protective against recurrent IgA. As decreasing or eliminating CSA will result in less overall immunosuppression, replacement with an alternative immunosuppressant may be required.

ACEis are safe to use in kidney transplant recipients and should be nephroprotective in the long term, with at least part of this nephroprotection due to the reduction in proteinuria that should occur (answer B correct). When introduced at this stage after transplantation, when there is small vessel disease within the kidney, some degree of deterioration in kidney function and elevation in serum potassium may be anticipated when this drug is commenced and these values should therefore be checked soon after starting treatment.

 Clinical pearl

- ACEis, and angiotensin receptor antagonists, are safe to use after kidney transplantation; however, the serum creatinine and potassium should be checked 2 to 5 days after commencement. If potassium rises above 6 mmol/L or serum creatinine increases by more that 25%, therapy should be suspended and re-evaluated.

Case history continued ...

Cyclosporin is withdrawn, azathioprine is switched to mycophenolate, prednisone dose is increased to 10 mg/day and perindopril is introduced. Over the next 12 months, serum creatinine remains between 120 and 140 µmol/L.

Question 7

The major risks to the future survival of this man's kidney transplant function are:
- **(a)** death from myocardial infarction
- **(b)** death from cancer
- **(c)** transplant failure due to chronic allograft nephropathy
- **(d)** transplant failure due to IgA nephropathy
- **(e)** acute rejection.

Answer
A, B, C and D

Explanation

Death with a functioning graft is the most common cause of late transplant failure in Australia, and cardiovascular disease and cancer are the leading causes of death (ANZDATA 2005) (answers A and B correct). CAN is the most common cause of graft failure for those with a primary diagnosis of glomerulonephritis (closely followed by death with a functioning graft, which is more common in those with a primary diagnosis other than glomerulonephritis according to ANZDATA's 2005 report) (answer C correct).

As this man has a documented recurrence and as treatment has not been proven to be effective, it is likely that he will lose his transplant function due to IgA, compounding the co-existing problem of CAN (ANZDATA 2005) (answer D correct). Acute rejection is unlikely at this stage, unless immunosuppression is stopped because of non-compliance or medical advice (e.g. if a cancer is diagnosed) (answer E incorrect).

LEVEL B

Question 8

The primary action of which of his immunosuppressant drugs is to inhibit the generation of interleukin-2 by T-cells?

(a) Prednisolone
(b) Cyclosporin
(c) Azathioprine

Answer

B

Explanation

Prednisolone has multiple mechanisms of action, the best characterised being inhibition of NF-kappa beta which is crucial in the generation of pro-inflammatory cytokines including IL-1beta and TNF-alpha (answer A incorrect). Cyclosporin inhibits calcineurin phosphatase which is required by T-cells for the generation of IL-2 in response to antigen exposure, a step known as signal 1 (answer B correct). Azathioprine inhibits purine synthesis, thereby inhibiting the proliferation of cells (answer C incorrect).

Question 9

Considering the clinical and lab findings presented earlier, why do you think his creatinine has increased after 6 years of stable transplant function?

(a) Acute rejection
(b) Chronic allograft nephropathy (CAN)
(c) Cyclosporin toxicity
(d) Hypertensive nephropathy

(e) Transplant renal artery stenosis
(f) Obstructive nephropathy due to benign prostatic hypertrophy
(g) Recurrent IgA nephropathy

Answers
B, C and G

Explanation

Acute rejection is quite rare beyond the first year after transplantation, except in instances of non-compliance or an intentional, major reduction in immuno-suppression (e.g. if a cancer is diagnosed) (answer A incorrect).

CAN is common and presents with a slow rise in serum creatinine, often accompanied by hypertension and proteinuria (answer B correct). CSA toxicity is almost universal among patients treated with solid maintenance doses of CSA (or tacrolimus) (Nankivell 2003) (answer C correct).

Hypertensive nephropathy is unlikely as his BP had been previously well controlled (answer D incorrect). Renal artery stenosis is also unlikely, though possible. Although he has become hypertensive, other causes of graft dysfunction and hypertension are far more common (answer E incorrect). Obstruction is uncommon in the absence of symptoms, though does require exclusion by ultrasound of the transplant kidney, as was the case here (answer F incorrect).

IgA nephropathy recurs histologically in over 50% of cases and graft dysfunction, though uncommon early after transplantation, becomes increasingly common over time. Approximately 10% of all patients with IgA who receive a transplant will lose their graft due to recurrence within the first 10 years after transplant (ANZDATA 2005) (answer G correct).

Question 10

A transplant kidney biopsy was performed (see Fig. 32.1). The likely diagnoses are:
(a) acute rejection
(b) recurrent IgA nephropathy
(c) cyclosporin nephrotoxicity
(d) BK nephropathy.

Answer
B and C

Explanation

The interstitium has a sparse infiltrate and no significant tubulitis, thus excluding acute rejection (answer A incorrect). The glomeruli are hypercellular, clustered

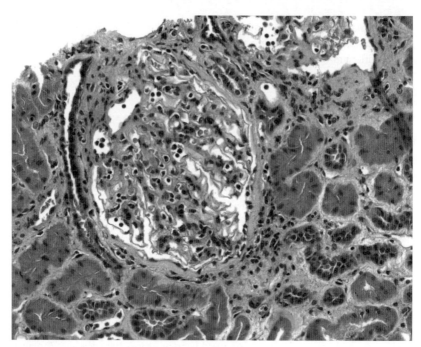

Figure 32.1 Transplant kidney biopsy of patient

around mesangial areas, which is typical for IgA (answer B correct). There are tracts of 'striped fibrosis' throughout the kidney which, together with the arteriolar hyalinosis, are suggestive of CSA toxicity (answer C correct). There are no atypical cells/nuclei to suggest viral activity (answer D incorrect).

Question 11

Given the clinical, lab and biopsy findings, which additional measures may be of use in managing this patient?
(a) Switch from cyclosporin to rapamycin
(b) Change from azathioprin to mycophenolate
(c) Change from cyclosporin to tacrolimus

Answer
B

Explanation

Had the patient been free from significant proteinuria (e.g. less than 300 mg/day total proteinuria or ACR <30 mg/mmol) and had the biopsy shown CSA toxicity only with no suggestion of a recurrence of IgA nephropathy, then a switch from cyclosporin to sirolimus (or everolimus) may have been recommended. However, the presence of proteinuria, particularly when that is due to recurrent glomerulonephritis, is a contraindication to the use of sirolimus/everolimus due to a high risk of accelerated graft dysfunction and increase in proteinuria (answer A incorrect).

Mycophenolate is non-nephrotoxic and a more potent immunosuppressant than azathioprine. In this case, a switch to mycophenolate may enable a substantial dose reduction in CSA, or possibly cessation, without risking under-immunosuppression. An additional theoretical advantage may be that mycophenolate may retard progression of the IgA nephropathy, although this is yet to be demonstrated for recurrent disease after transplantation (answer B correct). Tacrolimus is equally nephrotoxic to CSA (answer C incorrect).

Clinical pearls

- The mTOR inhibitors, sirolimus and everolimus, are relatively contraindicated if the patient has significant proteinuria: proteinuria 300 to 1000 mg/day is a relative contraindication and proteinuria >1000 mg/day is a strong contraindication.
- Patients managed with sirolimus or everolimus should be monitored for the development of proteinuria (e.g. every 3 months) and should proteinuria develop, strong consideration to ceasing that agent should be given.
- Considering patients managed with sirolimus or everolimus, proteinuria and progressive graft dysfunction appear to be most likely to develop in those with recurrent or de novo glomerular disease, such as glomerulonephritis or diabetic nephropathy.

LEVEL C

Question 12

What factors in the patient's history prior to and in the first year after transplantation indicate an increased chance of premature transplant failure?

(a) His primary diagnosis of IgA
(b) Donor characteristics
(c) A single episode of acute rejection at week 2 post-transplant which responded to therapy

(d) Use of cyclosporin

(e) Use of azathioprine

(f) Use of prednisone

Answer

B

Explanation

Individuals with glomerulonephritis, and IgA nephropathy in particular, incur the risk of graft failure due to recurrence of their original disease. However, the risk of this is approximately 10% in the first 10 years after transplantation (ANZDATA 2005) (answer A incorrect). This small risk is compensated for as patients with glomerulonephritis are on average less likely to die from vascular disease or cancer early after transplantation and therefore they are not at increased risk of premature transplant failure as compared to all other recipients (ANZDATA 2005).

The donor was deceased, and graft survival is on average inferior as compared to live donor recipients (answer B correct). As far as deceased donors go, this donor was ideal in that he was male, young and died from head trauma.

While acute rejection can cause graft failure, and can predispose the patient to developing chronic allograft nephropathy (Nankivell 2003), this is usually due to episodes of vascular rejection or severe or recurrent cellular rejection where initial treatment fails to restore transplant function to levels seen prior to the rejection episode (i.e. back to baseline). As this patient experienced a mild, cellular rejection (Banff 1A) and pulse steroid therapy caused creatinine to return to baseline, there should be no significant impact on the risk of transplant failure in the short to medium term (McDonald 2007) (answer C incorrect).

Although clinical trial evidence may suggest one immunosuppressant is superior to another, there is no convincing evidence that the risk of transplant failure is higher in the short to medium term (1 to 5 years post-transplant) among patients using cyclosporin (answer D incorrect). The 'pivotal' trials of mycophenolate demonstrated that this agent enabled less acute rejection, though produced no significant reduction in graft failure as compared to azathioprine (answer E incorrect). ANZDATA, and the majority of clinical trials examining this issue, have demonstrated that steroid avoidance (or steroid withdrawal if on cyclosporin and azathioprine) incurs a higher risk of premature transplant failure (answer F incorrect).

Case history continued ...

A kidney biopsy is performed and shows evidence of mesangial hypercellularity, tubulointerstitial fibrosis with a scant infiltrate (<10%), arteriolar hyalinosis and no significant areas of tubulitis.

Question 13

What additional information would you seek from the pathology lab?
- **(a)** Immunostaining for IgA deposits
- **(b)** T-cell staining
- **(c)** C4d staining
- **(d)** Electron microscopy

Answer
A and D

Explanation

Immunostaining (or immunofluoresence) would be important in considering recurrent IgA (answer A correct). T-cells may be present in a number of conditions and this would not discriminate between them (answer B incorrect).

C4d is best validated as a marker of antibody-mediated acute rejection in the first few months after transplantation, and neither the biopsy appearances nor the clinical context suggest this diagnosis. C4d deposition late after transplantation may suggest antibody-mediated chronic rejection; however, some evidence of C4d deposition may be seen in cases of glomerulonephritis and thus it would not help to differentiate in this case (answer C incorrect).

Electron microscopy is useful in distinguishing between IgA nephropathy and CAN (answer D correct).

Question 14

The patient asks about his prognosis and particularly whether he is likely to lose his graft. Which of the following statements are true?
- **(a)** He is more likely to die with a functioning graft than to experience graft failure.
- **(b)** Should his graft fail, he should not be offered re-transplantation due to the increased risk that recurrent IgA will cause the second graft to fail.
- **(c)** Should his graft fail, he should not accept a kidney from his father as IgA will be more likely to recur in a live-related, well-matched graft.

Answer
All are false

Explanation

Considering all renal transplant recipients, death with a functioning graft is the most common cause of graft failure. However, considering only patients with glomerulonephritis, graft loss due to CAN is more likely (Briganti et al. 2002). For those who experience recurrent glomerulonephritis, their risk of graft loss is double that of those without documented recurrence and this is mainly due to graft loss caused by the recurrent disease (answer A incorrect).

IgA is more likely to recur in a subsequent graft; however, considering the slow course of disease in the current graft (his graft will likely last at least 10 years), there is no reason to suspect the course in a subsequent graft will be any different and thus would provide a favourable outcome as compared to dialysis (answer B incorrect).

The impact of HLA matching on recurrence risk appears to be slight and should not preclude live-donor transplantation in this setting (answer C incorrect).

Bibliography

Levels A and B
1. Nankivell, B. (2003) The natural history of chronic allograft nephropathy. NEJM 2003. 349, 2326–33.
2. Briganti, E., Russ, G., McNeil, J., Atkins, R. and Chadban, S. NEJM 2002.
3. Australia and New Zealand Dialysis and Transplant Registry (ANZDATA) (2005) *The 28th Report.* McDonald, S. & Excell, L. (eds.).

Level C
4. Briganti, E., Russ, G., McNeil, J., Atkins, R. and Chadban, S. NEJM 2002.
5. Australia and New Zealand Dialysis and Transplant Registry (ANZDATA) (2005) *The 28th Report.* McDonald, S. & Excell, L. (eds.).
6. McDonald, S., Russ, G., Campbell, S. & Chadban, S. (2007) Kidney transplant rejection in Australia and New Zealand: relationships between rejection and graft outcome. Am J Transplantation.
7. Mathew, T.H. A blinded, long-term, randomized multicenter study of mycophenolate mofetil in cadaveric renal transplantation: results at three years. Tricontinental Mycophenolate Mofetil Renal Transplantation Study Group. (1998) Transplantation. 65, 1450–4.

Index